Taylor's Cardiovascular Diseases

T0235917

Taylor's Cardiovascular Diseases
A Handbook

Robert B. Taylor, M.D.   Editor
Professor Emeritus
Department of Family Medicine
Oregon Health & Science University
    School of Medicine
Portland, Oregon

Associate Editors

Alan K. David, M.D.
Professor and Chairman
Department of Family and
    Community Medicine
Medical College of Wisconsin
Milwaukee, Wisconsin

Scott A. Fields, M.D.
Professor and Vice Chairman
Department of Family Medicine
Oregon Health & Science University
    School of Medicine
Portland, Oregon

D. Melessa Phillips, M.D.
Professor and Chairman
Department of Family Medicine
University of Mississippi School
    of Medicine
Jackson, Mississippi

Joseph E. Scherger, M.D., M.P.H.
Clinical Professor
Department of Family and
    Preventive Medicine
University of California, San Diego
    School of Medicine
San Diego, California

With 10 Illustrations

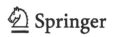 Springer

Robert B. Taylor, M.D.
Professor Emeritus
Department of Family Medicine
Oregon Health & Science University
  School of Medicine
Portland, OR 97201-3098, USA

Associate Editors

Alan K. David, M.D.
Professor and Chairman
Department of Family and
  Community Medicine
Medical College of Wisconsin
Milwaukee, WI 53226-0509, USA

Scott A. Fields, M.D.
Professor and Vice Chairman
Department of Family Medicine
Oregon Health & Science University
  School of Medicine
Portland, OR 97201-3098, USA

D. Melessa Phillips, M.D.
Professor and Chairman
Department of Family Medicine
University of Mississippi School
  of Medicine
Jackson, MS 39216-4500, USA

Joseph E. Scherger, M.D., M.P.H.
Clinical Professor
Department of Family and
  Preventive Medicine
University of California, San Diego
  School of Medicine
San Diego, CA 92103-0801

Library of Congress Cataloging-in-Publication Data
Taylor's cardiovascular diseases: a handbook/Robert B. Taylor, editor; associate
  editors, Alan K. David . . . [et al.].
      p.; cm.
    "This book is comprised of chapters from the sixth edition of the large reference book,
  Family medicine: principles and practice"—Pref.
    Includes bibliographical references and index.
    ISBN 0-387-22351-7 (alk. paper)
      1. Cardiovascular system—Diseases—Handbooks, manuals, etc.   I. Title: Cardiovascular
  diseases.   II. Taylor, Robert B.   III. Family medicine.
    [DNLM: 1. Cardiovascular Diseases. WG 120 T247 2005]
    RC669.15.T396 2005
    616.1—dc22   2004058950

ISBN 0-387-22351-7   Printed on acid-free paper.

© 2005 Springer Science+Business Media, Inc.
All rights reserved. This work may not be translated or copied in whole or in part without the
written permission of the publisher (Springer Science+Business Media, Inc., 233 Spring Street,
New York, NY 10013, USA), except for brief excerpts in connection with reviews or scholarly
analysis. Use in connection with any form of information storage and retrieval, electronic
adaptation, computer software, or by similar or dissimilar methodology now known or hereafter
developed is forbidden.
The use in this publication of trade names, trademarks, service marks and similar terms, even if
they are not identified as such, is not to be taken as an expression of opinion as to whether or not
they are subject to proprietary rights.
While the advice and information in this book are believed to be true and accurate at the date of
going to press, neither the authors nor the editors nor the publisher can accept any legal
responsibility for any errors or omissions that may be made. The publisher makes no warranty,
express or implied, with respect to the material contained herein.

Printed in the United States of America.   (MP/MVY)

9 8 7 6 5 4 3 2 1   SPIN 10994986

springeronline.com

Preface

In the end, most of our patients—and also most of us clinicians—will die a cardiovascular death. During life, many will experience discomfort and disability caused by diseases of the heart and blood vessels. This book is intended to be a primer on these causes of morbidity and mortality.

This book is comprised of chapters from the sixth edition of the large reference book, *Family Medicine: Principles and Practice*. Publishing chapters on selected topics provides volumes that are easy to carry in the pocket, are available at lower cost than large comprehensive volumes, and that allow clinicians to select books on areas that meet their specific needs.

This book on cardiovascular diseases includes the chapter on Hypertension, which afflicts approximately 60 million Americans and contributes to many instances of heart disease, stroke, and kidney disease. Chapters related directly to the heart are those on Ischemic Heart Disease, Cardiac Arrhythmias, Valvular Heart Disease, and Heart Failure. I included the chapter on Dyslipidemia, because elevated serum lipid levels contribute to many instances of cardiovascular disease. Venous Thromboembolism and Cerebrovascular Disease are the chief diseases of blood vessel. The chapter on Cardiovascular Emergencies includes what the primary care clinician needs to know when the unexpected strikes. When the primary care clinician provides Medical Care of the Surgical Patient, cardiovascular disease is often the main area of concern. Finally, Chapter 11 on Selected Disorders allows discussion of a variety of problems including pericarditis, myocarditis, endocarditis, the cardiomyopathies, pulmonary hypertension, and peripheral vascular disease.

I hope that you find this book useful in daily practice.

Robert B. Taylor, M.D.
Portland, Oregon, USA

Clinical Practice Notice

Everyone involved with the preparation of this book has worked very hard to assure that information presented here is accurate and that it represents accepted clinical practices. These efforts include confirming that drug recommendations and dosages discussed in this text are in accordance with current practice at the time of publication. Nevertheless, therapeutic recommendations and dosage schedules change with reports of ongoing research, changes in government recommendations, reports of adverse drug reactions, and other new information.

A few recommendations and drug uses described herein have Food and Drug Administration (FDA) clearance for limited use in restricted settings. It is the responsibility of the clinician to determine the FDA status of any drug selection, drug dosage, or device recommended to patients.

The reader should check the package insert for each drug to determine any change in indications or dosage as well as for any precautions or warnings. This admonition is especially true when the drug considered is new or infrequently used by the clinician.

The use of the information in this book in a specific clinical setting or situation is the professional responsibility of the clinician. The authors, editors, or publisher are not responsible for errors, omissions, adverse effects, or any consequences arising from the use of information in this book, and make no warranty, expressed or implied, with respect to the completeness, timeliness, or accuracy of the book's contents.

Contents

Contributors

David E. Anisman, M.D., Assistant Professor of Family Medicine, Uniformed Services University of the Health Sciences, Bethesda; Assistant Program Director, Family Practice Residency, Malcolm Grow Medical Center, Andrews Air Force Base, MD

Michael H. Bross, M.D., Medical Director, North Central County Health Center, Institute for Research and Education in Family Medicine, St. Louis, MO

Stephen A. Brunton, M.D., Director of Faculty Development, Stamford Hospital/Columbia University Family Practice Residency Program, Stamford, CT

David C. Campbell, M.D., M.Ed., Clinical Professor of Community and Family Medicine, St. Louis University School of Medicine; The Institute for Research and Education in Family Medicine, St. Louis, MO

Mel P. Daly, M.D., Family Physician, Greater Baltimore Medical Center, Baltimore, MD

A. Kesh Hebbar, M.D., Assistant Professor of Family Medicine, Medical University of South Carolina, Charleston, SC

Denise D. Hermann, M.D., Associate Clinical Professor of Medicine, Division of Cardiology, Department of Medicine, University of California–San Diego Medical Center, San Diego, CA

William J. Hueston, M.D., Professor and Chairman, Department of Family Medicine, Medical University of South Carolina, Charleston, SC

Michael S. Klinkman, M.D., M.S., Associate Professor of Family Medicine, University of Michigan School of Medicine, Ann Arbor, MI

Patrick E. McBride, M.D., M.P.H., Professor of Medicine, University of Wisconsin Medical School, Madison, WI

William A. Norcross, M.D., Professor of Clinical Family Medicine, University of California–San Diego School of Medicine, La Jolla, CA

Jim Nuovo, M.D., Associate Professor of Family and Community Medicine, University of California–Davis School of Medicine, Sacramento, CA

Glenn S. Rodriguez, M.D., Regional Medical Director of Quality Improvement and Health Services Integration, Providence Health System, Portland; Adjunct Associate Professor of Family Medicine, Oregon Health & Science University School of Medicine, Portland, OR

Thomas M. Schwartz, M.D., Clinical Assistant Professor of Family Medicine, Oregon Health and Science University School of Medicine; Faculty, Providence Milwaukie Family Practice Residency Program, Portland, OR

James H. Stein, M.D., Associate Professor of Medicine, University of Wisconsin Medical School, Madison, WI

Gail Underbakke, R.D., M.S., Nutrition Coordinator, Preventive Cardiology Program, University of Wisconsin Hospital and Clinics, Madison, WI

Eric Walsh, M.D., Associate Professor of Family Medicine, Oregon Health & Science University School of Medicine, Portland; Director, Oregon Health & Science University Family Practice Residency Program, Portland, OR

1
Hypertension

Stephen A. Brunton

Despite widespread efforts to improve education and enhance public awareness, up to 33% of persons with hypertension remain undiagnosed, and only about 50% of those known to have hypertension are adequately controlled. The percentages of patients who are aware that they have hypertension, who are treated, and who are controlled have increased since the 1970s (Table 1.1). Most have stage 1 hypertension, and controversy still exists concerning the appropriate approach to these patients. Nonpharmacologic therapy is often the first choice, and this approach continues to evolve.[1] Of the 20 to 30 million hypertensives who receive pharmacologic therapy, fewer than 50% adhere to their therapeutic regimen for more than 1 year, and 60% of these patients reduce the dosage of their drug owing to adverse effects. A negative impact on the patient's quality-of-life may occur as a result of just making the diagnosis. Effects such as increased absenteeism, sickness behavior, hypochondria, and decreased self-esteem have been noted in cohorts of previously well individuals who have been told they were hypertensive.[2] A 1987 survey of physicians revealed that they regarded quality-of-life changes to be the primary impediment to effective pharmacologic treatment of hypertension.

The challenge to the clinician is to provide patient education and develop a hypertension regimen that effectively lowers blood pressure or reduces cardiac risk factors, minimizes changes in concomitant disease states, and maintains or improves quality of life. Putting the patient first necessitates integrating the individual patient's lifestyle and current disease states with a thorough understanding of the effect of drug and nondrug therapy on quality of life.

Table 1.1. **Trends in the Awareness, Treatment, and Control of High Blood Pressure in Adults: United States, 1976–94[a]**

	NHANES II (1976–80)	NHANES III (Phase 1) 1988–91	NHANES III (Phase 2) 1991–94
Awareness	51%	73%	68.4%
Treatment	31%	55%	53.6%
Control[b]	10%	29%	27.4%

[a]Data are for adults age 18 to 74 years with SBP of 140 mm Hg or greater, DBP of 90 mm Hg or greater, or taking antihypertensive medication.
[b]SBP below 140 mm Hg and DBP below 90 mm Hg.
Source: National Institutes of Health.[1]

This chapter reviews nonpharmacologic and pharmacologic therapy, with special emphasis on individualizing patient regimens to improve adherence.

Detection

The diagnosis of hypertension should not be based on any single measurement but should be established on the basis of at least three readings with an average systolic blood pressure of 140 mm Hg and a diastolic pressure of 90 mm Hg. Mechanisms should be established to standardize the measurement process: (1) The patient should be seated comfortably with the arm positioned at heart level. (2) Caffeine or nicotine should not have been ingested within 30 minutes before measurement. (3) The patient should be seated in a quiet environment for at least 5 minutes. (4) An appropriate sphygmomanometer cuff should be used (i.e., the rubber bladder should encircle at least two-thirds of the arm). (5) Measurement of the diastolic blood pressure should be based on the disappearance of sound (phase V Korotkoff sound). Table 1.2 describes the classification of blood pressure for adults.

Evaluation

Evaluation is directed toward establishing the etiology of hypertension, identifying other cardiovascular risk factors, and evaluating the

Table 1.2. **Classification of Blood Pressure for Adults Aged 18 Years and Older**[a]

Category	Systolic (mm Hg)	Diastolic (mm Hg)
Optimal[b]	<120	<80
Normal	<130	<85
High normal	130–139	85–89
Hypertension[c]		
Stage 1	140–159	90–99
Stage 2	160–179	100–109
Stage 3	>180	>110

Source: National Institutes of Health.[1]

Note: In addition to classifying stages of hypertension based on average blood pressure levels, the clinician should specify the presence or absence of target organ disease and additional risk factors. For example, a patient with diabetes, a blood pressure of 142/94 mm Hg, and left ventricular hypertrophy should be classified as "stage 1 hypertension with target organ disease (left ventricular hypertrophy) and with another major risk factor (diabetes)." This specificity is important for risk classification and management.

[a]Not taking antihypertensive drugs and not acutely ill. When systolic and diastolic pressures fall into different categories, the higher category should be selected to classify the individual's blood pressure status. For instance, 160/92 mm Hg should be classified as stage 2 and 174/120 mm Hg as stage 3. Isolated systolic hypertension is defined as systolic pressure of 140 mm Hg or more and diastolic pressure of less than 90 mm Hg and staged appropriately (e.g., 170/82 mm Hg is defined as stage 2 isolated systolic hypertension).

[b]Optimal blood pressure with respect to cardiovascular risk is systolic pressure <120 mm Hg and diastolic pressure <80 mm Hg. However, unusually low readings should be evaluated for clinical significance.

[c]Based on the average of two or more readings taken at each of two or more visits after an initial screening.

possibility of target organ damage. Although most hypertension is considered "essential," primary, or idiopathic, it is necessary to eliminate secondary causes of hypertension, including renovascular disease, polycystic renal disease, aortic coarctation, Cushing syndrome, and pheochromocytoma. It is important to ensure that the patient is not on medications that may result in increased blood pressure, such as oral contraceptives, nasal decongestants, appetite suppressants, nonsteroidal antiinflammatory drugs (NSAIDs), steroids, and tricyclic antidepressants.

Medical History

The medical history should include a review of the family history for hypertension and cardiovascular disease, previous measurements of blood pressure, symptoms suggestive of secondary causes of hypertension, and other cardiovascular risk factors including smoking, hyperlipidemia, obesity, and diabetes. Environmental and psychosocial factors that may influence blood pressure control or the ability of the individual to comply with therapy should also be considered.

Physical Examination and Laboratory Tests

The physical examination should include more than one blood pressure measurement in both standing and seated positions with verification in the contralateral arm. (If a discrepancy exists, the higher value is used.) The rest of the physical examination includes (1) an evaluation of the optic fundi with gradation of hypertensive changes; (2) examination of the neck for bruits and thyromegaly; (3) a heart examination to evaluate for hypertrophy, arrhythmias, or additional sounds; (4) abdominal examination to search for evidence of aneurysms or kidney abnormalities; (5) examination of the extremities to check the pulses; and (6) a careful neurologic evaluation.

Some baseline laboratory tests may be helpful for the initial evaluation. They might include urinalysis and serum potassium, blood urea nitrogen, and creatinine levels. A lipid panel may help evaluate cardiovascular risk.

Treatment

The goal of therapy is not just to bring the blood pressure lower than 140 mm Hg systolic and 90 mm Hg diastolic, but rather to prevent the morbidity and mortality associated with hypertension. As such, the decision to treat hypertension is based on documentation that the blood pressure has remained elevated and on assessment of the risk for that particular patient.

In general, individuals with blood pressure ranges considered borderline high (i.e., systolic of 130 to 139 mm Hg or diastolic of 85 to 89 mm Hg) should have their blood pressures rechecked within 1 year. Blood pressures in the stage 1 range should be confirmed within 2 months by repeated measurements; however, certain lifestyle approaches are appropriate even at this level. Blood pressures that are markedly elevated (e.g., systolic >180 mm Hg or diastolic >110 mm Hg) or those associated with evidence of existing end-organ damage may require immediate pharmacologic intervention. In general, whether pharmacologic intervention is initiated, a nonpharmacologic approach is the foundation of any management strategy.[1]

Nonpharmacologic Therapeutic Approaches

Information concerning dietary modifications, exercise, weight reduction, the role of cations, and the possible role of relaxation and stress management techniques for reducing blood pressure have opened the door for greater acceptance of multiple nonpharmacologic approaches to the treatment of hypertension. The 1988 report of the Joint National Committee (JNC) on the Detection, Evaluation, and Treatment of High Blood Pressure recommended that "nonpharmacological approaches be used both as definitive intervention and as an adjunct for pharmacological therapy and should be considered for all antihypertensive therapy."

Several studies have shown positive correlation of increased blood pressure with alcohol consumption of more than 2 ounces/day.[3] Although smoking has not been shown to cause sustained hypertension, it is associated with increased cardiovascular, pulmonary, and hypertension risks, and therefore should be eliminated.[4]

Weight reduction has a strong correlation with decreased blood pressure in obese individuals. Stamler et al[5] reported that a 10-pound weight loss maintained over a 4-year period allowed 50% of participants previously on pharmacologic management to remain normotensive and free of medication.

Sodium restriction has been a mainstay of hypertension control, as a 100-mEq drop in daily intake can result in a 2- to 9-mm Hg decline in systolic blood pressure in salt-sensitive individuals. This goal is one of the easiest for a patient to accomplish, as moderate restriction can be accomplished by eliminating table salt for cooking, avoiding salty foods, and using a salt substitute.[6]

Regular aerobic exercise not only assists with weight reduction but also appears to lower diastolic blood pressure. Cade and associates[7] reported a decline from 117 to 97 mm Hg diastolic blood pressure after 3 months of daily walking or running for 2 miles. This effect appeared to be independent of weight loss, and some benefit persisted even if the patient became sedentary.

Vegetarian diets high in polyunsaturated fats, potassium, and fiber result in lower blood pressures than diets high in saturated fats. Dietary fat control also contributes to the reduction of cholesterol and coronary artery disease risk.[8] The role of cations such as potassium, magnesium, and calcium in lowering blood pressure has now been investigated. High potassium intake (>80 mEq/day) may result in a modest decline in blood pressure while offering a natriuretic and cardioprotective effect. These effects are more pronounced in hypokalemic individuals.[9] Magnesium and calcium supplementation of more than 300 mg/day and 800 mg/day, respectively, have been shown to lower the relative risk of developing hypertension in a large cohort of women. The impact of individual supplementation is less clear, and the role of these substances is still controversial.[10]

Stress management and relaxation techniques over a 4-year period have been shown to reduce systolic blood pressure 10 to 15 mm Hg and diastolic blood pressure 5 to 10 mm Hg. However, these results are variable and are largely dependent on the instructor–patient relationship.[11]

The effects of nonpharmacologic approaches can be additive and certainly are beneficial even if the patient requires drug therapy. Stamler and associates[12] documented that reducing weight and lowering salt and alcohol intake allowed 39% of patients previously on therapy to remain normotensive without medication over a 4-year period. In the mildly hypertensive individual, these lifestyle modifications should be tried for at least 6 months before initiating pharmacologic therapy.

Pharmacologic Therapy

The decision to initiate drug therapy requires consideration of individual patient characteristics, such as age, race, sex, family history, cardiovascular risk factors, concomitant disease states, compliance, and ability to purchase the prescribed therapeutic agent. Pharmacologic therapy is recommended when the systolic blood pressure is higher than 160 mm Hg and the diastolic blood pressure remains higher than 100 mm Hg. Treatment of stage 2 and 3 hypertension (systolic pressure >160 and diastolic pressure >100 mm Hg) has reduced cardiovascular morbidity and mortality dramatically since the 1960s. The incidence of stroke, congestive heart failure, and left ventricular hypertrophy has also decreased among treated stage 1 hypertensives, and therapy is recommended if patients have one or more cardiovascular risk factors and have not controlled their blood pressure after 6 months of lifestyle modification.

The ideal antihypertensive agent would improve quality of life, reduce coronary heart disease risk factors, maintain normal hemodynamic profiles, reduce left ventricular hypertrophy, have a positive impact on concomitant disease states, and reduce end-organ damage while effectively lowering blood pressure on a convenient dosing regimen at minimal cost to the patient. This "magic bullet" has yet to be synthesized, although several of the newer antihypertensive classes offer the possibility of many of these positive outcomes.

The selection of an appropriate antihypertensive agent may be based on the current recommendations of the JNC on the Detection, Evaluation, and Treatment of High Blood Pressure or individualized to the specific medical, social, psychological, and economic situation of each patient.[1] The previous stepped-care approach has been modified by the JNC into an algorithm that permits an individualized approach to the patient (Fig. 1.1). Many clinicians have moved away from the stepped-care philosophy toward a monotherapy approach, which maximizes the dose of one drug before substituting or adding another. Combination therapy with lower doses of several agents may also be utilized to minimize adverse effects. Therapeutic choices must be based on a sound understanding of the mechanism of action, pharmacokinetics, adverse effect profile, and cost of available agents.

Major Antihypertensive Classes

ACE Inhibitors

Angiotensin-converting enzyme (ACE) inhibitors (Table 1.3) block the conversion of angiotensin I to angiotensin II, resulting in decreased aldosterone production with subsequent increased sodium and water excretion. Renin and potassium levels are usually increased as a result of this medication. The hemodynamic response includes decreased peripheral resistance, increased renal blood flow, and minimal changes in cardiac output and glomerular filtration rate. There is little change in insulin and glucose levels or in the lipid fractions. The adverse effects of ACE inhibitors include cough (1–30%), headache, dizziness, first-dose syncope in salt- or volume-depleted patients, acute renal failure in patients with renal artery stenosis, angioedema (0.1–0.2%), and teratogenic effects in the human fetus. Thus, ACE inhibitors should not be used during the second and third trimesters of pregnancy. Captopril (Capoten) has a higher incidence of rash, dysgeusia, neutropenia, and proteinuria than the others due to a sulfhydryl group in the ring structure.[13]

The ACE inhibitors are good first-line agents for patients with diabetes, congestive heart failure, peripheral vascular disease, elevated lipids, and renal insufficiency. This class is effective in all races and ages, although black patients respond better with the addition of a diuretic.[14,15]

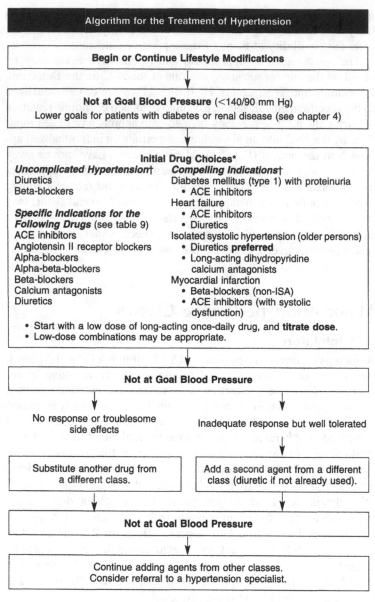

Algorithm for the Treatment of Hypertension

Begin or Continue Lifestyle Modifications

↓

Not at Goal Blood Pressure (<140/90 mm Hg)
Lower goals for patients with diabetes or renal disease (see chapter 4)

↓

Initial Drug Choices*

Uncomplicated Hypertension†	*Compelling Indications†*

Uncomplicated Hypertension†
Diuretics
Beta-blockers

*Specific Indications for the
Following Drugs* (see table 9)
ACE inhibitors
Angiotensin II receptor blockers
Alpha-blockers
Alpha-beta-blockers
Beta-blockers
Calcium antagonists
Diuretics

Compelling Indications†
Diabetes mellitus (type 1) with proteinuria
 • ACE inhibitors
Heart failure
 • ACE inhibitors
 • Diuretics
Isolated systolic hypertension (older persons)
 • Diuretics **preferred**
 • Long-acting dihydropyridine
   calcium antagonists
Myocardial infarction
 • Beta-blockers (non-ISA)
 • ACE inhibitors (with systolic
   dysfunction)

 • Start with a low dose of long-acting once-daily drug, and **titrate dose**.
 • Low-dose combinations may be appropriate.

↓

Not at Goal Blood Pressure

↓   ↓

No response or troublesome   Inadequate response but well tolerated
side effects

↓   ↓

Substitute another drug from   Add a second agent from a different
a different class.   class (diuretic if not already used).

↓   ↓

Not at Goal Blood Pressure

↓

Continue adding agents from other classes.
Consider referral to a hypertension specialist.

*Unless contraindicated. ACE indicates angiotensin-converting enzyme; ISA, intrinsic sympathomimetic activity.
†Based on randomized controlled trials (see chapters 3 and 4).

Fig. 1.1. Algorithm for the treatment of hypertension. (From National Institutes of Health.[1])

Angiotensin Receptor Antagonists

Angiotensin receptor antagonists, a newer class of antihypertensive agents, binds to the angiotensin II receptors, resulting in blockade of the vasoconstrictor and aldosterone-secreting effects of angiotensin II. In addition, bradykinin production is not stimulated. The first agent available in the United States was losartan (Cozaar). The physiologic effects of losartan include a rise in plasma renin and angiotensin II levels and a decrease in aldosterone production. There is no significant change in plasma potassium levels and no effect on glomerular filtration rate, renal plasma flow, heart rate, triglycerides, total cholesterol, high-density lipoprotein (HDL) cholesterol, or glucose. Losartan use does produce a small uricosuric effect with lowering of plasma uric acid levels.

These agents are effective antihypertensives in adults and the elderly. Blood pressure–lowering effects are not as significant in black patients. Adverse effects include muscle pain, dizziness, cough, insomnia, and nasal congestion. As with ACE inhibitors, angiotensin receptor antagonists should not be used during the second and third trimesters of pregnancy.

At this time the role of angiotensin receptor antagonists is not completely defined. Further study of the hemodynamic effects in large populations is needed to determine the role in cardiac patients. These agents are an alternative antihypertensive agent for patients experiencing adverse effects from ACE inhibitors.

Calcium Entry Antagonists

Calcium entry antagonists (CEAs) inhibit the movement of calcium across cell membranes in myocardial and smooth muscles. This action dilates coronary arteries, and additional peripheral arteriole dilation reduces total peripheral resistance, resulting in decreased blood pressure. Although the mechanism of action for lowering blood pressure is similar for these agents, structural differences result in varying effects on cardiac conduction and adverse effect profiles. Verapamil (Calan, Covera, Isoptin, Verelan) and diltiazem (Cardizem, Dilacor, Tiazac) slow atrioventricular (AV) node conduction and prolong the effective refractory period in the AV node. Cardiac output is increased by nifedipine (Procardia), nicardipine (Cardene), isradipine (DynaCirc), and felodipine (Plendil).

The calcium entry antagonists are contraindicated in patients with heart block, cardiogenic shock, or acute myocardial infarction. Common adverse effects include peripheral edema, dizziness, headache, asthenia, nausea, constipation, flushing, and tachycardia. Calcium entry antagonists have no significant impact on lipid profiles or glucose metabolism.[1]

These agents are effective at all ages and in all races. They are good choices for patients with diabetes, angina, migraine, chronic obstructive pulmonary disease (COPD)/asthma, peripheral vascular disease, renal insufficiency, and supraventricular arrhythmias.[14,15]

Diuretics

Thiazide, loop, and potassium-sparing diuretics have been the mainstay of antihypertensive therapy since the 1960s. They remain as first-line agents in the JNC VI approach, although the ACE inhibitors and calcium entry antagonists are rapidly replacing diuretics as monotherapy for hypertension.

Thiazide diuretics increase renal excretion of sodium and chloride at the distal segment of the renal tubule, resulting in decreased plasma volume, cardiac output, and renal blood flow and increased renin activity. Potassium excretion is increased, and calcium and uric acid elimination is decreased.[13] Thiazides adversely affect lipid metabolism by increasing the total cholesterol level 6% to 10% and the low-density lipoprotein (LDL) cholesterol 6% to 20%, and by causing a possible 15% to 20% rise in triglycerides.[15] Plasma glucose levels increase secondary to a decrease in insulin secretion. Clinical adverse effects include nausea, vomiting, diarrhea, dizziness, headache, fatigue, muscle cramps, gout attacks, and impotence. Thiazides are inexpensive choices for initial therapy, but caution must be exercised in patients with preexisting cardiac dysfunction, lipid abnormalities, diabetes mellitus, and gout. The lowest effective dose is recommended to minimize these potential adverse effects. Suggested daily doses are hydrochlorothiazide (HydroDIURIL) 25 mg, chlorthalidone (Hygroton) 25 mg, and indapamide (Lozol) 2.5 mg daily. Indapamide is unique among thiazides in that it has minimal effects on glucose, lipids, and uric acid. Thiazides are good choices for volume/salt-dependent, low-renin hypertensives. Thiazides improve blood pressure control when added to ACE inhibitors, beta-blockers, vasodilators, and alpha-blockers.

The loop diuretics—furosemide (Lasix), torsemide (Demadex), and bumetanide (Bumex)—inhibit sodium and chloride reabsorption in the proximal and distal tubules and the loop of Henle. These diuretics are effective in patients with decreased renal function. The primary adverse effects include ototoxicity with high doses in patients with severe renal disease and in combination with an aminoglycoside, photosensitivity, excess potassium loss, increased serum uric acid, decreased calcium levels, and impaired glucose metabolism. Patients may experience nausea, vomiting, diarrhea, headache, blurred vision, tinnitus, muscle cramps, fatigue, or weakness. Furosemide and bumetanide are utilized in patients with compromised renal function or congestive heart failure (CHF) and as adjuncts to volume-retaining agents such as hydralazine (Apresoline) and minoxidil (Loniten).

The potassium-sparing diuretics spironolactone (Aldactone), triamterene (Dyrenium), and amiloride (Midamor) are useful for preventing potassium wastage from thiazide and loop diuretics. Spironolactone competitively inhibits the uptake of aldosterone at the receptor site in the distal tubule, thereby reducing aldosterone effects. It is used for treatment of primary aldosteronism, CHF, cirrhosis with ascites, hypertension, and hirsutism. Triamterene is used in combination with hydrochlorothiazide as Dyazide or Maxzide and effectively prevents potassium loss. Amiloride inhibits potassium excretion at the collecting duct. Adverse reactions associated with spironolactone include gynecomastia, nausea, vomiting, diarrhea, muscle cramps, lethargy, and hyperkalemia. Triamterene and amiloride have adverse effects similar to those seen with the thiazide diuretics.[13-15]

Antiadrenergic Agents

Beta-Blockers

β-adrenergic blocking agents compete with β-agonists for B_1 receptors in cardiac muscles and B_2 receptors in the bronchial and vascular musculature, inhibiting the dilator, inotropic, and chronotropic effects of β-adrenergic stimulation. Clinical responses to β-adrenergic blockade include decreased heart rate, cardiac output, blood pressure, renin production, and bronchiolar constriction; there is also an initial increase in total peripheral resistance, which returns to normal with chronic use.

Beta-blockers are contraindicated for sinus bradycardia, second- or third-degree heart block, cardiogenic shock, cardiac failure, and severe COPD/asthma. The adverse effect profile of beta-blocking agents is partially dependent on their receptor selectivity (Table 1.3). Acebutolol (Sectral), penbutolol (Levatol), carteolol (Cartrol), and pindolol (Visken) have intrinsic sympathomimetic activity (ISA), resulting in less effect on cardiac output and lipid profiles. Beta-blockers without ISA slow the heart rate, decrease cardiac output, increase peripheral vascular resistance, and cause bronchospasm. Common adverse effects include fatigue, impotence, depression, short-

Table 1.3. **Antihypertensive Drugs**

Drug class	Available doses (mg)	Usual dose/schedule (mg/day)	Half-life (hours)	Peak (hours)	Pregnancy class
ACE inhibitors					
Benazepril (Lotensin)	5, 10, 20, 40	10–40 qd	10	2–4	C (1st trimester) D (2nd and 3rd trimester)
Captopril (Capoten)	12.5, 25, 50, 100	25–50 bid–tid	2	1–2	C (1st trimester) D (2nd and 3rd trimester)
Enalapril (Vasotec)	2.5, 5, 10, 20	5–40 qd	11	4	C (1st trimester) D (2nd and 3rd trimester)
Fosinopril (Monopril)	10, 20	10–40 qd	12	2–6	C (1st trimester) D (2nd and 3rd trimester)
Lisinopril (Prinivil, Zestril)	2.5, 5, 10, 20, 40	10–40 qd	12	6	C (1st trimester) D (2nd and 3rd trimester)
Moexipril (Univasc)	7.5, 15	7.5–30 qd	2–10	1.5	C (1st trimester) D (2nd and 3rd trimester)
Quinapril (Accupril)	5, 10, 20, 40	10–80 qd	2	2–4	C (1st trimester) D (2nd and 3rd trimester)

				Selectivity	
Perindopril (Aceon)	2, 4, 8,	3–10	4–8qd	3–7	C (1st trimester) D (2nd and 3rd trimester)
Ramipril (Altace)	1.25, 2.5, 5, 10	2	2.5–20 qd	3–6	C (1st trimester) D (2nd and 3rd trimester)
Trandolapril (Mavik)	1, 2, 4	10	2–4 mg qd	4–10	C (1st trimester) D (2nd and 3rd trimester)
β-Blockers					
Atenolol (Tenormin)	25, 50, 100	9	50–100 qd	B_1	C
Acebutolol (Sectral)	200, 400	4	400–800 qd	B_1, ISA	B
Betaxolol (Kerlone)	10, 20	22	10–20 qd	B_1	C
Bisoprolol (Zebeta)	5, 10	11	5–20 qd	B_1	C
Carteolol (Cartrol)	2.5, 5	6	2.5–10 qd	B_1, B_2, ISA	C
Labetalol (Normodyne)	100, 200, 300	6	100–400 bid	B_1, B_2, α	C
Nadolol (Corgard)	20, 40, 80, 120, 160	24	40–80 qd	B_1, B_2	C
Metoprolol (Lopressor)	50, 100	3	100–450 qd	B_1	C
Penbutolol (Levatol)	20	5	20–80 qd	B_1, B_2, ISA	C
Pindolol (Visken)	5, 10	4	10–30 qd	B_1, B_2, ISA	B
Propranolol (Inderal)	60, 80, 120, 160, SR; 10, 20, 40, 60, 80, 90	10	80–160 SR qd 20–120 bid	B_1, B_2	C
Timolol (Blocadren)	5, 10, 20	4	10–30 bid	B_1, B_2	C

(continued)

Table 1.3 (Continued).

Drug class	Available doses (mg)	Usual dose/schedule (mg/day)	Half-life (hours)	Peak (hours)	Pregnancy class
Calcium entry antagonists					
Amlodipine (Norvasc)	2.5, 5, 10	2.5–10		6–12	C
Diltiazem (Cardizem)	SR 60, 90, 120	SR 60–120 bid		6–11	C
	CD 120, 180, 240, 300	CD 180–360 qd		12	
(Dilacor XR)	30, 60, 90, 120,	30–90 qid	6	2–3	C
	120, 180, 240	120–360 qd	4	4–6	C
Felodipine (Plendil)	SR 2.5, 5, 10	5–20 qd	16	2–5	C
Isradipine (DynaCirc)	2.5, 5	2.5–5 bid	8	1.5	C
Nicardipine	SR 30, 45, 60	SR 30–60 bid			
(Cardene)	20, 30	20–40 tid	4	0.5–2	C
Nifedipine	SR 10, 20, 30, 60, 90	30–120 qd	5	0.5–6	C
(Adalat Procardia)					
Nisoldipine (Sular)	10, 20, 30, 40	20–40 qd	10	6–12	C
Verapamil (Calan,	SR 120, 180, 240	240–480 qd	7	1–2	C
Covera, Isoptin,	40, 80, 120				
Verelan)					
α_1-blockers					
Doxazosin (Cardura)	1, 2, 4, 8	1–16 mg qd	22	2–3	B
Prazosin (Minipress)	1, 2, 5	1–5 bid–tid	3	3	C
Terazosin (Hytrin)	1, 2, 5, 10	1–10 qd	12	1–2	C
Central α_2-agonists					
Clonidine (Catapres)	0.1, 0.2, 0.3	0.2–1.2 qd	16	3–5	C
	TTS 1, 2, 3	1 patch weekly	19	2–3 days	

Guanabenz (Wytensin)	4, 8	4–8 bid	6	2–4	C
Guanfacine (Tenex)	1, 2	1–3 qd	17	3	B
Methyldopa (Aldomet)	125, 250, 500	250–500 tid–qid	2	2–4	B
Vasodilators					
Hydralazine (Apresoline)	10, 25, 50, 100	10–50 qid	7	0.5–2	C
Minoxidil (Loniten)	2.5, 10	10–40 qd	4	2–3	C
αβ-Blockers					
Carvedilol (Coreg)	6.25, 12.5, 25	6.25–12.5 bid	7	3–4	C
Labetalol (Normodyne)	100, 200, 300	100 mg–400 bid	6	2–4	C
Selected thiazide diuretics					
Chlorothiazide (Diuril)	250–500	500–2000 qd	6–12	4	
Hydrochlorothiazide (HydroDIURIL)	25, 50, 100	25–50 qd	6–12	4–6	
Chlorthalidone (Hygroton)	25, 50, 100	25–100 qd	24–72	2–6	
Indapamide (Lozol)	1.25, 2.5	2.5–5 qd	36	2	B
Metolazone (Zaroxolyn)	0.5, 2.5, 5, 10	2.5–5 qd	12–24	2.6	B
Loop diuretics					
Bumetanide (Bumex)	0.5, 1, 2	0.5–2 qd	4–6	1–2,	C
Furosemide (Lasix)	20, 40, 80	20–40 qd–bid	6–8	1–2	C
Potassium-sparing diuretics					
Amiloride (Midamor)	5	5–20 qd	24	6–10	B

(continued)

Table 1.3 (Continued).

Drug class	Available doses (mg)	Usual dose/schedule (mg/day)	Half-life (hours)	Peak (hours)	Pregnancy class
Spironolactone (Aldactone)	25, 50, 100	25–100 qd	48–72	48–72	D
Triamterene (Dyrenium)	50, 100	100 bid	12–16	6–8	B
Angiotensin receptor antagonists					
Eprosartan (Teveten)	400, 600	400–800 qd	5–9	3–6	C (1st trimester) D (2nd and 3rd trimester)
Irbesartan (Avapro)	75, 150, 300	150–300 qd	11–15	3–6	C (1st trimester) D (2nd and 3rd trimester)
Losartan (Cozaar)	25, 50	25–100 qd	2–9	1–4	C (1st trimester) D (2nd and 3rd trimester)
Telmisartan (Micardis)	20, 40, 80	20–80 qd	24	0.5–1	C (1st trimester) D (2nd and 3rd trimester)
Valsartan (Diovan)	80, 160	80–320 qd	6	2–4	C (1st trimester) D (2nd and 3rd trimester)

ISA = Intrinsic sympathomimetic activity; D = positive evidence of human fetal risk; C = fetal risk documented in animals; B = low fetal risk; SR = slow release; CD = controlled delivery.

ness of breath, cold extremities, cough, drowsiness, and dizziness. The more lipid-soluble agents, such as propranolol and metoprolol, have a higher incidence of central nervous system (CNS) effects. In diabetic patients beta-blockers may mask the usual symptoms of hypoglycemia, such as tremor, tachycardia, and hunger.[13] Increased triglycerides (30%) and decreased HDL cholesterol (1–20%) occur with non-ISA agents.[15] Beta-blockers are effective agents in the young and white populations. Black patients may not respond as well to monotherapy because of their lower renin levels. Beta-blockers are good choices for patients with supraventricular tachycardia, high cardiac output, angina, recent myocardial infarction, migraine, and glaucoma. Caution should be exercised in those with diabetes, CHF, peripheral vascular disease, COPD/asthma, and an elevated lipid profile.[14]

Central Acting Drugs

Methyldopa (Aldomet), clonidine (Catapres), guanfacine (Tenex), and guanabenz (Wytensin) are central α_2-agonists. These agents decrease dopamine and norepinephrine production in the brain, resulting in a decrease in sympathetic nervous activity throughout the body. Blood pressure declines with the decrease in peripheral resistance. Methyldopa exhibits a unique adverse effect profile as it induces autoimmune disorders, such as those with positive Coombs' and antinuclear antibody (ANA) tests, hemolytic anemia, and hepatic necrosis. The other agents produce sedation, dry mouth, and dizziness. Abrupt clonidine withdrawal may result in rebound hypertension. These drugs are good choices for patients with asthma, diabetes, high cholesterol, and peripheral vascular disease.

Peripheral Acting Drugs

Guanadrel (Hylorel), reserpine (Serpasil), and guanethidine (Ismelin) are peripheral antiadrenergic agents. Their mechanism of action is at the storage granule level of norepinephrine release. They are infrequently chosen because of their significant side effects, which include profound hypotension, sedation, depression, and impotence.

α_1-Blockers

α_1-Receptor blockers have an affinity for the α_1-receptor on vascular smooth muscles, thereby blocking the uptake of catecholamines by smooth muscle cells. This action results in peripheral vasodilation. The currently available agents are prazosin (Minipress), terazosin (Hytrin), and doxazosin (Cardura). There is a marked reduction in blood pressure with the first dose of these drugs. It is recommended that they be started with 1 mg at bedtime and titrate slowly upward over 2 to 4 weeks. When adding a second antihypertensive the α-blocker dose should be decreased and titrated upward again. Often a diuretic is added to α_1-blocker therapy to reduce sodium and water retention. The primary adverse effects of these three drugs are dizziness, sedation, nasal congestion, headache, and postural effects. They do not significantly affect lipids, glucose, electrolytes, or exercise tolerance. α_1-Blockers are good choices for young active adults and patients with diabetes, renal insufficiency, CHF, peripheral vascular disease, COPD/asthma, or elevated lipids.

The Antihypertensive and Lipid Lowering Treatment to Prevent Heart Attack Trial (ALLHAT) was initiated in 1994 to evaluate the impact of various classes of antihypertensives on outcomes. In early 2000 the doxazosin treatment arm was discontinued because a twofold higher incidence of CHF was noted compared to those on chlorthalidone.[16]

Vasodilators

The two direct vasodilators, hydralazine (Apresoline) and minoxidil (Loniten), dilate peripheral arterioles, resulting in a significant fall in blood pressure. A sympathetic reflex increase in heart rate, renin and catecholamine release, and venous constriction occur. The renal response includes sodium and water retention. The patient often experiences tachycardia, flushing, and headache. Addition of a diuretic and a beta-blocker relieves the major adverse effects of the vasodilators. Hydralazine may cause a lupuslike reaction with fever, rash, and joint pain. Chronic use of minoxidil often results in hirsutism with increased facial and arm hair. These drugs are third- or fourth-line agents because of their adverse side-effect profile.[13–15]

Quality-of-Life Issues

The need for lifestyle changes and probable drug therapy increases the possibility that the patient's quality of life will be altered. The adverse physical, mental, and metabolic effects of antihypertensive therapy results in significant nonadherence to prescribed regimens. In 1982 Jachuck and associates[17] investigated the effect of medications on their patients by asking them, their closest relatives, and their physicians a series of questions concerning their quality of life since starting the blood pressure medications. The physicians and patients thought there was either no change or improvement, whereas 99% of the relatives thought the patients were worse. They cited side effects such as memory loss, irritability, decreased libido, hypochondria, and decreased energy as major problems.[17] Other studies during the 1980s confirm that nonselective beta-blockers, diuretics, and methyldopa compromised quality of life to a far greater extent than ACE inhibitors or calcium entry antagonists.[17–19] Further research in this area is necessary to assist the physician in determining the optimum strategy for blood pressure control to improve adherence and quality of life.

Antihypertensive Selection

It is important to consider the patient's lifestyle, economic status, belief systems, and concerns about treatment when selecting an antihypertensive agent. Therapy should be initiated with one drug in small doses to minimize adverse effects. It is important to educate the patient about the long-term benefits of therapy, including the decreased incidence of stroke and renal and cardiac disease. Adequate follow-up visits are scheduled to assess adherence and adverse effects. During these visits the patient is asked to describe the mental, physical, and emotional changes that have occurred as a result of therapy. If adverse effects are bothersome, consider an alternative selection from a different drug class and attempt to maintain monotherapy. If a second drug is needed, agents can be combined that improve efficacy without significantly altering the adverse-effect profile (e.g., adding a diuretic to an ACE inhibitor).

There are some special considerations when prescribing medications. Concomitant disease states must be considered and drugs selected that either improve or at least maintain the current clinical condition. Hypertension is a major risk factor for thrombotic and hemorrhagic strokes; smoking, CHF, diabetes, and coronary artery disease increase the risk. Patients with coronary artery disease may benefit from a calcium entry antagonist or beta-blocker with ISA to decrease anginal pain while resulting in minimal changes in lipid profiles. CHF and hypertension respond well to ACE inhibitors and diuretic therapy. Diabetes may be adversely affected by thiazide diuretics and beta-blockers. ACE inhibitors, calcium entry antagonists, and central α_2-agonists are appropriate choices.

Patients with severe renal disease are most effectively treated with loop diuretics, whereas ACE inhibitors and CEAs may decrease proteinuria and slow the progress of renal failure. As renal function declines, ACE inhibitors must be used with some caution as increased potassium and decreased renal perfusion may occur. A few agents such as methyldopa, clonidine, atenolol, nadolol, and captopril need dosage reduction in the presence of renal failure.

Asthma and COPD patients may be effectively treated with calcium entry antagonists, central α_2-agonists, and α_1-blockers. Beta-blockers and possibly diuretics should be avoided because they might exacerbate bronchospasm.

The elderly are of special concern when selecting an antihypertensive. They have decreased receptor sensitivity, changing baroreceptor response, atherosclerosis, decreased myocardial function, declining total body water, decreased renal function, and memory loss. Blood pressure should be lowered cautiously using smaller than normal doses that are slowly titrated upward. Calcium entry antagonists, ACE inhibitors, and diuretics are possible choices for the elderly. Beta-blockers are effective in the elderly especially in conjunction with diuretics. Larger doses may result in declining mental function, depression, fatigue, and impotence. α_1-Blockers and central α_2-agonists may be used with caution. First-dose syncope and sedation are the major concerns.

Black patients may not respond as well to ACE inhibitors or beta-blockers as other races, perhaps due in part to low renin, salt/volume-dependent hypertension. Thiazide diuretics may adversely affect diabetes, gout, and lipids. Calcium entry antagonists, α_1-blockers, central α_2-agonists, and ACE inhibitors are possible choices.

Young women with hyperdynamic hypertension may respond best to a beta-blocker to slow the heart rate and relieve symptoms of stress. An active young man would be better served with an ACE inhibitor, calcium entry antagonist, or alpha-blocker, as beta-blockers and diuretics may cause impotence and exercise intolerance.[14]

Severe Hypertension and Emergencies

Patients with a diastolic blood pressure (DBP) over 115 mm Hg must be treated upon diagnosis. The blood pressure should be lowered in 5- to 10-mm Hg increments with a goal of lowering it to less than 100 mm Hg after several weeks of therapy. Often more than one drug must be used initially to control the blood pressure. A hypertensive emergency exists if the DBP is over 130 mm Hg and evidence of end-organ damage exists, such as retinal hemorrhage, encephalopathy, pulmonary edema, myocardial infarction, or unstable angina. Drugs available for treatment in this situation include sodium nitroprusside, nitroglycerin, hydralazine, phentolamine, labetalol, and methyldopa. Patients must be hospitalized for appropriate monitoring. Hypertensive urgency exists when the DBP is over 115 mm Hg without evidence of end-organ damage. Oral agents such as clonidine, captopril, and minoxidil may be used to lower the DBP 10 to 15 mm Hg over several hours.[1] Nifedipine should not be used in this situation as many serious adverse events have been reported including severe hypotension, acute myocardial infarction, and death.[20]

Conclusion

Pharmacologic management of hypertension challenges the physician to understand the patient's social, psychological, and economic status in order to select an antihypertensive regimen that effectively lowers the blood pressure, alleviates concomitant disease states, and allows easy adherence to the regimen. Continual assessment of therapy is necessary to determine the effectiveness of the regimen, adverse side effects, and the patient's quality-of-life issues.

Acknowledgment

The assistance of Janet Pick-Whitsitt, Pharm. D., with Table 1.3 is gratefully acknowledged.

References

1. National Institutes of Health. Sixth Report of the Joint National Committee on Detection, Evaluation, and Treatment of High Blood Pressure. National High Blood Pressure Education. NIH publication no. 98-4080. Bethesda: National Heart, Lung and Blood Institute, 1997.
2. Haynes RB, Sackett DL, Taylor DW, et al. Increased absenteeism from work after detection and labeling of hypertensive patients. N Engl J Med 1978;297:741–4.
3. Gordon T, Doyle JT. Alcohol consumption and its relationship to smoking, weight, blood pressure, and blood lipids. Arch Intern Med 1986;146:262–5.
4. Pooling Project Research Group. Relationship of blood pressure, serum cholesterol, smoking habit, relative weight and ECG abnormalities to incidence of major coronary events. J Chronic Dis 1978;31:201–6.
5. Stamler J, Farinaro E, Majonnier LM, et al. Prevention and control of hypertension by nutritional-hygienic means. JAMA 1980;243:1819–23.
6. Rose G, Stamler J. The Intersalt Study: background, methods and main results: Intersalt Cooperative Research Group. J Hum Hypertens 1989;3:283–8.

7. Cade R, Mars D, Wagemaker H, et al. Effect of aerobic exercise training on patients with systemic arterial hypertension. Am J Med 1984;77:785–90.

8. Margetts BM, Beilin LJ, Armstrong BK. A randomized control trial of a vegetarian diet in the treatment of mild hypertension. Clin Exp Pharmacol Physiol 1985;12:263–6.

9. Kaplan NM. Non-drug treatment of hypertension. Ann Intern Med 1985;102:359–73.

10. Witteman JC, Willett WC, Stampfer MJ, et al. A prospective study of nutritional factors and hypertension among US women. Circulation 1989;80:1320–7.

11. Patel C, Marmot MG. Stress management, blood pressure and quality of life. J Hypertens 1987;5(suppl 1):521–8.

12. Stamler R, Stamler J, Grimm R, et al. Nutritional therapy for high blood pressure. JAMA 1987;257:1484–91.

13. American Hospital Formulary Service Drug Information. Bethesda: American Society of Hospital Pharmacists, 2001.

14. Kaplan NM. Clinical hypertension, 7th ed. Baltimore: Williams & Wilkins, 1998.

15. Houston MC. New insights and new approaches for the treatment of essential hypertension: selection of therapy based on coronary heart disease, risk factor analysis, hemodynamic profiles, quality of life and subsets of hypertension. Am Heart J 1989;117:911–51.

16. ALLHAT Collaborative Research Group. Major cardiovascular events in hypertensive patients randomized to doxazosin vs. chlorthalidone: the antihypertensive and lipid-lowering treatment to prevent heart attack trial (ALLHAT) JAMA 1999;283(15):1967–75.

17. Jachuck SJ, Brierly H, Jachuck S, et al. The effect of hypotensive drugs on quality of life. J R Coll Gen Pract 1982;32:103–5.

18. Croog SH, Levine S, Testa MA, et al. The effects of antihypertensive therapy on the quality of life. N Engl J Med 1986;314:1657–64.

19. Steiner SS, Friedhoff AJ, Wilson BL, et al. Antihypertensive therapy and quality of life: a comparison of atenolol, captopril, enalapril and propranolol. J Hum Hypertens 1990;4:217–25.

20. Grossman E, Messerli FH, Grodzicki T. Should a moratorium be place on sublingual nifedipine capsules given for hypertensive emergencies and pseudoemergencies? JAMA 1996;276(16):1328–31.

2

Ischemic Heart Disease

Jim Nuovo

Cardiovascular disease remains the most significant cause of morbidity and mortality in the United States. In 1998 approximately 1.3 million Americans experienced a myocardial infarction (MI) and 700,000 of them died.[1] It is estimated that 12.4 million Americans are alive today with a history of MI, angina, or both. The financial impact of this disease is enormous. The cost estimate for cardiovascular disease in 1998 was over $110 billion. It is important for all primary care providers to implement screening and preventive care programs to reduce the burden of cardiovascular disease. Because of the high morbidity and mortality it is also important to recognize the early manifestations of this disease.

Unfortunately, in up to 20% of patients the first manifestation of ischemic heart disease (IHD) is sudden cardiac arrest.[2] Most deaths from IHD occur outside the hospital and within 2 hours of the onset of symptoms. Since the 1960s a great deal of effort has been directed toward the practice of cardiopulmonary resuscitation and emergency cardiac care. These efforts have been directed toward minimizing the number of cardiac deaths. Recently revised evidence-based guidelines present a summary of the collaborative effort of the American Heart Association and the International Liaison Committee on Resuscitation.[2] Furthermore, there has been a substantial undertaking to identify and treat individuals with significant cardiovascular risk factors with the goal of lowering morbidity and mortality. This effort has been successful as noted by the decline in death rates from myocardial ischemia and its complications. This chapter discusses three issues, relevant to the family physician, regarding IHD: the evaluation of patients with chest pain, the diagnosis and management of angina pectoris, and the diagnosis and management of MI.

Chest Pain

Chest pain is one of the common reasons for patients visiting primary care physicians.[3] The major diagnostic considerations for chest pain are listed in Table 2.1. Of the diagnostic considerations, which are the most commonly seen by family physicians? A Family Practice Research Network investigated this issue. Over 1 year the Michigan Research Network (MIRNET) prospectively collected information on 399 patients with episodes of chest pain. The most common diagnostic findings were (1) musculoskeletal pain (20.4%); (2) reflux esophagitis (13.4%); (3) costochondritis (13.1%); and (4) angina pectoris (10.3%).[4] The highest priority is generally given to distinguishing cardiac from noncardiac chest pain. Of the many diseases listed, the most common differential diagnostic considerations are of esophageal and psychiatric etiologies.

Table 2.1. **Common Causes of Chronic and Recurrent Chest Pain**

Cardiac causes
  Hypertrophic cardiomyopathy
  Ischemic heart disease
  Mitral valve prolapse
  Pericarditis

Chest wall problems
  Costochondritis
  Myofascial syndrome

Gastrointestinal causes
  Esophageal motility disorders
  Gastroesophageal reflux

Neurologic causes
  Radiculopathy
  Zoster (postherpetic neuralgia)

Psychiatric causes
  Anxiety
  Depression
  Hyperventilation
  Panic disorder

Noncardiac Chest Pain

Noncardiac chest pain remains a complex diagnosis and management problem. Studies have demonstrated that 10% to 30% of patients with chest pain who undergo coronary arteriography have no arterial abnormalities.[5,6] Follow-up studies of these patients have shown that the risk of subsequent myocardial infarction is low.[7,8] Fifty to seventy-five percent of these patients have persistent complaints of chest pain and disability.[9,10] The most common noncardiac problems in the differential are esophageal disorders, hyperventilation, panic attacks, and anxiety disorders.

Esophageal Chest Pain

Of the patients who have undergone coronary arteriography and have been found to have normal coronary arteries, as many as 50% have demonstrable esophageal abnormalities.[11] Richter et al[12] critically reviewed 117 articles on recurring chest pain of esophageal origin to clarify issues related to this disease. They paid specific attention to the following controversial issues: potential mechanisms of esophageal pain, differentiation of cardiac and esophageal causes, evaluation of esophageal motility disorders, use of esophageal tests for evaluating noncardiac chest pain, usefulness of techniques for prolonged monitoring of intraesophageal pressure and pH, and the relation of psychological abnormalities to esophageal motility disorders. They concluded that (1) specific mechanisms that produce chest pain are not well understood; (2) esophageal chest pain has usually been attributed to the stimulation of chemoreceptors (acid and bile) or mechanoreceptors (spasm and distention); and (3) studies done to confirm direct associations between these factors and pain have not been consistent in their findings.

It appears that the triggers for esophageal chest pain are multifactorial and often idiosyncratic to the individual. Differentiating cardiac from esophageal disease can be frustrating. As many as 50% of patients with coronary disease have esophageal disease.[13] There are many esophageal disorders that produce pain mimicking myocardial ischemia. Areskog et al[14] have shown that esophageal abnormalities are common in patients who are admitted to a coronary care unit and are later found to have no evidence of cardiac disease. The clinical history frequently does not differentiate between cardiac and esophageal chest pain, although features may be helpful in this process. Features suggesting esophageal origin include pain that continues for hours, pain that interrupts sleep or is meal-related, pain relieved by antacids, or the presence of other esophageal symptoms (heartburn, dysphagia, regurgitation). Conversely, it is well documented that gastroesophageal reflux may be triggered by heavy exercise and may produce exertional chest pain mimicking angina even during treadmill testing.

Tests that can be done to determine the presence of esophageal disease include esophageal motility testing, continuous ambulatory esophageal pH monitoring, and provocative testing (e.g., acid perfusion and balloon distension).[15] Although findings from these tests have produced a better understanding of the pathologic conditions leading to the development of chest pain with esophageal disorders, there is no consensus as to the usefulness of these tests for the specific patient with chest pain. As noted by Pope,[16] "What is needed is a simple and safe provocative esophageal maneuver to turn on chest pain that possesses a high degree of sensitivity."

There is clearly an interaction between psychological abnormalities and esophageal disorders. Patients with esophageal disorders have been shown to have significantly higher levels of anxiety, somatization, and depression.[17] It is not clear if there is a cause-and-effect relation. Given the aforementioned difficulties in the diagnosis of esophageal chest pain, the differentiation of this pain from cardiac disease, and the close relation between cardiac, esophageal, and psychiatric disease, it is wise to maintain a consistent approach to the evaluation of these patients. Richter et al.[12] developed a stepwise approach for patients with recurring chest pain. They recommended exclusion of cardiac disease, with the subsequent evaluation to rule out structural abnormalities of the upper gastrointestinal (GI) tract (barium swallow, upper GI series, and endoscopy). Also recommended is a trial of antireflux therapy for 1 to 2 months. In those patients who fail to respond, specialized testing may then be appropriate (esophageal motility, 24-hour pH monitoring, provocative testing, and psychological evaluation).[15]

Psychiatric Illness

There has long been a connection between psychiatric disorders and noncardiac chest pain. Katon et al[18] reported the results of an evaluation of 74 patients with chest pain and no history of organic heart disease. Each patient underwent a structured psychiatric interview immediately after coronary arteriography. Patients with chest pain and negative coronary arteriograms were significantly younger, more likely to be female, more apt to have a higher number of autonomic symptoms (tachycardia, dyspnea, dizziness, paresthesias) associated with chest pain, and more likely to describe atypical chest pain. These patients also had significantly higher scores on indices of anxiety and depression that met *Diagnostic and Statistical Manual of Mental Disorders*, 3rd edition (DSM-III) criteria for panic disorder, major depression, and phobias.

The strong association between anxiety and depression disorders in patients with noncardiac chest pain has been observed in many other studies. Specific medical therapy directed at anxiety and depression may help some of these patients. Cannon et al[19] reported a study on a group of patients with chest pain despite normal coronary angiograms. Imipramine was shown to improve their symptoms. Patients who were given 50 mg nightly had a statistically significant reduction (52%) in episodes of chest pain.

Cardiac Chest Pain: Angina Pectoris

Angina is not simply one type of pain; it is a constellation of symptoms related to cardiac ischemia. The description of angina may fit several patterns:

1. *Classic angina.* Classic angina presents as an ill-defined pressure, heaviness (feeling like a weight), or squeezing sensation brought on by exertion and relieved by rest. The pain is most often substernal and left-sided. It may radiate to the jaw, interscapular area, or down the arm. Angina usually begins gradually and lasts only a few minutes.
2. *Atypical angina.* Similar symptoms are experienced but with the absence of one or more of the criteria for classic angina. For example, the pain may not be consistently related to exertion or relieved by rest. Conversely, the pain may have an atypical character (sharp, stabbing), but the precipitating factors are clearly anginal.
3. *Anginal equivalent.* The sensation of dyspnea is the sole or major manifestation.
4. *Variant (Prinzmetal's) angina.* This angina occurs at rest and may manifest in stereotyped patterns, such as nocturnal symptoms or symptoms that appear only after exercise. It is thought to be caused by coronary artery spasm. Its symptoms often occur periodically, with characteristic pain-free intervals, and are associated with typical electrocardiographic (ECG) changes, most commonly ST segment elevation.
5. *Syndrome X (microvascular angina).* Some patients with the clinical diagnosis of coronary artery disease have no evidence of obstructive atherosclerosis. Several reports investigating this population have found a subset with metabolic evidence for ischemia

(myocardial lactate during induced myocardial stress as evidence for ischemia). The term *syndrome X* has been proposed.[20] It has been suggested that some of these patients have microvascular angina.

It is important for clinicians to recognize the factors that may confound the clinical diagnosis of angina pectoris: (1) The severity of pain is not necessarily proportional to the seriousness of the underlying illness. (2) The physical examination is not generally helpful for differentiating cardiac from noncardiac disease. A normal examination cannot be counted on to rule out significant cardiac disease. (3) The ECG is normal in more than 50% of patients with IHD. A normal ECG cannot be used to rule out significant cardiac disease. (4) Denial is a significant component in the presentation of chest pain caused by MI. (5) Some of the diseases common in the differential diagnosis of chest pain may present concurrently. Major depressive disorder and panic disorder are known to be prevalent in patients with esophageal disorders. Colgan et al[21] reported that of 63 patients with chest pain and normal angiograms 32 (51%) had evidence of an esophageal disorder, and 19 of the 32 (59%) had a current psychiatric disorder (anxiety or depression). Patients with concurrent disorders are particularly challenging to the clinician sorting out the cause of the chest pain.

Clinical Tools Used to Distinguish Cardiac from Noncardiac Chest Pain

Despite the difficulties noted above, there are important clinical tools that can be used to distinguish cardiac from noncardiac chest pain.

History

Despite the cited difficulties, the history is key to distinguishing cardiac from noncardiac etiologies of chest pain. Noncardiac chest pain is often fleeting, brief, sharp, or stabbing. The pain may be reproduced by palpating the chest wall. The duration of pain is also important. Symptoms that last many hours or days are not likely to be anginal. A great deal of work has been done to assess the probability of IHD in a given patient based on the clinical presentation. In 1979 Diamond and Forrester[22] presented such an approach. Using data from the clinical presentation correlated with autopsy and angiographic information, they presented a pretest likelihood of coronary artery disease in symptomatic patients according to age, sex, and type of chest pain (nonanginal, atypical angina, or typical angina).

Table 2.2. **Pretest Likelihood of Significant Ischemic Heart Disease (IHD) Based on Symptoms**

Age (years)	Likelihood of IHD, M/F (%)		
	Nonanginal	Atypical angina	Typical angina
30–39	5.0/0.8	22/4	69/26
40–49	14/3	46/13	87/55
50–59	21/8	59/32	92/79
60–69	28/18	67/54	94/90

Source: Diamond and Forrester[22] Copyright© 1979 Massachusetts Medical Society. Reprinted with permission. All rights reserved.

Several observations can be made from this chart (Table 2.2): Men have a substantially greater risk than women for any given type of chest pain and at any given age. A middle-aged man with atypical chest pain is at high risk for having significant coronary artery disease. Young women (ages 30–40 years) with classic angina have a relatively low risk of having significant coronary artery disease.

Diagnostic Testing

After establishing a pretest probability of IHD, there are a variety of tests available to help establish an accurate diagnosis. Although many tests are now firmly established in clinical practice, none is particularly suited to wide-scale, cost-effective application because each has limitations concerning sensitivity and specificity.

Exercise Tolerance Testing. In 1997 the American College of Cardiology and the American Heart Association Task Force on Assessment of Cardiovascular Procedures set guidelines for exercise treadmill testing (ETT).[23] For patients with symptoms suggestive of coronary artery disease there are five basic indications for undertaking exercise stress testing: (1) as a diagnostic test for patients with suspected IHD, (2) to assist in identifying those patients with documented IHD who are potentially at high risk due to advanced coronary disease or left ventricular dysfunction, (3) to evaluate patients after coronary artery bypass surgery, (4) to quantify a patient's functional capacity or response to therapy, and (5) to follow the natural course of the disease at appropriate intervals. The purpose of ETT for the patient with chest pain is to help establish whether the pain is indeed due to IHD.

Although there are many exercise protocols available, the protocols proposed by Bruce in 1956 remain appropriate. A review of the

ETT for family physicians has been published.[24,25] In the standard ETT (Bruce protocol) the patient is asked to exercise for 3-minute intervals on a motorized treadmill device while being monitored for the following: heart rate and blood pressure response to exercise, symptoms during the test, ECG response (specifically ST segment displacement), dysrhythmias, and exercise capacity. Contraindications to ETT include unstable angina, MI, rapid atrial or ventricular dysrhythmias, poorly controlled congestive heart failure (CHF), severe aortic stenosis, myocarditis, recent significant illness, and an uncooperative patient. A significant (positive) test includes an ST segment depression of 1.0 mm below the baseline. Many factors influence the results of an ETT and can lead to false-positive or false-negative findings. Factors leading to false-positive results include (1) the use of medications such as digoxin, estrogens, and diuretics; and (2) conditions such as mitral valve prolapse, cardiomyopathy, and hyperventilation. Factors leading to false-negative results include (1) the use of medications such as nitrates, beta-blockers, calcium channel blockers; and (2) conditions such as a prior MI or a submaximal effort.[26] The sensitivity of the ETT has been estimated to range from 56% to 81% and the specificity from 72% to 96%.[26] The key point is that given the vagaries of the ETT for diagnosing IHD (generally low sensitivity and specificity) a patient with a high pretest likelihood of IHD (e.g., a 50-year-old man with typical angina) still has a high probability of having significant disease even in the face of a normal (negative) test. Furthermore, a patient with a low probability of IHD (e.g., a 40-year-old woman with atypical chest pain) still has a low chance of significant disease even if the test is positive.[22] The optimal use of diagnostic testing is for those patients with moderate pretest probabilities (e.g., a 40- to 50-year-old man with atypical pain).

In addition to the diagnostic implications of an ETT, there are prognostic implications. The following are considered to be parameters associated with poor prognosis or increased disease severity: failure to complete stage 2 of a Bruce protocol, failure to achieve a heart rate over 120 bpm (off beta-blockers), onset of ST segment depression at a heart rate of less than 120 bpm, ST segment depression over 2.0 mm, ST segment depression lasting more than 6 minutes into recovery, ST segment depression in multiple leads, poor systolic blood pressure response to exercise, ST segment elevation, angina with exercise, and exercise-induced ventricular tachycardia.[26]

Radionuclide Perfusion Imaging. There are patients in whom the standard ETT is not a useful diagnostic tool and in whom a radionuclide procedure would be more appropriate. Patients with baseline ECG abnormalities due to digitalis or left ventricular hypertrophy with strain or those with bundle branch block (especially left bundle branch block) cannot have proper evaluation of the ST segment for characteristic ischemic changes. In these patients a radionuclide stress test is appropriate. The principle behind radionuclide testing is as follows: Myocardial thallium 201 chloride uptake is proportional to the coronary blood flow. A myocardial segment supplied by a stenotic coronary artery receives less flow relative to normal tissue, causing a thallium perfusion defect. Thallium washout is also slower in stenotic areas. With perfusion imaging, both stress and rest images are compared for perfusion. As a general rule, a defect is visible on thallium imaging if there is 50% or greater stenosis in a coronary artery. In the standard exercise thallium test, repeat imaging is performed 3 to 4 hours after completion of the ETT. Some investigators advocate 24-hour imaging in patients with perfusion defects to look for delayed reversibility.

For patients unable to exercise, thallium imaging can be performed using dipyridamole (Persantine) as a coronary vasodilator. Adenosine may also be used. Its advantages over dipyridamole include an ultrashort half-life (less than 10 seconds) and better coronary vasodilation. Two technetium radiopharmaceuticals [technetium sestamibi (Cardiolyte) and technetium teboroxime (Cardiotec)] have been approved for myocardial perfusion imaging. These agents may eventually replace thallium because of more favorable imaging characteristics.[27]

Compared to the standard ETT, the thallium 201 ETT has the advantage of increased sensitivity (80–87%) and specificity (85–90%).[27] Dipyridamole, adenosine, and technetium perfusion testing has a sensitivity ranging from 70% to 95% and specificity from 60% to 100%. Unfortunately, the cost of these procedures is more than five times as great as a standard ETT ($1000–$1400 versus $175–$250).[25]

Stress Echocardiography. Ischemic heart disease can be detected with stress echocardiography. During stress-induced myocardial ischemia, the affected ventricular walls become hypokinetic. Studies suggest that physical exercise and dobutamine may be the preferable means of provoking ischemia in patients undergoing stress echocardiography.[28,29] Preliminary data suggest a higher sensitivity and specificity than for the standard ETT and increased usefulness for predicting subsequent myocardial events; however, the primary utility of this test appears to be for detection of ischemia in patients who are unable to exercise adequately. Similar values for sensitivity and specificity between stress echocardiography and perfusion imaging have been reported. Stress echocardiography may be particularly valuable in patients who have a questionable defect on perfusion imaging.

The advantages and disadvantages of each of these diagnostic tests for IHD, as well as gender-specific issues, are presented in a summary by Redberg.[30]

Response to Nitroglycerin. Another approach employs clinical information to determine the probability of coronary artery disease based on response to treatment. One such study involved the use of sublingual nitroglycerin to determine the likelihood of disease. Horwitz et al[31] evaluated the usefulness of nitroglycerin as a diagnostic aid for IHD. They found a sensitivity of 76% and a specificity of 80% in 70 patients with chest pain of anginal type. It was concluded that 90% of patients with recurrent, angina-like chest pain who exhibit a prompt response to nitroglycerin (within 3 minutes) have IHD; however, a delayed or absent response paradoxically indicates either an absence of IHD or unusually severe disease. Therefore failure to respond to nitroglycerin should not be used to exclude the diagnosis of IHD.

Angina Pectoris

Once the diagnosis of angina is established, there are several important management considerations for this disease. The first is related to disease prognosis, the second to drug therapy, and the third to further investigative tests and invasive therapeutic interventions. Comprehensive management guidelines were prepared in 1999 by the American College of Cardiology and American Heart Association Task Force.[32]

Prognosis

Three major factors determine the prognosis of patients with angina pectoris: the amount of viable but jeopardized left ventricular myocardium, the percentage of irreversibly scarred myocardium, and the severity of underlying coronary atherosclerosis. A number of studies were reported before invasive therapies were available that assess the prognosis of patients with stable angina. Most of them appeared between 1952 and 1973 and reported an annual mortality of 4%. Since cardiac catheterization has come into general use, the prognosis has been modified and is based on the number of diseased vessels. Currently, the annual mortality rates for patients with one-vessel disease, two-vessel disease, three-vessel disease, and left main coronary artery disease (CAD) are 1.5%, 3.5%, 6.0%, and 8.0% to 10.0%, respectively.[33]

Exercise tolerance testing has been used to establish the prognosis in patients with symptomatic IHD. The exercise test parameters associated with a poor outcome have been described above.[26]

When does angina signal severe coronary disease? Pryor et al[34] developed a nomogram based on a point scoring system to help answer this question. They based the nomogram on the following factors: type of chest pain (typical, atypical, nonanginal), sex, selective cardiovascular risk factors (hypertension, smoking, hyperlipidemia, diabetes mellitus), anginal duration (months), and the presence of carotid bruits. By applying the nomogram for the individual patient one can determine the probability of severe disease (i.e., 75% narrowing of the left main coronary artery or three-vessel disease).

Drug Therapy

In patients with stable exertional angina who do not have severe disease, the goal of therapy is to abolish or reduce anginal attacks and myocardial ischemia and to promote a normal lifestyle. For the relief of angina, the treatment strategy is to lower myocardial oxygen demand and increase coronary blood flow to the ischemic regions.

Patients are screened for the presence of significant cardiovascular risk factors and are advised to modify any that are present. Three classes of antianginal drugs are commonly used: nitrates, beta-blockers, and calcium channel blockers. Each reduces myocardial oxygen demand and may improve blood flow to the ischemic regions. The mechanisms by which these agents reduce myocardial oxygen demand or increase coronary blood flow to ischemic areas differ from one class of drug to another. No greater efficacy in relieving chest pain or decreasing exercise-induced ischemia has been shown for one or another group of drugs.

Nitrates

Nitrates are potent venous and arterial dilators. At low doses venous dilation predominates, and at higher doses arterial dilation occurs as well. Nitrates decrease myocardial oxygen demand in the following ways: Decreased venous return reduces left ventricular end-diastolic volume and ventricular wall stress. Increased arterial compliance and cardiac output lowers systolic blood pressure and decreases peripheral resistance (afterload). It also enhances myocardial oxygen supply by preventing closure of stenotic coronary arteries during exercise, dilating epicardial coronary arteries, and decreasing left ventricular end-diastolic pressure, thereby enhancing subendocardial blood flow and inhibiting coronary artery spasm. Nitrates are inexpensive and have a well documented safety record. Both short- and long-acting nitrates are available. Short-acting preparations are used for relief of an established attack, whereas long-acting nitrates are used for prevention. The most significant concern about the long-acting nitrates is tolerance. Most studies have shown that tolerance develops rapidly when long-acting nitrates are given for anginal prophylaxis.[34]

With nitroglycerin patches tolerance can develop within 24 hours, and further therapy can lead to complete loss of the antianginal effect.[35] Various dosing strategies with oral and transdermal formulations have been used to overcome the development of nitroglycerin tolerance. Patch-free intervals of 10 to 12 hours are commonly used to retain the antianginal effectiveness. For oral administration, nitroglycerin isosorbide dinitrate three times daily at 7 A.M., noon, and 5 P.M. appears to prevent the development of tolerance. Because of the concern for intervals during which patients remain unprotected, it is common to add another antianginal agent to the nitroglycerin regimen. Other problems with nitroglycerin include the fact that 10% of patients do not respond and 10% have associated intolerable headaches that may necessitate discontinuation.[35]

Beta-Blockers

The antianginal effect of beta-blockers is well established.[36] These agents improve exercise tolerance and reduce myocardial ischemia. The effect produces a reduction in myocardial oxygen demand through a reduction in heart rate and contractility. Many beta-blockers are available. They may be divided into those that are nonselective (β_1 and β_2) (i.e., propranolol, timolol, nadolol), those that are β_1 selective (i.e., atenolol, metoprolol, acebutolol), and those that are nonselective and produce vasodilatory effects through the ability to block α_1-receptors and dilate blood vessels directly (i.e., labetalol). All beta-blockers, irrespective of their selective properties, are equally effective in patients with angina.[36]

Some 20% of patients do not respond to beta-blockers. Those who do not respond are more likely to have severe IHD. Furthermore, some patients do not tolerate the adverse side effects, such as fatigue, depression, dyspnea, and cold extremities. Other concerns include a small but significant aggravation of hyperlipidemia and precipitation of CHF and bronchospasm in susceptible individuals. Generally, beta-blockers are dose-adjusted to achieve a heart rate of 50 to 60 bpm. Patients should be cautioned to not stop beta-blockers abruptly, thereby avoiding a rebound phenomenon.

Calcium Channel Blockers

Calcium channel blockers are a diverse group of compounds, all of which impede calcium ion influx into the myocardium and smooth muscle cells. These agents relieve myocardial ischemia by reducing myocardial oxygen demand secondary to decreased afterload and myocardial contractility. In addition, they dilate coronary arteries. There are three classes of calcium channel blockers: papaverine derivatives (verapamil), dihydropyridines (nifedipine, nicardipine), and benzothiaze-pines (diltiazem). Each of the drugs in the three classes has different effects on the atrioventricular (AV) node, heart rate, coronary vasodilation, diastolic relaxation, cardiac contractility, systemic blood pressure, and afterload. All three classes are effective for the management of patients with stable angina.[37] Most studies have shown them to have effects equal to those of beta-blockers. Calcium channel blockers may be preferred in patients with obstructive airway disease, hypertension, peripheral vascular disease, or supraventricular tachycardia. In general, they are well tolerated. The most troublesome side effects include constipation, edema, headache, and aggravation of congestive heart failure.

Concern has developed that short-acting calcium channel blockers may be associated with an increased risk of MI. There has been evidence of a 58% to 70% increase in risk of MI compared to that in patients on beta-blockers or diuretics. The phenomenon has been noted to be dose-related. At present the National Heart, Lung, and Blood Institute has issued a statement recommending caution with the use of short-acting calcium channel blockers.[38]

Combination Therapy

It is important to maximize therapy with any one class of antianginal drug before considering it a failed trial. If monotherapy fails, it is appropriate to add another agent. Generally beta-blockers and nitrates or calcium channel blockers and nitrates complement each other. Calcium channel blockers and beta-blockers can be used together. Combination therapy may be more effective than either agent alone. It is important to be cautious, as some combinations produce deleterious effects. For example, verapamil and beta-blockers may produce extreme bradycardia or heart block.

Aspirin

Aspirin is effective for primary and secondary prevention of MI, presumably by inhibiting thrombosis. Although there is controversy as to the ideal therapeutic dose, low-dose therapy (81–325 mg) is generally recommended.[39] Alternative antiplatelet regimens to aspirin include ticlopidine and clopidogrel. A 1994 review found no evidence that any antiplatelet regimen was more effective than medium-dose aspirin alone in the prevention of vascular events.[40] Another review of randomized trials comparing either ticlopidine or clopidogrel with aspirin found several trials showing a small additional benefit of these two drugs over aspirin in reducing the odds of a vascular event.[41]

Invasive Testing

Cardiac catheterization is not routinely recommended for initial management of patients with stable angina. Patients who warrant such an evaluation are those who exhibit evidence of severe myocardial ischemia on noninvasive testing or who have symptoms refractory to antianginal medications. In patients who undergo catheterization, the most important determinant of survival is left ventricular function followed by the number of diseased vessels. Patients with left main artery disease or three-vessel disease with diminished left ventricular function are candidates for a coronary artery bypass graft procedure. Others (those with one- or two-vessel disease) are managed medically or considered for percutaneous transluminal coronary angioplasty (PTCA).

Unstable Angina Pectoris

Unstable angina manifests clinically either as an abrupt onset of ischemic symptoms at rest or as an intensification or change in the pattern of ischemic symptoms in a patient with a history of IHD. This intensification may be manifested by an increase in the frequency, severity, and duration of symptoms as well as an increasing ease of provocation (symptoms at rest or with minimal effort). Recurrence of ischemic symptoms soon after an MI (usually within 4 weeks) is also considered a sign of unstable angina. Unstable angina is generally diagnosed on clinical grounds alone. Because of the episodic nature of ischemia in unstable angina, however, transient ECG abnormalities (ST segment depression or elevation or T wave abnormalities, i.e., inversion, flattening, or peaking) may not be documented in 50% to 70% of patients with the clinical diagnosis of unstable angina. In studies in which prolonged Holter monitoring was used during the in-hospital phase of unstable angina, transient ischemic ST segment deviations have been described in 60% to 70% of cases, more than 70% of them being clinically unsuspected or silent.[42]

Prognosis

The prognosis of patients with unstable angina is not as good as those with chronic stable angina. Mortality is increased in those who fail to respond to initial therapy, who have severe left ventricular dysfunction, and who have multivessel CAD (particularly left main artery disease).

Management Strategy

An important development in the management of unstable angina was the 1994 report of the Agency for Health Care Policy and Research.[43] This report includes clinical practice guidelines that are based on a consensus panel of experts. The guidelines allow physicians to consider outpatient management for a select subgroup of patients with unstable angina, specifically those who are thought to be at low risk for MI. According to the report, in the initial management physicians should use the information in Table 2.3 to determine whether a particular patient has high, intermediate, or low likelihood of having significant CAD. For example, the patient with low likelihood might be nondiabetic, have atypical chest pain, be younger (<60 years for men, <70 years for women), and have a normal ECG. The next step is to determine the level of risk for MI. The information in Table 2.4 allows a similar stratification of risk. For example, a low-risk patient is one with a history of angina that is now provoked at a lower threshold but not at rest, and the ECG is normal or unchanged. Low-risk patients may be treated with aspirin, nitroglycerin, beta-blockers, or a combination. Follow-up should be no later than 72 hours. High- or moderate-risk patients should be admitted for intensive medical management. Intensive medical management includes consideration of aspirin, heparin, nitrates, beta-blockers, calcium channel blockers (if the patient is already on adequate doses of nitrates and beta-blockers or unable to tolerate them), and morphine sulfate.

Once patients are stable, they should be considered for noninvasive exercise testing to further define the prognosis and direct the treatment plan. Low-risk patients can be managed medically. Those at intermediate risk should be considered for additional testing (either a cardiac catheterization, radionuclide stress test, or echocardio-

Table 2.3. **Likelihood of Significant Coronary Artery Disease (CAD) in Patients with Symptoms Suggesting Unstable Angina**

High likelihood (any of the listed features)	Intermediate likelihood (absence of high-likelihood features and any of the listed features)	Low likelihood (absence of high- or intermediate-likelihood features but may have the listed features)
Known history of CAD	Definite angina: men <60, women <70	Chest pain, probably not angina
Definite angina: men ≥60 women ≥70	Probable angina: men >60 or women >70	One risk factor but not diabetes
Hemodynamic changes or ECG changes with pain	Probably not angina in diabetics or in nondiabetics with ≥two other risk factors[a]	T wave flat or inverted <1 mm in leads with dominant R waves
Variant angina	Extracardiac vascular disease	Normal ECG
ST increase or decrease ≥1 mm	ST depression 0.05 to 1.00 mm	
Marked symmetric T wave inversion in multiple precordial leads	T wave inversion ≥1 mm in leads with dominant R waves	

Source: Braunwald et al.[43]

[a]CAD risk factors include diabetes, smoking, hypertension, and elevated cholesterol.

Table 2.4. Short-Term Risk of Death or Nonfatal Myocardial Infarction in Patients with Symptoms Suggesting Unstable Angina

High risk (at least one of the listed features must be present)	Intermediate risk (no high-risk feature but must have any of the listed features)	Low risk (no high- or intermediate-risk feature but may have any of the listed features)
Prolonged ongoing (>20 min) rest pain	Rest angina now resolved but not low likelihood of CAD	Increased angina frequency, severity, or duration
Pulmonary edema	Rest angina (>20 min or relieved with rest or nitroglycerin)	Angina provoked at a lower threshold
Angina with new or worsening mitral regurgitation murmurs	Angina with dynamic T wave changes	New-onset angina within 2 weeks to 2 months
Rest angina with dynamic ST changes ≥1 mm	Normal or unchanged ECG	Nocturnal angina
Angina with S$_3$ or rales	New onset of CCSC III or IV angina during past 2 weeks but not low likelihood of CAD	
Angina with hypotension	Q waves or ST depression ≥1 mm in multiple leads	
Age >65 years		

Source: Braunwald et al.[43]

CCSC = Canadian Cardiovascular Study Class.

graphic stress test). Those at high risk should be referred for cardiac catheterization.[43]

Since the publication of the 1994 report, efforts have been directed at the use of markers of cardiac injury, i.e., cardiac troponins (troponin T and troponin I). Their detection, even at low levels, is highly sensitive and specific for injury. Troponin elevation in patients otherwise considered to have unstable angina identifies a subset of patients requiring more aggressive intervention. Hamm and Braunwald[44] have proposed a risk-stratification algorithm that incorporates troponin testing.

Antiplatelet Therapy

Antiplatelet therapy is an important addition for patients with unstable angina. A number of studies have demonstrated that a common cause of crescendo angina is platelet aggregation and thrombus formation on the surface of an ulcerated plaque. In the Veterans Administration Cooperative Study, men with unstable angina who received aspirin (325 mg/day) had a 50% reduction in subsequent death from MI.[45] As noted previously, ticlopidine and clopidogrel are alternative antiplatelet regimens to aspirin.

Percutaneous Transluminal Coronary Angioplasty

There has been a marked increase in the use of angioplasty over the past 20 years. The American College of Cardiology and the American Heart Association Task Force have published guidelines for the selection of patients for coronary angioplasty.[46] Among patients with unstable angina, PTCA is recommended for those who do not show an adequate response to medical treatment (continued chest pain or evidence of ongoing ischemia during ECG monitoring) or who are intolerant of medical therapy because of uncontrollable side effects.

The long-term outcome after successful angioplasty has been reported to be excellent even when compared with patients undergoing bypass surgery.[47] Further research is important in the areas of long-term outcome for multiple lesions, extensive disease, and avoidance of complications. Technologies such as stents, laser angioplasty, and atherectomy await further evaluation.

Coronary Artery Bypass Graft

Large randomized trials have shown that surgical revascularization is more effective than medical therapy for relieving angina and improving exercise tolerance for at least several years. Development of atherosclerosis in the coronary artery bypass graft resulting in angina generally occurs within 5 to 10 years. However, patients with internal mammary artery grafts have substantially fewer problems with graft occlusion (90% patency rate at 10 years). Improved survival with surgical versus medical therapy is seen only in the subset of patients with severe CAD or left ventricular dysfunction.[48]

Silent Ischemia

Many investigations have established that most ischemic episodes in patients with stable angina are not accompanied by chest pain (silent ischemia). What remains unclear is the precise nature of events that accompany ischemic events that do or do not produce pain. Patients with predominantly silent ischemia may be hyposensitive to pain in general; denial may play a role, or they may experience pain but attribute the symptoms to a less significant event. It is well documented that personality-related, emotional, and social factors can modulate the perception of pain. It is not surprising that the symptoms among cardiac patients with the same degree of disease vary greatly. Personality inventory studies have shown that patients with reproducible angina have higher scores on indices of nervousness and excitability than do those who are free of symptoms. Many studies have shown that stress of various types can influence the frequency and duration of ischemic episodes in patients with angina.[49]

Silent ischemia is prevalent. Seventy percent of ischemic episodes in patients with IHD are estimated to be asymptomatic. Among patients with stable angina who undergo 24-hour Holter monitoring, 40% to 72% of the episodes are painless. Among patients with unstable angina, more than half manifest painless ST segment depression.

In 1988 Cohn[50] proposed classifying silent ischemia into three clinical types to help clarify the prevalence, detection, prognosis, and management of this syndrome. Type 1 includes persons with ischemia who are asymptomatic, never having had any signs or symptoms of cardiovascular disease. Type 2 includes persons who are asymptomatic after an MI but still show painless ischemia. Type 3 includes patients with both angina and silent ischemia. From Cohn's data 2.5% to 10.0% of middle-aged men have type 1 silent ischemia. Among middle-aged men known to have CAD, 18% have type 2 and 40% have type 3.

Methods of Detection

Certain tests can be used to assess the presence of silent ischemia: ETT, ambulatory ECG for ST segment changes (Holter monitor), radionuclide tests including thallium scintigraphy and gated pooled [multiple gated acquisition (MUGA)] scan, and stress echocardiography. Of these tests, the most commonly considered are ETT and Holter monitoring.

For Holter monitoring, when ST segment changes that meet strict criteria are seen in a patient with known IHD, it is generally accepted that they represent episodes of myocardial ischemia. Ischemic criteria include at least 1.0 mm of horizontal or down-sloping ST segment depression that lasts for at least 1 minute and is separated from other discrete episodes by at least 1 minute of a normal baseline. The methodology has limitations, including difficulty reading ST segment changes in patients with an abnormal baseline (left ventricular hypertrophy with strain) or in those with a left bundle branch block.

It is not thought at this time that any of the methods to detect silent ischemia are useful for screening for the presence of IHD in apparently healthy populations. Although this subject remains controversial, it may be wise to screen those patients at high risk (i.e., diabetics or patients with two or more cardiac risk factors).

Prognostic Implications

The presence of frequent, prolonged ischemic episodes despite medical therapy in patients with stable and unstable angina has been associated with a poor prognosis. Using Cohn's classification system, those patients with type 2 silent ischemia have the worst prognosis, especially those with left ventricular dysfunction and three-vessel disease. Exercise tests done 2 to 3 weeks after an MI have shown an adverse 1-year prognosis associated with silent ischemia.[50] It is unclear whether those with type 3 have a worse prognosis.

Management

Antiischemic medical and revascularization therapies have been shown to reduce asymptomatic ischemia. It is prudent to consider patients with persistent asymptomatic ischemia to be at higher risk for subsequent events and therefore to warrant more aggressive therapy. Patients with type 1 are advised to modify risk factors and avoid activities known to produce ischemia. Those with strongly positive tests can be considered for angiography. For patients with types 2 or 3, treatment with beta-blockers for a cardioprotective effect should be considered. It remains unresolved whether asymptomatic ischemia has a causal relation with subsequent MI and cardiac death or is merely a marker of high risk.[51]

Myocardial Infarction

Clinical Presentation

The classic initial manifestations of an acute MI include prolonged substernal chest pain with dyspnea, diaphoresis, and nausea. The pain may be described as a crushing, pressing, constricting, vise-like, or heavy sensation. There may be radiation of the pain to one or both shoulders and arms or to the neck, jaw, or interscapular area. Only a few patients have this classic overall picture. Although 80% of patients with an acute MI have chest pain at the time of initial examination, only 20% describe it as crushing, constricting, or vise-like.[52] The pain may also be described atypically, such as sharp or stabbing, or it can involve atypical areas such as the epigastrium or the back of the neck. "Atypical" presentations are common in the elderly.

Pathy[53] found that the initial manifestations of an acute MI were more likely to include symptoms such as sudden dyspnea, acute confusion, cerebrovascular events (e.g., stroke or syncope), acute CHF, vomiting, and palpitations. There is strong evidence that a substantial proportion of MIs are asymptomatic. In an update of the Framingham Study, Kannel and Abbott[54] reported that 28% of infarcts were discovered only through the appearance of new ECG changes (Q waves or loss of R waves) observed on a routine biennial study. These infarctions had been previously unrecognized by both patient and physician.

Physical Examination

For the patient with an "uncomplicated MI" there are few physical examination findings. The main purpose of the examination is to assess the patient for evidence of complications from the MI and to establish a baseline for future comparisons. Signs of severe left ventricular dysfunction include hypotension, peripheral vasoconstriction, tachycardia, pulmonary rales, an S_3, and elevated jugular venous pressure (see Chapter 5). Preexisting murmurs should be verified. A new systolic murmur can result from a number of causes: papillary muscle dysfunction, mitral regurgitation as a result of ventricular dilatation, ventricular septal rupture, and acute severe mitral regurgitation due to papillary muscle rupture.

Electrocardiography

The classic ECG changes of acute ischemia are peaked, hyperacute T waves, T wave flattening or inversion with or without ST segment depression, horizontal ST segment depression, and ST segment elevation. Changes associated with an infarction are (1) the fresh appearance of Q waves or the increased prominence of preexisting ones; (2) ST segment elevations; and (3) T wave inversions. It is important to recognize that with acute MI the ECG may be entirely normal or contain only "soft" ECG evidence of infarction.

In the past infarcts were classified as transmural or subendocardial, depending of the presence of Q waves. This terminology has now been replaced by the terms *Q-wave* and *non–Q-wave* MI. This distinction has more clinical relevance, as several studies have indicated differences in etiology and outcome. The key differences between these two groups are as follows: (1) Q-wave infarctions account for 60% to 70% of all infarcts and non–Q-wave infarctions for 30% to 40%. (2) ST segment elevation is present in 80% of Q-wave infarctions and 40% of non–Q-wave infarctions. (3) The peak creatine kinase tends to be higher in Q-wave infarctions. (4) Postinfarction ischemia and early reinfarction are more common with non–Q-wave infarctions. (5) In-hospital mortality is greater with Q-wave infarctions (20% versus 8% for non–Q-wave infarctions). In general, it is thought that the non–Q-wave infarction is a more unstable condition because of the higher risk of reinfarction and ischemia.

Laboratory Findings

Elevation of the creatine kinase muscle and brain subunits (CK-MB) isoenzyme is essential for the diagnosis of acute MI. In general, acute elevations of this enzyme are accounted for by myocardial necrosis. Detectable CK-MB from noncardiac causes is rare except during trauma or surgery. The peak level appearance of CK-MB is expected within 12 to 24 hours after the onset of symptoms; normalization is expected in 2 to 3 days. Therefore patients should have a CK-MB level determined on admission and every 8 to 12 hours thereafter (repeated twice). Reliance on a single CK assay in an emergency room setting to rule out MI is not sensitive and should be discouraged. Cardiac troponins (T and I) are newer markers for cardiac injury. The troponins first become detectable after the first few hours following the onset of myocardial necrosis, and they peak after 12 to 24 hours. Normalization of troponin T levels requires 5 to 14 days; troponin I levels requires 5 to 10 days.[55]

Management Guidelines

Comprehensive management guidelines were prepared in 1999 by the American College of Cardiology and American Heart Association Task Force.[46] The main priority for patients with an acute MI is relief of pain. The frequent clinical observation of rapid, complete relief of pain after early reperfusion with thrombolytic therapy has made it clear that the pain of an acute MI is due to continuing ischemia of living jeopardized myocardium rather than to the effects of completed myocardial necrosis.

Effective analgesia should be administered at the time of diagnosis. Analgesia can be achieved by the use of sublingual nitroglycerin or intravenous morphine (or both). Sublingual nitroglycerin is given immediately unless the systolic blood pressure is less than 90 mm Hg. If the systolic blood pressure is under 90 mm Hg, nitroglycerin may be used after intravenous access has been obtained. Long-acting oral nitrate preparations are avoided for management of early acute MI. Sublingual or transdermal nitroglycerin can be used, but intravenous infusion of nitroglycerin allows more precise control. The intravenous dose can be titrated by frequently measuring blood pressure and heart rate. Morphine sulfate is also highly effective for the relief of pain associated with an acute MI. In addition to its analgesic properties, morphine exerts favorable hemodynamic effects by increasing venous capacitance and reducing systemic vascular resistance. The result is to decrease myocardial oxygen demand. As with nitroglycerin, hypotension may occur. The hypotension may be treated with intravenous fluids or leg elevation.

Oxygen

Supplemental oxygen is given to all patients with an acute MI. Hypoxemia in a patient with an uncomplicated infarction is usually caused by ventilation-perfusion abnormalities. When oxygen is used it is administered by nasal cannula or mask at a rate of 4 to 10 L/min. In patients with chronic obstructive pulmonary disease it may be wise to use lower flow rates.

Thrombolytic Therapy

In addition to relieving pain and managing ischemia, thrombolytic therapy must be considered. Thrombosis has a major role in the development of an acute MI. Approximately 66% of patients with MIs have ST segment elevation, making it likely that the process is caused by an occlusive clot. The goal of thrombolytic therapy is reperfusion with a minimum of side effects. The most commonly used thrombolytic agents are streptokinase, anisoylated plasminogen streptokinase activator complex (APSAC), recombinant tissue-type plasminogen activator (rt-PA), urokinase, and pro-urokinase.

Early administration of thrombolytic therapy, within 6 to 12 hours from the onset of symptoms, has been associated with a reduction in mortality. Indications for thrombolytic therapy include typical chest pain >30 minutes but <12 hours that is unrelieved by nitroglycerin, and ST segment elevation in more than two contiguous leads (>1 mm in limb leads or >2 mm in chest leads) or ST segment depression in only V_1 and V_2 or a new left bundle branch block. Relative contraindications for thrombolytic therapy include history of stroke, active bleeding, blood pressure >180 mm Hg systolic, major surgery/ trauma in the last 3 to 6 months, recent noncompressible vascular puncture, and possible intracranial event/unclear mental status.[56] Wright and colleagues[56] present a summary of the major thrombolytic trials. Advances in this therapeutic modality during the past 5 years include new third-generation fibrinolytic agents and various strategies to enhance administration and efficacy of these agents. A number of ongoing trials are attempting to determine whether the combination of fibrinolytic therapy with low molecular weight heparin enhances coronary reperfusion and reduces mortality and late reocclusion. Also presented is a dose and cost summary of the available fibrinolytic agents.[56]

Complications (Mechanical)

The most common complications of an acute MI are mechanical and electrical. Mechanical complications include those that are quickly reversible and those that are clearly life-threatening. Reversible causes of hypotension include hypovolemia, vasovagal reaction, overzealous therapy with antianginal or antiarrhythmic drugs, and brady- and tachyarrhythmias. Other, more serious etiologies include primary left ventricular failure, cardiac tamponade, rupture of the ventricular septum, acute papillary muscle dysfunction, and mitral regurgitation (see Chapter 9).

Killip and Kimball[57] developed a classification of patients with acute MI.

Class 1: Patients with uncomplicated infarction without evidence of heart failure as judged by the absence of rales and an S_3.
Class 2: Patients with mild to moderate heart failure as evidenced by pulmonary rales in the lower half of the lung fields and an S_3.
Class 3: Patients with severe left ventricular failure and pulmonary edema.
Class 4: Patients with cardiogenic shock, defined as systolic blood pressure less than 90 mm Hg with oliguria and other evidence of poor peripheral perfusion.

Cardiogenic shock has emerged as the most common cause of in-hospital mortality of patients with an acute MI. Despite advances in medical therapy, cardiogenic shock has a dismal prognosis (80–90% mortality). The management of patients with cardiogenic shock includes adequate oxygenation, reduction in myocardial oxygen demands, protection ofischemic myocardium, and circulatory support (see Chapter 9). The potential for myocardial salvage with emergency reperfusion should be considered in all cases.

Complications (Electrical)

The past 30 years has seen major developments in the recognition and treatment of arrhythmias (see Chapter 4). The most common include the brady- and tachyarrhythmias, AV conduction disturbances, and ventricular arrhythmias. Organized treatment protocols have been developed for each of these dysrhythmias.[58]

Post-MI Evaluation

Recommendations for pre- and postdischarge evaluations of patients with an acute MI have been outlined by the American College of Cardiologists, the American Heart Association, and the American College of Physicians.[46] They include recommendations for testing exercise tolerance and strategies to determine those who would benefit from medical or surgical intervention. These recommendations include a submaximal ETT at 6 to 10 days and at 3 weeks to determine functional capacity.

Rehabilitation

The goal of cardiac rehabilitation includes maintenance of a desirable level of physical, social, and psychological functioning after the onset of cardiovascular illness.[59] Specific goals of rehabilitation include risk stratification, limitation of adverse psychological and emotional consequences of cardiovascular disease, modification of risk factors, alleviation of symptoms, and improved function. Risk stratification is accomplished by exercise tolerance testing. Additionally, high-risk patients include those with CHF, silent ischemia, and ventricular dysrhythmias. All patients should undergo an evaluation to reduce risk factors (smoking, hyperlipidemia, and hypertension). Risk modification of these factors has been associated with significant reduction in subsequent cardiac events. Enrollment in a cardiac rehabilitation program with particular emphasis on exercise has been shown to reduce cardiovascular mortality.[60]

References

1. 2001 Heart and Stroke Statistical Update. American Heart Association. *http://www.americanheart.org.*
2. Guidelines 2000 for cardiopulmonary resuscitation and emergency cardiovascular care. An international consensus on science. The American Heart Association in Collaboration with the International Liaison Committee on Resuscitation. *http://www.americanheart.org/ECC/index.html.*
3. Fulp SR, Richter JE. Esophageal chest pain. Am Fam Physician 1989;40: 101–16.
4. Klinkman MS, Stevens D, Gorenflo DW. Episodes of care for chest pain: a preliminary report from MIRNET. J Fam Pract 1994;38:345–52.
5. Kemp HG, Vokonas PS, Cohn PF, Gorlin R. The anginal syndrome associated with normal coronary arteriograms: report of a six-year experience. Am J Med 1973;54:735–42.
6. Marchandise B, Bourrassa MG, Chairman BR, Lesperance J. Angiographic evaluation of the natural history of normal coronary arteries and mild coronary atherosclerosis. Am J Cardiol 1978;41:216–20.
7. Proudfit WL, Bruschke AVG, Sones FM. Clinical course of patients with normal or slightly or moderately abnormal coronary arteriograms: 10-year follow-up of 521 patients. Circulation 1980;62:712–17.
8. Kemp HG, Kronmal RA, Vlietstra RE, Frye RL. Seven year survival of patients with normal or near normal coronary arteriograms: a CASS registry study. J Am Coll Cardiol 1986;7:479–83.
9. Ockene IS, Shay MJ, Alpert JS, Weiner BH, Dalen JE. Unexplained chest pain in patients with normal coronary arteriograms: a follow-up study of functional status. N Engl J Med 1980;303:1249–52.
10. Lavey EB, Winkle RA. Continuing disability of patients with chest pain and normal coronary arteriograms. J Chronic Dis 1979;32:191–6.
11. Davies HA, Jones DB, Rhodes J. Esophageal angina as the cause of chest pain. JAMA 1982;248:2274–8.
12. Richter JE, Bradley LA, Castell DO. Esophageal chest pain current controversies in pathogenesis, diagnosis and therapy. Ann Intern Med 1989; 110:66–78.
13. Schofield PM, Bennett DH, Whorwell PJ, et al. Exertional gastro-oesophageal reflux: a mechanism for symptoms in patient with angina pectoris and normal coronary angiograms. BMJ 1987;294:1459–61.
14. Areskog M, Tibbling L, Wranne B. Noninfarction in coronary care unit patients. Acta Med Scand 1981;209:51–7.
15. Glade MJ. Continuous ambulatory esophageal pH monitoring in the evaluation of patients with gastrointestinal reflux: Diagnostic and therapeutic technology assessment (DATTA). JAMA 1995;274:662–8.
16. Pope CE. Chest pain: heart? gullet? both? neither? [editorial]. JAMA 1992;248:2315.
17. Clouse RE, Lustman PJ. Psychiatric illness and contraction abnormalities of the esophagus. N Engl J Med 1983;309:1337–42.
18. Katon W, Hall ML, Russo J, et al. Chest pain: relationship of psychiatric illness to coronary arteriographic results. Am J Med 1988;84:1–9.
19. Cannon RO, Quyyumi AA, Mincemoyer R, Stine AM, Gracely RH,

Smith WB. Imipramine in patients with chest pain despite normal coronary angiograms. N Engl J Med 1994;330:1411–17.

20. Cannon RO. Angina pectoris with normal coronary angiograms. Cardiol Clin 1991;9:157–66.

21. Colgan SM, Schofield PJ, Whorwell DH, Bennett DH, Brook NH, Jones PE. Angina-like chest pain: a joint medical and psychiatric investigation. Postgrad Med J 1988;64:743–6.

22. Diamond GA, Forrester JS. Analysis of probability as an aid in the clinical diagnosis of coronary-artery disease. N Engl J Med 1979;300: 1350–8.

23. ACC/AHA guidelines for exercise testing: a report of the American College of Cardiology/American Heart Association Task Force on Practice Guidelines (Committee on Exercise Testing). J Am Coll Cardiol 1997;30:260–311.

24. Evans CH, Karunaratne HB. Exercise stress testing for the family physician. Part 1. Performing the test. Am Fam Physician 1992;45:121–32.

25. Evans CH, Karunaratne HB. Exercise stress testing for the family physician. Part 2. Am Fam Physician 1992;45:679–88.

26. Ellestad MH. Stress testing: principles and practice, 4th ed. Philadelphia: FA Davis, 1995.

27. Botvinick EH. Stress imaging: current clinical options for the diagnosis, localization, and evaluation of coronary artery disease. Med Clin North Am 1995;79:1025–61.

28. Afridi I, Quinones MA, Zoghbi WA, Cheirif J. Dobutamine stress echocardiography: sensitivity, specificity, and predictive value for future cardiac events. Am Heart J 1994;127:1510–15.

29. Beleslin BD, Ostojic M, Stepanovic J, et al. Stress echocardiography in the detection of myocardial ischemia: head-to-head comparison of exercise, dobutamine, and dipyridamole tests. Circulation 1994;90:1168–76.

30. Redberg RF. Diagnostic testing for coronary artery disease in women and gender differences in referral for revascularization. Cardiol Clin 1998;16:67–77.

31. Horwitz LD, Herman MV, Gorlin R. Clinical response to nitroglycerin as a diagnostic test for coronary artery disease. Am J Cardiol 1972;29:149–53.

32. 1999 update: ACC/AHA guidelines for the management of patients with chronic stable angina. A report of the American College of Cardiology/American Heart Association Task Force on Practice Guidelines (Committee on Management of chronic stable angina). J Am Coll Cardiol 1999;33:2092–197.

33. Hilton TC, Chaitman BR. The prognosis in stable and unstable angina. Cardiol Clin 1991;9:27–39.

34. Pryor DB, Shaw L, Harrell FE, et al. Estimating the likelihood of severe coronary artery disease. Am J Med 1991;90:553–62.

35. Bomber JW, Detullio PL. Oral nitrate preparations: an update. Am Fam Physician 1995;52:2331–6.

36. Howard PA, Ellerbeck EF. Optimizing beta-blocker use after myocardial infarction. Am Fam Physician 2000;62:1853–60.

37. Opie LH. Calcium channel antagonists. Part II. Use and comparative properties of prototypical calcium antagonists in ischemic heart disease,

including recommendations based on analysis of 45 trials. Rev Cardiovasc Drug Ther 1987;1:4461–75.

38. Psaty BM, Heckbert ER, Koepsell TD, et al. The risk of myocardial infarction associated with antihypertensive drug therapies. JAMA 1995; 274:670–5.
39. Hennekens CH, Buring JE. Aspirin in the primary prevention of cardiovascular disease. Cardiol Clin 1994;12:443–50.
40. Antiplatelet Trialists' Collaboration. Collaborative overview of randomized trials of antiplatelet therapy—I. Prevention of death, myocardial infarction, and stroke by prolonged antiplatelet therapy in various categories of patients. BMJ 1994;308:81–106.
41. Hankey GJ, Sudlow CLM, Dunbabin DW. Thienopyridine derivatives (ticlopidine, clopidogrel) versus aspirin for preventing stroke and other serious vascular events in high vascular risk patients. In: The Cochrane Library, issue 1. Oxford: Cochrane Library, 2000.
42. Shah PK. Pathophysiology of unstable angina. Cardiol Clin 1991;9: 11–26.
43. Braunwald E, Mark DB, Jones RH, et al. Diagnosing and managing unstable angina: quick reference guide for clinicians, number 10. AHCPR publication no. 94-0603. Rockville, MD: US Department of Health and Human Services, Public Health Service, Agency for Health Care Policy and Research and National Heart, Lung, and Blood Institute, 1994.
44. Hamm CW, Braunwald E. A classification of unstable angina revisited. Circulation 2000;102:118–22.
45. Lewis HD, Davis JW, Archibald DG, et al. Protective effects of aspirin against acute myocardial infarction and death in men with unstable angina: results of a Veterans Administration cooperative study. N Engl J Med 1983;309:396–403.
46. 1999 update: ACC/AHA guidelines for the management of patients with acute myocardial infarction. A report of the American College of Cardiology/American Heart Association Task Force on Practice Guidelines (Committee of Management of Acute Myocardial Infarction). J Am Coll Cardiol 1999;34:890–911.
47. Faxon DP. Percutaneous coronary angioplasty in stable and unstable angina. Cardiol Clin 1991;9:99–113.
48. Sherman DL, Ryan TJ. Coronary angioplasty versus bypass grafting: cost-benefit considerations. Med Clin North Am 1995;79:1085–95.
49. Barsky AJ, Hochstrasser B, Coles A, et al. Silent myocardial ischemia: is the person or the event silent? JAMA 1990;264:1132–5.
50. Cohn PF. Silent myocardial ischemia. Ann Intern Med 1988;109:312–17.
51. Gottlieb SO. Asymptomatic or silent myocardial ischemia in angina pectoris: pathophysiology and clinical implications. Cardiol Clin 1991;9: 49–61.
52. Lavie CJ, Gersh BJ. Acute myocardial infarction: initial manifestations, management, and prognosis. Mayo Clin Proc 1990;65:531–48.
53. Pathy MS. Clinical presentation of myocardial infarction in the elderly. Br Heart J 1967;29:190–9.
54. Kannel WB, Abbott RD. Incidence and prognosis of unrecognized myocardial infarction: an update on the Framingham study. N Engl J Med 1984;311:1144–7.

55. Mair J, Morandell D, Genser N. Equivalent early sensitivities of myoglobin, creatine kinase MB mass, creatine kinase isoform ratios, and cardiac troponins I and T for acute myocardial infarction. Clin Chem 1995;41:1266–72.
56. Wright, RS, Kopecky SL, Reeder GS. Update on intravenous fibrinolytic therapy for acute myocardial infarction. Mayo Clin Proc 2000;75:1185–92.
57. Killip T, Kimball JT. Treatment of myocardial infarction in a coronary care unit: a two-year experience with 250 patients. Am J Cardiol 1967;20:457–61.
58. Guidelines 2000 for cardiopulmonary resuscitation and emergency cardiovascular care. International consensus on science. Circulation 2000;102:1–384.
59. Squires RW, Gau GT, Miller TD, Allison TG, Lavie CJ. Cardiovascular rehabilitation: status 1990. Mayo Clin Proc 1990;65:731–55.
60. O'Connor GT, Buring JE, Yusuf S, et al. An overview of randomized trials of rehabilitation with exercise after myocardial infarction. Circulation 1989;80:234–44.

3
Cardiac Arrhythmias

Michael S. Klinkman

Cardiac arrhythmias are frequently seen in routine primary care practice, and "palpitations" or patient concerns about "skipped heartbeats" are among the most common presenting complaints in primary care. However, in this area the linkage between symptom and disease is tenuous: symptomatic patients often do not have significant cardiac arrhythmias, whereas many clinically significant arrhythmias are detected in asymptomatic patients. This creates a difficult balancing act for the primary care clinician, whose job it is to effectively uncover treatable disease while avoiding unnecessary health care utilization or specialty consultation.

Although diagnosis and treatment are rapidly moving from the office to the electrophysiology laboratory, many cardiac arrhythmias can still be diagnosed and managed within the primary care setting. This chapter focuses on identification and outpatient management of these common arrhythmias and includes a primer of relevant physiology and pharmacology. Because of the specialized and complex nature of cardiac electrophysiology in children, discussion is limited to the adult and older adolescent patient. The goals of this chapter are threefold: to assist family physicians in the diagnosis of common arrhythmias, to provide basic management advice for conditions treatable in the office, and to point to conditions for which more specialized diagnostic testing and referral are indicated.

Basic Electrophysiology of the Heart

All cardiac cells share the ability to automatically contract (automaticity) at an inherent rate (rhythmicity). Myocardial cells contract when a transmembrane action potential (AP) develops. Fully polarized cells have a transmembrane electrical potential (TEP) of −90 mV. After stimulation by an electrical impulse, the membrane allows a slow inward leak of sodium ions. When the TEP has been reduced to a critical level of −60 mV, a "fast" sodium ion channel opens momentarily to actively transport ions across the membrane and depolarize the cell (phase 0 of the AP of the cell). Following depolarization the sodium channel closes, and a complex exchange of sodium, potassium, and calcium ions occurs during phases 1 and 2 of the AP. During phase 3 potassium ions are pumped out of the cell, the TEP returns to slightly below baseline, and the cell cannot contract (absolute refractory period). During phase 4 potassium moves in and sodium out of the cell through specific ion channels, and a strong electrical stimulus can cause depolarization and contraction (relative refractory period). The cell is now ready for its next beat in response to an impulse. If no electrical impulse occurs, the slow inward transport of positive ions eventually results in spontaneous depolarization and contraction at a rate specific to the type of cell (e.g., 40 per minute for ventricular myocardial cells). The protein structures of the ion channels are controlled by several recently identified genes on chromosomes 3, 4, 7, 11, and 21.[1]

Normal cardiac rhythm depends on the automaticity and conductivity of the specialized group of cells that compose the conduction system, and the receptivity of individual myocardial cells to impulses conducted over the system. The sinoatrial (SA) node, located high in the left atrium, controls the normal heart rate. Cells in the SA node spontaneously "fire" (transmit electrical impulses) at regular intervals owing to increased membrane permeability to sodium and calcium. The AP is transmitted as an electrical impulse from the SA node through the atria to the atrioventricular (AV) node, then through the His system and bundle branches to the Purkinje fibers in the ventricle, then to ventricular myocardial cells. This cell-to-cell communication is controlled by connexins, specialized proteins functioning in the gap junction between cardiac cells. A slight delay occurs at the AV node, which has a pattern of automaticity similar to that of the SA node. Cells in the two nodes also have an absolute and relative refractory period, which is an important factor in the genesis of reentrant arrhythmias.

General Causes of Arrhythmias

The identification of several mutations in the genes that encode the protein structures of sodium and potassium ion channels[1–3] has rev-

Table 3.1. **General Causes of Arrhythmias**

Autonomic nervous system input
  Sympathetic input through stellate ganglion
  Parasympathetic input through vagus nerve
Autonomic response to stressful external factors
Autonomic response to mental health conditions (e.g., anxiety
  disorder)
Autonomic response to physical factors (e.g., carotid sinus pressure)
Anatomic alterations in the conduction system (bypass tracts)
Alterations in extracellular electrolyte concentrations
Alterations in circulating endocrine mediators (e.g., thyroid hormone)
Decreased tissue oxygenation
Decreased extracellular pH
Destruction of or damage to myocardial cells
Endocrine mediators (e.g., thyroid hormone)
Genetic mutations
Ingested substances
  Stimulants (e.g., caffeine) and sympathomimetics
  Depressants (e.g., alcohol)
  Prescription drugs
  Illicit drugs
Senescence in cardiac conduction system or myocardial cells

olutionized our understanding of arrhythmias. It is increasingly clear that mutations in any of the genes responsible for ion channel, connexin, or myosin protein structure can either directly cause arrhythmias or predispose individuals to an arrhythmia under any of the circumstances described below. We are entering the era of "molecular epidemiology," in which genotyping and variable gene expression will be important parts of diagnosis and treatment.

Anything that can influence cardiac automaticity or conductivity can cause an arrhythmia (Table 3.1) in a susceptible heart. Autonomic nervous system input can greatly influence both automaticity and conductivity. Sympathetic input through the stellate ganglion stimulates cardiac β_1-receptors and increases automaticity and conductivity, and parasympathetic input through the vagus nerve stimulates muscarinic receptors and inhibits β_1-receptors, decreasing automaticity and conductivity. The presence of stressful external events or circumstances commonly stimulates sympathetic activity and can cause arrhythmias, whereas some mental health conditions (e.g., anxiety, panic attacks, panic disorder) are also associated with increased sympathetic activity. The central nervous system (CNS) can also alter baseline sympathetic and parasympathetic tone and predispose to arrhythmias. Local or mechanical factors can influence conductivity and automaticity through the autonomic nervous system. For example, pressure on the neck can stimulate the carotid sinus and increase parasympathetic output, and placing an extremity or the face in ice water can greatly stimulate parasympathetic activity.

Anatomic alterations in the conduction system may also cause arrhythmias. Accessory or alternate pathways for the conduction of cardiac impulses can be present from birth or develop over time. Under certain circumstances these pathways can provide a bypass tract that replaces the normal sinus node–generated rhythm with a reentrant rhythm. This process is believed to cause most supraventricular arrhythmias.

Alterations in extracellular electrolyte concentrations, particularly potassium, calcium, magnesium, and sodium, can alter automaticity and conductivity by affecting TEP generation and recovery. Extracellular oxygen content can greatly influence cardiac rhythm; low oxygen tension can decrease conductivity and contractility of myocardial cells and promote arrhythmia, as seen with myocardial infarction (MI), cardiac ischemia, and some cases of congestive heart failure (CHF). Decreased extracellular pH, often seen with MI or cardiac ischemia, can cause similar decreases in conductivity and result in arrhythmia. Endocrine mediators can also have direct or indirect effects on cardiac rhythm. Increased amounts of circulating catecholamines or thyroid hormone can increase contractility and automaticity through the sympathetic nervous system and by direct effect on myocardial cells, whereas decreases in circulating thyroid hormone or corticosteroid concentrations can decrease contractility and automaticity.

Ingested substances can also have profound effects on cardiac rhythm. Caffeine and other sympathomimetic substances can increase conductivity, whereas CNS depressants such as alcohol have the opposite effect. Illicit drugs such as amphetamines and cocaine have strong, well-known stimulatory effects on cardiac rhythm, but other street drugs can also precipitate arrhythmias. A multitude of prescription and nonprescription drugs have been associated with cardiac rhythm disturbances. Cardiac medications (e.g., digoxin and all classes of antiarrhythmics) and tricyclic antidepressants are perhaps the best known groups of medications with proarrhythmic effects, but combinations of medications (astemizole and ketoconazole) and some over-the-counter medications (pseudoephedrine) can also affect conductivity and automaticity.

Localized damage to cardiac muscle, such as the destruction of myocardial and conduction system cells seen with MI or damage from surgery to repair congenital anomalies, can result in decreased conductivity and contractility and create reentrant circuits.

Finally, senescence of cardiac conduction system cells and myocardial cells may affect automaticity and conductivity in elderly individuals. This phenomenon can occur directly, through fibrotic degradation in the conduction system, or indirectly, through the increased susceptibility of cardiac cells to the agents mentioned above.

Approach to the Diagnosis of Cardiac Arrhythmias

The initial step in managing arrhythmias in the primary care setting is to determine if the patient is hemodynamically stable. Unstable patients require immediate management and may benefit from transfer to an emergency or inpatient facility. Stable patients can be evaluated in the office using a stepwise approach (Table 3.2). Although the diagnosis of specific cardiac arrhythmia rests on the presence of specific electrocardiographic (ECG) or electrophysiologic (EP) study findings, valuable clues regarding the clinical significance and cause of the arrhythmia can be obtained by a careful clinical history and physical examination.

History

Patients may present with nonspecific symptoms suggestive of cardiac arrhythmia, such as palpitations, sensation of a racing heart, dizziness, or sudden fatigue. In these circumstances four key questions help determine the clinical significance of the symptoms and sometimes point to likely cause(s):

1. *When did the symptom(s) start?* After starting a new medication? A long time ago? Yesterday?
2. *What sets it off?* Exertion? Emotional stress? Ingestion of a meal or certain foods such as coffee? Taking a dose of medication? Lying down or sudden position change? A tight shirt collar or tie?
3. *How long does it last?* Moments? Or does it go on for hours or days?
4. *What else happens?* Chest pain? Dyspnea? Orthopnea? Nausea? Tingling in the hands or around the mouth?

Clinicians who discover arrhythmias in asymptomatic patients may get little help from patients' answers to these questions. However, a

Table 3.2. **Diagnostic Approach for Patients with Arrhythmias**

Determine whether patient is hemodynamically stable and triage
  appropriately
Obtain clinical history
  Circumstances surrounding onset of symptoms, duration of
  symptoms
  Brief review of systems
  Complete substance use and diet history
  Past medical history
  Brief mental health screen
Perform physical examination as directed by history
  Search for evidence of medical conditions associated with
    arrhythmias
  Cardiac auscultation
Obtain electrocardiogram (ECG)
Consider other laboratory tests (serum chemistries and electrolytes) as
  directed by history
Options for additional diagnostic studies
  Graded exercise test (GXT, "stress test")
  24- or 48-hour ambulatory ECG monitoring
  Long-term, continuous-loop, event monitoring
  Echocardiography
  Electrophysiologic (EP) study
  Cardiac catheterization

complete drug history, including prescription, nonprescription, and illicit drug use, should be obtained for all patients, as well as a smoking, alcohol, and brief dietary history. A brief review of systems should also be completed, focusing on symptoms of cardiac or endocrine conditions. Reviewing the patient's medical history for the presence of conditions associated with arrhythmia may reveal a likely cause. Finally, screening for mental health problems such as anxiety, panic, or depression provides valuable clues in some cases.

Physical Examination

The physical examination should look for evidence of medical conditions associated with arrhythmias. For example, sudden weight gain, the presence of bibasilar rales on pulmonary examination, ankle edema, and an audible S_3 on cardiac auscultation may indicate the presence of congestive heart failure, whereas moist skin, the presence of a fine tremor, hypertension, and lid lag suggest the hyperthyroid stage of Graves' disease. Cardiac auscultation alone can point to specific arrhythmias, as an irregularly irregular rhythm almost always signifies atrial fibrillation.

Electrocardiogram

The ECG is necessary to establish a specific diagnosis and may be the point at which evaluation of arrhythmia begins for asymptomatic patients. Lead II is the best single lead for evaluation of cardiac rhythm in most patients, as the P and QRS electrical vectors in patients without axis deviation are most positive in this lead. A long rhythm strip is often valuable for evaluating arrhythmias, particularly in the case of AV conduction defects. Although an increasing number of primary care offices use ECG equipment that prints out a computerized diagnostic assessment on the tracing, these algorithm-based diagnoses are often incomplete or inaccurate. Clinicians are urged to read and interpret the ECG themselves, paying particular attention to P wave appearance, intervals (PR, PP, and QT) and the relation between the P wave and QRS complex. Several reference books are available to assist clinicians in ECG interpretation.

Other Diagnostic Studies

Depending on the type of arrhythmia and its clinical presentation, additional diagnostic evaluation may be helpful. Simple graded exercise testing (GXT) can sometimes reproduce arrhythmia patterns in patients with exercise-induced symptoms. If the clinical history is suspicious for arrhythmia but the physical examination and ECG do not confirm its presence, 24- or 48-hour continuous ambulatory ECG monitoring (Holter monitoring) or long-term, continuous-loop, event recorder monitoring may be performed to capture occasional periods of cardiac arrhythmia.[4] However, studies have shown that rhythm abnormalities noted in the monitor tracing often have little temporal correspondence with patient symptoms as recorded in a symptom diary,[5,6] and the clinical significance of this pattern of results is not clear. Echocardiography, particularly transesophageal echocardiography (TEE), can also be useful to look for structural changes that may predispose to arrhythmias or affect management decisions, such as an enlarged left atrium or left atrial appendage in patients with atrial fibrillation.[7–9] Electrophysiologic studies are a powerful diagnostic tool, although they require the patient to undergo cardiac catheterization. Programmed electrical stimulation of specific areas of the conduction system or cardiac tissue via catheter can uncover ectopic pacemakers, find accessory or bypass tracts responsible for reentry arrhythmias, and in combination with radiofrequency ablation (RFA) eliminate the cause of many arrhythmias.[10–14] Although most family physicians do not perform these tests, it is important that they know the appropriate indications for each test and how to interpret test results.

Approach to Therapy for Cardiac Arrhythmias

Many cardiac arrhythmias are of little clinical significance and do not require therapy other than careful discussion with the patient and reassurance. For other arrhythmias, clinicians should begin by searching for and treating any reversible underlying causes or medical conditions. If the arrhythmia persists, four types of treatment are available: drug therapy, cardioversion, radiofrequency or surgical ablation, and implantable devices (pacemakers and defibrillators).

Correction of Underlying Problems

Medication use or ingestions (e.g., caffeine) are the most commonly seen reversible causes of arrhythmias, and changing or discontinuing medications or discontinuing use of caffeine or other substances may eliminate the problem. Correction of electrolyte imbalances can also eliminate arrhythmias. In patients with CHF or ischemic heart disease and arrhythmia, effective therapy for the underlying condition may improve tissue oxygen delivery and local pH and result in return to sinus rhythm. Clinicians should look for and correct all potentially reversible causes before initiating drug or ablative therapy.

Drug Therapy

Antiarrhythmic drugs have been assigned to classes based on their mode of action. Table 3.3 lists examples of drugs in each of the Vaughan-Williams classes.[15] Class I agents act on the sodium ion channel, with slight differences between IA, IB, and IC agents in specific actions. Randomized controlled trials of drug therapy for ventricular arrhythmia have shown no improvement in survival, and in some cases excess mortality, in patients using class I antiarrhythmics. Use of these agents is declining,[16–19] although there may be a role for class IC agents propafenone and flecainide in supraventricular arrhythmias.[19–21] The use of class II drugs (beta-blockers) has been shown to have a beneficial effect on survival in post-MI patients, presumably due to suppression of lethal ventricular arrhythmia. They are also useful as adjunctive treatment to implantable cardiac defib-

Table 3.3. Dosing, Indications, and Contraindications for Common Antiarrhythmic Drugs Listed by Vaughan-Williams Class

Name	Dosing	Indications	Contraindications • clinical notes
Class IA			
Disopyramide		VT	CHF (relative); 2nd- or 3rd-degree AV block prolonged QT interval
Norpace	100–200 mg po q6–8h		• Proarrhythmic effects
Norpace CR	200–400 mg po q12h		
Procainamide		Primary: VT	CHF relative; complete heart block
Pronestyl	375–500 mg q3–4h	Secondary: VT, AT in	• Drug-induced lupus
Pronestyl SR	500–1000 mg q6–8h	WPW syndrome	• Blood dyscrasias
Procan SR	500–750 mg q6–8h		• Proarrhythmic effects
Quinidine		VT	2nd- or 3rd-degree AV block prolonged QT interval
Quinidine sulfate	200–300 mg q6–8h		• Proarrhythmic effects
Quinidex Extentabs	300–600 mg q8–12h		
Quinaglute	324–648 mg q8–12°		
Class IB			
Lidocaine	IV: 1 mg/kg bolus followed by 1–4 mg/min infusion	VT, VF	• CNS side effects
Mexiletine		Primary: VT	2nd- or 3rd-degree AV block
Mexitil	150–300 mg po q8–12h	Secondary: SVT in WPW syndrome	• ?Hepatic toxicity
			• CNS side effects
			• Proarrhythmic effects

Drug	Dosage	Indications	Contraindications/Side effects
Tocainide Tonocard	400–600 mg po q8h	VT	2nd- or 3rd-degree AV block • Blood dyscrasias • Pulmonary fibrosis • Proarrhythmic effects
Class IC			
Flecainide Tambocor	IV: 2 mg/kg over 5–10 min 50–200 mg po q12h	Primary: VT Secondary: SVT, paroxysmal AF, atrial flutter	CHF (relative) 2nd- or 3rd-degree AV block; bifascicular block • Proarrhythmic effects
Propafenone Rythmol	150–300 mg po q8h	Primary: VT Secondary: SVT in WPW syndrome	CHF; 2nd- or 3rd-degree AV block; severe asthma • Proarrhythmic effects
Moricizine Ethmozine	200–300 mg po q8h	Primary: VT Secondary: SVT	Cardiogenic shock; 2nd-3rd-degree AV block; bifascicular block • Proarrhythmic effects
Class II (β-blockers)			
Propranolol Inderal Inderal LA	20–80 mg po q6h 20–160 mg po q12h	AT; sinus tachycardia; SVT; VT prophylaxis; SVT in WPW syndrome; VPB post-MI	CHF; severe asthma; severe bradycardia; 2nd- or 3rd-degree AV block
Acebutolol Sectral	200–600 mg po BID	Same as propranolol	CHF; severe bradycardia; 2nd- or 3rd-degree AV block
Atenolol Tenormin	50–100 mg po q12h	Same as propranolol	CHF; severe bradycardia; 2nd- or 3rd-degree AV block

(continued)

Table 3.3 (Continued).

Name	Dosing	Indications	Contraindications • clinical notes
Bisoprolol Zebeta	2.5–20 mg po qd	Same as propranolol	CHF; severe asthma; severe bradycardia; 2nd- or 3rd-degree AV block
Esmolol Brevibloc	IV: 0.5 mg/kg bolus, 0.05 to 0.2 mg/min infusion	SVT; VT; AF	CHF; severe asthma; severe bradycardia; 2nd- or 3rd-degree AV block
Labetalol	IV: 1–2 mg/kg bolus, 0.5–2 mg/min infusion	SVT	CHF (relative); severe asthma; severe bradycardia; 2nd- or 3rd-degree AV
Normodyne Trandate	100–400 mg po q8–12h 100–400 mg po q8–12h	Same as propranolol	
Metoprolol	IV: 2.5–5.0 mg over 2 min, up to 15 mg total	SVT	CHF; severe bradycardia; 2nd- or 3rd-degree AV block
Toprol XL Lopressor	50–200 mg po qd 50–100 mg po q8–12h	Same as propranolol	
Nadolol Corgard	40–240 mg po qd	Same as propranolol	CHF; severe asthma; severe bradycardia; 2nd- or 3rd-degree AV block
Timolol Blocadren	10–20 mg po q12h	Same as propranolol	CHF; severe asthma; severe COPD; severe bradycardia; 2nd- or 3rd-degree AV block
Pindolol Visken	2.5–30 mg po q12h	Same as propranolol	CHF; severe asthma; severe bradycardia; 2nd- or 3rd-degree AV block

	Dosage	Indication	Contraindications/Adverse effects
Class III			
Amiodarone Cordarone	IV: 5 mg/kg over 10–15 min bolus, then 0.5–1 mg/min 800–1600 mg po qd or q12h for 1–2 weeks (loading dose); 200–400 mg po qd (maintenance)	Primary: VT; VF prophylaxis Secondary: AF; VPB post-MI	Severe bradycardia; 2nd- or 3rd-degree AV block (unless pacemaker capability) • proarrhythmic effects • pulmonary toxicity • hepatic toxicity • corneal deposits • thyroid abnormalities
Sotalol Betapace	IV: 1–1.5 mg/kg over 10 min 80–160 mg po q12h	VT; VF prophylaxis	CHF; severe asthma; severe bradycardia; 2nd- 3rd-degree AV block; prolonged QT interval • Proarrhythmic effects
Ibutilide Corvert	IV: 1–2 mg over 10 min	AF (termination); SVT	• Proarrhythmic effects
Dofetilide Tikosyn	125–500 mg po q12h	AF	Prolonged QT interval; renal impairment; use with verapamil, cimetidine, trimethoprim or ketoconazole
Class IV (calcium channel blockers)			
Diltiazem Cardizem	IV: 0.25 mg/kg bolus followed by 10–15 mg/hr infusion 30–90 mg po q6h	AT; sinus tachycardia; SVT; AF; atrial flutter	Sick sinus syndrome severe bradycardia; 2nd- or 3rd-degree AV block
Cardizem Cardizem SR	60–180 mg po q12h		

(continued)

Table 3.3 (Continued).

Name	Dosing	Indications	Contraindications • clinical notes
Verapamil			
Isoptin	IV: 5–10 mg over 2 min, repeat in 30 min if needed	AT; sinus tachycardia; SVT; AF; atrial flutter	Sick sinus syndrome; severe bradycardia; 2nd- or 3rd-degree AV block; concomitant use of IV and IV beta-blockers; AF in WPW
Isoptin	80–120 mg q6–8h		
Isoptin SR	180–480 mg po q12h to qd		
Calan	80–120 mg q6–8h		
Calan SR	180–180 mg po q12h to qd		
Miscellaneous			
Adenosine Adenocard	IV: 6 mg over 1–2 sec, may repeat bolus twice with 12 mg over 1–2 min if needed	SVT; SVT in WPW syndrome	Sick sinus syndrome; AV block 2nd or 3rd-degree • may cause dyspnea, chest pain, flushing
Digoxin Lanoxin	IV: 0.5 mg bolus followed by 0.1–0.3 mg q4–6h Loading dose: 0.5–0.75 mg po followed by 0.125–0.25 mg q6h 0.125–0.25 mg po qd	AF; atrial flutter; AT	VF • proarrhythmic effects

AF = atrial fibrillation; AT = (paroxysmal) atrial tachycardia; CHF = congestive heart failure; CNS = central nervous system; COPD = chronic obstructive pulmonary disease; MI = myocardial infarction; SVT = supraventricular tachycardia; VPB = ventricular premature beat; VT = ventricular tachycardia; WPW syndrome = Wolff-Parkinson-White syndrome.

Note: VPBs are not included in list of indications, as treatment is generally not indicated for VPBs.

rillators (ICDs), as an alternative to RFA for AV nodal reentrant tach-yarrhythmias, and to control rate in atrial fibrillation.[13,19,22] Class III drugs prolong the AP by increasing refractoriness. Amiodarone has emerged as an effective agent for both ventricular and supraventric-ular arrhythmias.[23,24] Dofetilide and ibutilide have also shown promise in recent clinical trials, while sotalol (a combined class II and III agent) appears to be less effective than other class III agents.[19,25–27] Class IV agents (calcium channel blockers) are effec-tive for many supraventricular arrhythmias.[19,28]

The major drawback to the use of any of these agents is their po-tential for inducing complex arrhythmias (proarrhythmic ef-fect).[19,29,30] The best known example is the emergence of torsades de pointes arrhythmia in patients with prolonged QT intervals treated with class I antiarrhythmics,[31] but all antiarrhythmic drugs have proarrhythmic potential and their use must be carefully monitored.

Cardioversion

Urgent or emergent direct current (DC) cardioversion is most com-monly used in hemodynamically unstable patients with atrial or ven-tricular arrhythmias, but elective cardioversion can be an effective treatment for selected supraventricular arrhythmias. It has been suc-cessfully employed either before or after medication to convert atrial fibrillation or flutter to sinus rhythm,[14] and it has a place in the non-pharmacologic management of other supraventricular tachyarrhyth-mias.[32] Microcurrent catheter-based cardioversion is currently being studied.

Ablative Therapy

The ablative approach rests on identification and localization of an aberrant conduction pathway responsible for the arrhythmia, usually through an EP study. Ablation is clearly effective in treating supraventricular tachyarrhythmias. Physical interruption of aberrant pathways via sharp surgical dissection during open-heart surgical procedures became common during the 1980s; the maze procedure (named for the procedure that creates a pattern that looks like a maze and traps the reentrant circuit) and its variants are the best example of this approach.[33,34] More recently, cryoablation and RFA tech-niques have become the nonpharmacologic treatment of choice for selected supraventricular tachyarrhythmias.[10–12] In RFA, application of radiofrequency energy to a portion of the aberrant pathway pro-duces thermal injury and a permanent refractory state in the tissue, preventing any further aberrant conduction. High success rates have been reported for RFA in most settings,[10-12] and it may prove to be the most cost-effective approach to management of many supraventricular tachyarrhythmias.[35-37] RFA also has a growing role in treatment of monomorphic ventricular tachycardia refractory to drug therapy.[10]

Pacemakers and Defibrillators

Implantable cardiac pacemakers have been available for many years and provide effective therapy for many bradyarrhythmias and other conduction disturbances. Although pace-makers have been developed for use in supraventricular tachyarrhythmias, they are infrequently used.[38] Implantable cardiac defibrillators have evolved rapidly in size, sophistication, and ease of insertion over the past decade. Recent clinical trials have confirmed their superior effectiveness as compared to drug therapy in reducing mortality in survivors of cardiac arrest and patients at high risk for sudden cardiac death (SCD).[39-42] ICDs are now considered the treatment of choice for secondary prevention of SCD, and an emerging standard for primary prevention of SCD in high-risk patients, despite the absence of good data on their relative cost-effectiveness.[43]

Automatic external defibrillators (AEDs) combine computerized detection of ventricular fibrillation with low-energy biphasic waveform defibrillation.[44] They have also evolved rapidly over the past decade in size, cost, and ease of use, and have emerged as a central part of new emergency and "public access" defibrillation protocols employed by first-response emergency personnel.[44-46]

Specific Cardiac Arrhythmias: Diagnosis and Management

This section describes the salient clinical features and management options for the most common cardiac arrhythmias, including sample ECG tracings where appropriate. Table 3.4 lists arrhythmias by class in the order addressed in the text, and Table 3.5 lists treatments of choice and alternative treatments for specific arrhythmias.

Sinus Bradycardia

Sinus bradycardia consists of normally conducted cardiac impulses originating in the sinus node at a rate less than 60 beats per minute (bpm). It occurs in individuals at a high level of athletic condition-

Table 3.4. **Common Cardiac Arrhythmias**

Supraventricular arrhythmias—slow to moderate rate
  Sinus bradycardia
  Sinus pause/sinus arrest
  Atrial premature beats (premature atrial complexes)
Supraventricular tachyarrhythmias
  Sinus tachycardia
  Atrial tachycardia
  Multifocal atrial tachycardia
  AV nodal reentrant tachycardias (paroxysmal supraventricular
    tachycardia)
  AV reciprocating tachycardias ("preexcitation" syndromes)
  Atrial fibrillation
  Atrial flutter
Other atrioventricular conduction abnormalities
  1st-degree AV block
  2nd-degree AV block, Mobitz type I (Wenckebach block)
  2nd-degree AV block, Mobitz type II
  3rd-degree AV block
Ventricular arrhythmias
  Ventricular premature beats (premature ventricular complexes)
  Ventricular tachycardia—nonsustained and sustained
  Ventricular fibrillation

AV = atrioventricular.

ing, as a result of vagal hyperactivity or pain, and during sleep. It can be a symptom of hypothyroidism and is often associated with medication use (e.g., narcotic analgesics, calcium channel antagonists, beta-blockers, digoxin, quinidine, procainamide). It can also occur in the setting of an inferior wall MI. It can present significant problems when it appears in elderly patients, if it is the result of sinus node disease or fibrosis, or if it is associated with an acute inferior wall MI.

The clinical history may vary from no symptoms to fatigue, dizziness, syncope or near-syncope, or chest pain (if associated with MI). Clinicians should look for signs or symptoms of hypothyroidism, CHF, and MI. The ECG appears normal except for a slow heart rate. No other tests are necessary, unless an associated medical condition is suspected.

Treatment is not necessary unless the patient is symptomatic or is at high risk for complications related to slow heart rate (e.g., an elderly patient at risk for falls). In general, treat an underlying cause first whenever possible: if associated with medication use, discontinue the offending medication; if due to hypothyroidism, begin treat-

Table 3.5. **Treatment of Choice and Alternative Treatments for Common Cardiac Arrhythmias**

Arrhythmia	Treatment(s) of choice	Alternative treatment
Sinus bradycardia	Atropine (emergent) Pacemaker	Isoproterenol
Sinus pause/arrest	Atropine (emergent) Pacemaker	
Atrial premature beats, junctional premature beats	Treatment often not necessary	Beta-blockers, verapamil
Sinus tachycardia	Beta-blockers	Verapamil
Atrial tachycardia	Beta-blockers RFA (curative)	Verapamil
Multifocal atrial tachycardia	IV verapamil (conversion) Beta-blockers, verapamil	RFA of AV node plus pacemaker
AV nodal reentrant tachycardias (SVT) and AV reciprocating tachycardias ("preexcitation")	IV adenosine (conversion) IV verapamil (conversion) Carotid sinus pressure, vagal maneuvers (conversion) Beta-blockers (prophylaxis) Calcium channel blockers (prophylaxis) RFA (curative)	IV esmolol (conversion) DC cardioversion Pacemaker Class IC antiarrhythmics (prophylaxis) Class III antiarrhythmics (prophylaxis) Digoxin (conversion and prophylaxis; use with caution)
Atrial fibrillation	DC cardioversion Amiodarone Beta-blockers Calcium-channel blockers Digoxin Aspirin, coumadin (CVA prevention)	Class I antiarrhythmics Class III antiarrhythmics RFA of ectopic focus (if present) RFA of AV node plus pacemaker Surgical ablation (Cox maze procedure)

Atrial flutter	DC cardioversion Rapid atrial pacing (conversion) Beta-blockers Calcium channel blockers RFA of reentrant circuit (curative)	Ibutilide (conversion) Class IA antiarrhythmics RFA of AV node plus pacemaker
1st-degree AV block and 2nd-degree (Mobitz type I)	Treatment often not necessary	Pacemaker (symptomatic Mobitz type I)
2nd-degree (Mobitz type II) and 3rd-degree AV block	Pacemaker	
Ventricular premature beats	Treatment often not necessary	Beta-blockers Amiodarone With heart disease: amiodarone EP study with RFA of ectopic focus
Ventricular tachycardia, nonsustained	With no heart disease: no treatment necessary With heart disease and VT on EP study: implantable cardiac defibrillator With heart disease and no VT on EP study: treat heart disease (see text)	
Ventricular tachycardia, sustained	ACLS protocol, transfer for definitive care Postevent: implantable cardiac defibrillator	
Ventricular fibrillation	ACLS protocol, automatic external defibrillator, transfer for definitive care Postevent: implantable cardiac defibrillator	

ACLS = advanced cardiac life support; AV = atrioventricular; CVA = cerebrovascular accident; EP = electrophysiologic; RFA = radiofrequency ablation; VT = ventricular tachycardia.

ment with thyroid hormone. Patients who do not have a likely cause or who do not respond to treatment may require pacemaker insertion. Emergent treatment for unstable patients can be initiated in the office with atropine until definitive care can be arranged.

Sinus Pause/Sinus Arrest

As its name suggests, sinus pause/sinus arrest consists of an unexpected pause in an otherwise normal pattern of cardiac impulses. The sinus node does not fire, and a pause of up to several seconds may occur followed by resumption of a regular rhythm or emergence of a nodal or idioventricular "escape" rhythm. It commonly occurs in individuals during deep sleep, but when frequent and associated with escape rhythms it may also indicate a fibrotic and malfunctioning SA node, sick sinus syndrome, or medication effect (digoxin, quinidine, calcium channel blocker, or beta-blocker overdosing).

The condition may be asymptomatic or associated with recurrent dizziness, near-syncope, or syncope, and resumption of cardiac impulses may be perceived by the patient as palpitations. The ECG shows normal sinus rhythm with a sudden pause during which P waves are absent, followed either by resumption of P waves and normal sinus rhythm or appearance of a junctional or ventricular QRS complex. With sick sinus syndrome, other types of arrhythmia or conduction disturbance are seen as well.

Treatment is not always necessary, but in light of the potential for significant symptoms and the possibility of significant underlying cardiac disease, referral for cardiac evaluation is warranted. If symptomatic patients do not respond to correction of known underlying causes, cardiac pacemaker insertion may be necessary. Emergent office-based treatment for full sinus arrest consists of intravenous atropine or isoproterenol until definitive care can be arranged.

Premature Atrial Complexes

The terms *premature atrial complexes* (PACs) and *atrial premature beats* (APBs) are both used, and they represent the same phenomenon. Cardiac impulses are initiated in one or more ectopic atrial foci but are otherwise conducted as for a normal beat. They often occur in individuals with a normal heart and can be precipitated by anxiety, fatigue, ingestion of a number of substances (alcohol, tobacco, caffeine, sympathomimetic drugs), and possibly sleep deprivation. They can also occur in the presence of atrial enlargement, CHF, myocardial ischemia and infarction, pericarditis, or as a response to hypoxia, elevated local pH, or electrolyte imbalance.

Figure 1a: Premature atrial complexes (atrial premature beats) [beats #3,6,9]

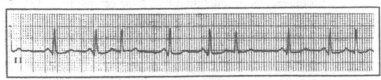

Figure 1b: Sinus tachycardia

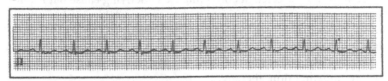

Figure 1c: Multifocal atrial tachycardia

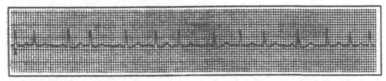

Figure 1d: Supraventricular tachycardia

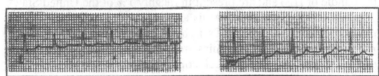

Figure 1e: AV reciprocating tachycardias ("preexcitation" syndromes)
      [example: Wolff-Parkinson-White syndrome]

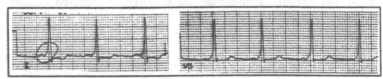

Fig. 3.1. Selected supraventricular arrhythmias: sample electrocardiogram (ECG) tracings. ECG leads from which tracings were obtained are listed in the lower left corner. See text for discussion of specific ECG features of each arrhythmia.

The APBs are usually asymptomatic, but patients may present with palpitations. Physical examination is nonspecific, except for signs of underlying conditions. On ECG (Fig. 3.1a), the amplitudes and axes of ectopic P waves differ from that seen in sinus rhythm, as a different part of the atrium is depolarizing. The PR interval of the APB is usually prolonged, as conduction between the ectopic focus to the AV node is slowed. A prolonged PP interval is often seen between the APB and a subsequent normal beat. The QRS complex appears normal, unless aberrant conduction bypassing the AV node or ventricular conduction disturbance is also present. APBs may occur in patterns such as bigeminy or trigeminy, in couplets, or as short runs.

Treatment is directed at correcting the underlying cause but is otherwise not necessary. In patients with an unacceptable level of symptoms, verapamil or beta-blockers can be used to suppress APBs with relatively mild side effects. However, clinicians should carefully consider the risk/benefit ratio of drug therapy for this benign condition before initiating drug therapy.

Supraventricular Tachyarrhythmias

Increased experience with EP studies and our growing knowledge of molecular genetics have combined to fundamentally change our understanding of the supraventricular tachyarrhythmias (SVTs). SVTs include all tachyarrhythmias that originate above the bifurcation of the bundle of His, and are present in roughly 1% of the United States population.[13] Terminology in this area is evolving and confusing. A practical way to stratify SVTs is by involvement of the AV node: AV-node–*dependent* arrhythmias are more responsive to medications or procedures that slow or block conduction at the AV node than are *independent* arrhythmias that bypass the node. Reentry is now believed to be the underlying mechanism of most SVTs, with a smaller proportion caused by abnormal automaticity or triggered activity without a bypass tract.

Sinus Tachycardia

Sinus tachycardia consists of normally conducted cardiac impulses originating in the sinus node at a rate of over 100 bpm. It may be asymptomatic or symptomatic, often described by patients as "palpitations" or a "racing heart." This rhythm is an appropriate response to the need for increased cardiac output and can be a normal finding in distressed or exercising individuals. However, its occurrence at rest is not normal and should lead to a search for an underlying cause. Possible causes include hyperthyroidism, fever, anemia, hypoxia, CHF, hypovolemia, anxiety, caffeine or other stimulants, illicit drug ingestion, and medication use (common nonprescription medications such as cold preparations with sympathomimetic effects, as well as tricyclic antidepressants, prazosin, and theophylline). In some cases a reentrant process at the SA node may be the cause.

Symptoms are generally nonspecific, although in patients with underlying ischemic heart disease sinus tachycardia can precipitate acute ischemia. The ECG (Fig. 3.1b) is normal except for the rate; all waves and complexes have normal morphology. Evaluation depends on the likelihood of significant underlying illness.

Treatment is directed at the underlying cause. Treatment with rate-lowering drugs is indicated only for relief of hemodynamically significant symptoms (syncope, near-syncope, ischemia) when no underlying cause can be found.

Atrial Tachycardia

Atrial tachycardia (also known as automatic or paroxysmal atrial tachycardia) might be considered a variant of sinus tachycardia, in which an ectopic atrial pacemaker or an intraatrial reentry mechanism initiates a rapid regular rhythm using the normal conduction system. The heart rate may vary from 100 to 300 bpm, depending on whether AV block is present. Atrial tachycardia with AV block is strongly associated with digoxin intoxication; otherwise, it has many of the same precipitating factors as sinus tachycardia. It can be distinguished from sinus tachycardia by the appearance of abnormal P waves or by retrograde or nonconducted P waves when some degree of AV block is present.

Treatment depends on the cause. If symptoms are significant, treatment with rate-lowering drugs may be indicated. Referral to a cardiologist for an EP study may allow identification and ablation of a causative intraatrial reentry tract.

Multifocal Atrial Tachycardia

Multifocal atrial tachycardia (MAT) is characterized by the appearance of multiple ectopic atrial foci, with a rapid and slightly irregular rhythm the result of transmission of these multiple foci through the AV node. It is usually associated with respiratory failure due to chronic pulmonary disease, although it is also seen with chronic heart disease and with the use of thioxanthene drugs. Hypoxia and hypokalemia have been hypothesized as the major causative mechanisms.[47]

The arrhythmia itself rarely causes symptoms, but the underlying condition is usually all too clear. Because the pulse is often irregularly irregular, MAT can be mistaken for atrial fibrillation on clinical examination. The ECG (Fig. 3.1c) shows an atrial rate over 100 bpm with at least three distinct P wave morphologies. The PP, PR, and RR intervals are irregular due to the varying conduction pathways, and some P waves are not conducted. If the ectopic P waves are of low amplitude, the ECG can also resemble that seen with atrial fibrillation.

Treatment is directed at correcting the presumed metabolic abnormalities. Administration of supplemental oxygen for pulmonary failure or treatment of associated CHF may alleviate hypoxia. Intravenous bolus administration of verapamil has been shown to convert MAT to sinus rhythm, and oral verapamil or beta-blockers can slow the ventricular rate. However, these medications are often poorly tolerated in MAT patients with severe cardiac or pulmonary disease, and drug therapy is usually reserved for patients who develop ischemia or hemodynamic instability. Patients refractory to drug therapy may benefit from AV nodal ablation followed by pacemaker insertion.[10,12]

AV Nodal Reentrant Tachycardias

Many clinicians recognize AV nodal reentrant tachycardia (AVNRT) by the commonly used term *paroxysmal supraventricular tachycardia* (PSVT). It consists of a regular and rapid rhythm, usually between 140 and 220 bpm, caused by a reentry mechanism dependent on a dual conduction pathway within the AV node. Regular beats are transmitted through the node along a "fast" pathway. A premature atrial beat initiates the arrhythmia; it is blocked from antegrade passage through the fast pathway during its refractory period but transmitted antegrade through a "slow" pathway in the node. This impulse is then transmitted both antegrade to the ventricles and retrograde through the fast pathway (now nonrefractory) back to the slow pathway, where the process is repeated. This arrhythmia is often seen in young, healthy individuals with otherwise normal hearts, but it may occur with myocarditis, cardiac ischemia, chronic obstructive pulmonary disease (COPD), or other conditions potentially affecting AV nodal function.

Many patients are asymptomatic during episodes. Young patients may note only palpitations but may also have associated weakness, dizziness, or mild dyspnea; they are usually hemodynamically stable during an episode. Older patients, particularly those with underlying cardiac or pulmonary disease, may develop angina, CHF, or cerebrovascular insufficiency during episodes; syncope is rarely reported. Cardiac auscultation reveals a regular, rapid rhythm. The ECG (Fig. 3.1d) shows a regular rhythm with normal QRS complexes (unless aberrant ventricular conduction is also present), but P waves are abnormal owing to retrograde conduction. In many cases of AVNRT,

P waves are absent as atria depolarize at the same time as the ventricles. In other cases, a slight difference in depolarization timing creates slurs in the normal QRS due to atrial activity.

Treatment depends in large part on the level of symptoms and the patient's hemodynamic stability. Unstable patients require emergent conversion by DC cardioversion or intravenous bolus administration of adenosine, verapamil, or esmolol. Intravenous adenosine is currently the treatment of choice in many centers, as it terminates SVT in more than 90% of cases.[48] Other class I antiarrhythmics may produce conversion to sinus rhythm at high rates, but their high risk/benefit ratios essentially preclude their use in this setting. Rapid digitalization has been used for urgent conversion in the past with high success rates, but it does not result in immediate correction and may predispose to the development of other arrhythmias.[13] Nonpharmacologic techniques such as carotid sinus massage, Valsalva maneuver, or other vagal maneuvers such as facial ice bag application or ice bucket immersion prolong AV node refractory periods and can produce conversion to sinus rhythm in selected situations.

Once converted to sinus rhythm, several drugs are effective in preventing recurrence, including oral verapamil, diltiazem, beta-blockers, and digoxin. Because digoxin appears to exert its effect indirectly through the vagus nerve, exercise may lead to recurrence of SVT in patients treated with this drug. Class IC and class III agents have shown some success in preventing recurrence of SVT but in general are less desirable because of their high incidence of side effects.

Asymptomatic SVT in young, healthy patients generally does not require treatment. Infrequent symptomatic episodes may be treated with the nonpharmacologic techniques described above as well as by preventive pharmacotherapy. Some patients may be able to administer self-treatment at the onset of SVT, using either the Valsalva maneuver or a single dose of medication (oral propranolol or verapamil or sublingual verapamil).

Nonpharmacologic therapeutic interventions aimed at eliminating the reentrant pathway have developed rapidly in recent years. RFA has been widely and successfully employed and may be the most cost-effective approach to therapy for patients with breakthrough SVT while on medication.[36]

AV Reciprocating Tachycardias

Atrioventricular reciprocating tachycardias (AVRTs), also known as "preexcitation" syndromes or accessory pathway arrhythmias, are characterized by a regular, rapid rhythm, usually between 140 and

220 bpm. They are caused by an anatomically distinct accessory pathway that conducts in retrograde fashion from ventricle to atrium, establishing a reentry circuit between the AV node and the pathway that causes paroxysmal bursts of supraventricular tachycardia. The reentry can be either orthodromic (antegrade transmission to the ventricles through the normal pathway for a normal QRS complex during tachycardia, retrograde transmission to the atria through the accessory pathway) or antidromic (antegrade transmission to the ventricles through the accessory pathway, which may alter the QRS). It is technically more correct to say that preexcitation syndromes cause AVRTs, as tachycardia is the intermittently occurring consequence of the presence of the pathway. The two best known examples of AVRT are the Wolff-Parkinson-White (WPW) and Lown-Ganong-Levine (LGL) syndromes.

This condition is often seen in young adults with otherwise normal hearts, but it is also associated with hypertrophic cardiomyopathy, several congenital cardiac anomalies, and possibly mitral valve prolapse. Patients have the same range of symptoms as seen with other types of SVT. Unlike most AVNRTs, preexcitation syndromes can be diagnosed between episodes by their ECG appearance. The classic ECG appearance of WPW between episodes of tachycardia is a short PR interval (<0.12 second) and a widened QRS complex with a slurred up-sloping initial component called the delta wave (Fig. 3.1e). With orthodromic conduction, episodes of tachycardia will have an ECG appearance indistinguishable from other types of SVT; however, delta waves can be seen during tachycardia in antidromic conduction, and if large can cause a widened QRS complex easily mistaken for ventricular tachycardia. LGL syndrome is less unique in its ECG appearance, consisting of a short PR interval (<0.12 second) and a normal QRS, leading some experts to question whether it simply represents a short but otherwise normal atrial conduction process in patients with AVNRT from other causes.

Treatment follows the same general principles as for SVT. Digoxin should be used with caution, as it may cause emergence of other arrhythmias, and verapamil may cause heart rate acceleration rather than conversion in those with WPW syndrome. Surgical ablation of the accessory pathway has largely given way to RFA as the curative therapy of choice.[10,13]

Atrial Fibrillation

Atrial fibrillation (AF) is the most common sustained supraventricular arrhythmia and is primarily a disease of elderly patients, by one estimate currently affecting over 2.3 million U.S. adults, including

4% of adults over 60 years of age and 9% of those over 80.[49] It represents a major cause of morbidity and mortality in the United States, particularly due to its association with embolic stroke. A tremendous research effort has been targeted to determine its mechanism and optimal management. It now appears that AF represents a chaotic form of intraatrial reentry involving multiple circuits generating 350 to 700 wavelets per minute with variable conduction through the atrium and the rest of the conduction system. In some patients, an ectopic focus in or near the pulmonary veins has been identified as the source of the reentrant activity.[50] Over time, these reentrant circuits alter the electrical milieu to promote maintenance of the arrhythmia in a process called electrical remodeling, leading to the new aphorism that "AF begets AF."[51] Although a few cases may occur in elderly patients with otherwise normal hearts ("lone AF"), it is most commonly seen in patients with increased atrial mass, valvular heart disease, and other types of chronic cardiac or pulmonary disease. In patients with underlying cardiac or pulmonary disease, any of the general causes of arrhythmias listed in Table 3.1 can precipitate AF.

Atrial fibrillation can present as either a sustained or intermittent arrhythmia. Symptoms may or may not be present and range from palpitations to dizziness to exacerbation of associated chronic conditions; in the elderly, syncope and falls may occur as a consequence of poor perfusion. Cardiac auscultation reveals an irregularly irregular rhythm, a first heart sound of variable intensity, often a variable pulse, and other clinical findings consistent with underlying disease(s). The ECG (Fig. 3.2a,b) is characterized by an irregular, wavy baseline representing chaotic atrial depolarization, the absence of P waves, and irregularly appearing QRS complexes. A ventricular rate of more than 100 bpm is labeled a "rapid" ventricular response, between 60 and 100 bpm a "moderate" response, and less than 60 bpm a "slow" response. Slow ventricular rates suggest AV nodal disease, hypothyroidism, or the presence of drugs that increase AV node refractory time (digoxin, beta-blockers, calcium channel blockers, and possibly class I antiarrhythmics).

A detailed discussion of the management of atrial fibrillation is beyond the scope of this chapter, but important management principles for common clinical situations can be described. If AF precipitates acute CHF, hypotension, syncope, cerebral hypoperfusion, or angina at rest, or if patients are otherwise hemodynamically unstable, urgent treatment (usually in the hospital or emergency department setting) is required. This situation is most likely to occur with AF with a rapid ventricular response. Because a significant proportion of unstable AF patients may have had an acute MI, clinicians

Figure 2a: Atrial fibrillation with slow ventricular response

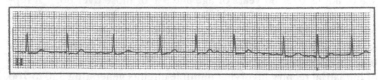

Figure 2b: Atrial fibrillation with rapid ventricular response

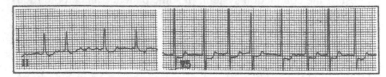

Figure 2c: Atrial flutter

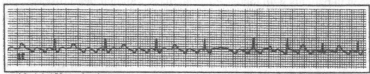

with 4:1 AV conduction

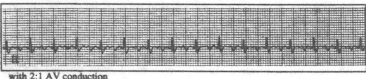

with 2:1 AV conduction

Fig. 3.2. Atrial fibrillation and flutter. Sample ECG tracings for atrial fibrillation with slow and rapid ventricular response and atrial flutter. ECG leads from which tracings were obtained are listed in the lower left corner.

should carefully consider this possibility when evaluating the patient. Cardioversion can be attempted in the emergency or inpatient setting for unstable patients, but caution is needed to minimize the risk of embolism at the time of conversion. When time allows, drug therapy can be initiated with digoxin, beta-blockers, verapamil, or diltiazem to help control the ventricular rate and increase the likelihood of successful cardioversion.

In the clinically stable patient with newly diagnosed AF, the duration of the episode and the presence of underlying cardiac disease are the main factors determining treatment. In patients with good cardiac function, spontaneous conversion to sinus rhythm (SR) within 24 hours of onset is common.[52] In patients with known duration of AF less than 48 hours and no significant cardiac disease, active treatment is also likely to result in conversion to SR; after acute anticoagulation, either DC cardioversion or medication (IV ibutilide or oral propafenone, flecainide, or quinidine) has shown good success in terminating AF.[50] For patients with over 48 hours or unknown duration of AF or with underlying cardiac disease, TEE can be used to guide therapy. If TEE shows no evidence of atrial thrombus or stasis, heparinization and DC cardioversion followed by 4 weeks of anticoagulation with warfarin has been shown to be safe and effective in restoring SR in the short term.[8] If thrombus or stasis is present on TEE, 3 weeks of therapeutic anticoagulation with warfarin, followed by DC cardioversion and at least 4 more weeks of anticoagulation, is the current recommendation.

The long-term success of cardioversion depends primarily on the patient's age, duration of AF, underlying disease, and left atrial diameter, but in most patients AF recurs after cardioversion.[50,53] Despite the theoretical appeal of maintenance drug therapy to prevent recurrence, its role is controversial. Clinical trials have shown both improved success in maintaining SR and excess mortality from proarrhythmic side effects.[17,54,55] Amiodarone appears to offer the best combination of effectiveness and safety in this role, although 12-month recurrence rates are still high.[55] Some experts recommend DC cardioversion alone for a first AF episode, with cardioversion followed by amiodarone for a first relapse.[56] For patients with an ectopic focus near the pulmonary veins, RFA to eliminate the focus offers a potential cure for AF, but preliminary reports have yielded inconsistent results.[56,57] RFA of the AV node followed by permanent pacemaker insertion may be necessary in symptomatic patients refractory to other treatment.

Paroxysmal AF can be considered a special case of symptomatic recurrent AF, and results of clinical trials of drug therapy mirror those for maintenance drug therapy. Several sdrugs, including propafenone, flecainide, and sotalol, increase the length of time between paroxysms but do not abolish them, and may predispose to proarrhythmia.[19,50]

In general, management of persistent or recurrent AF should not focus on restoring and maintaining sinus rhythm but on maximizing ventricular function and reducing the risk of stroke, which approaches 6% per year in AF patients.[58] Three types of antiarrhythmic drug can be used to block AV node conduction, slow a rapid ventricular rate, and improve ventricular function: digoxin, beta-blockers, and calcium channel blockers. Digoxin has been used extensively in elderly patients because of its effectiveness in enhancing left ventricular contractility, but it may be less effective in controlling the rate than either of the other two medications. Digoxin and atenolol have been used in combination with some success.[56] Unfortunately, beta-blockers and calcium channel blockers (particularly verapamil) may precipitate or worsen CHF.

Reducing the risk of stroke is the major goal of treatment of AF. The results of several clinical trials of stroke prevention in AF support the use of warfarin in most clinical circumstances.[59-63] Pooled analysis of clinical trial data highlights several risk factors for stroke: mitral stenosis, hypertension (treated or untreated), previous transient ischemic attack or stroke, CHF, left ventricular dysfunction, and age over 75 years.[63-65] Unless contraindicated, warfarin is recommended for all patients with one or more risk factors, with either warfarin or aspirin recommended for those between 65 and 75 years of age with no risk factors. Aspirin is recommended for those under 65 with no additional risk factors, but there is little data on the effectiveness of aspirin in this group. Aspirin is indicated for those unable to use warfarin, although its effectiveness is unknown. The risk of hemorrhagic complications from warfarin can be minimized by dosing adjustment to maintain an international normalized ratio (INR) between 2.0 and 3.0.[65]

Atrial Flutter

Atrial flutter is virtually always caused by a reentry circuit in the right atrium, which creates a wavefront of depolarization most often moving in a counterclockwise direction across the atria ("typical," "common," or "counterclockwise" atrial flutter), but occasionally traveling clockwise ("atypical," "uncommon," "rare," or "clockwise" flutter). It is associated with underlying cardiac disease such as myocarditis, myocardial infarction, coronary artery disease, or acute ischemia. The underlying atrial rate is approximately 300 bpm (250–350 bpm, although it can be higher), with the ventricular rate dependent on the degree of AV block present. If an AV bypass tract is present, 1:1 conduction occurs for a ventricular rate of about 300 bpm, and conduction through a healthy AV node results in a 2:1 block and ventricular rate of about 150 bpm. A higher degree of block (3:1 or 4:1) may occur with a diseased or fibrotic AV node, resulting in a ventricular rate of 70 to 100 bpm.

Patients may be asymptomatic, or symptoms may resemble those seen with SVT or atrial fibrillation. Physical examination most often reveals a rapid heart rate, and hypotension or CHF may be seen if ventricular filling is low due to the rapid rate. Pulses may be variable and irregular if variable AV block is present. On ECG (Fig. 3.2c), the atrial rate is regular, usually between 250 and 350 bpm, and has a wave-like or sawtooth pattern ("flutter waves") seen best in leads II, III, and aVF. If 1:1 conduction occurs, these waves are hidden by QRS complexes; they may still be difficult to appreciate with a 2:1 block but can be seen more easily with a 3:1 or greater block. If atrial flutter is suspected in the setting of rapid ventricular rates, vagal maneuvers such as carotid sinus massage or an intravenous bolus of adenosine may increase the AV block and reveal the sawtooth pattern.

Atrial flutter is considered an unstable rhythm, and its termination is indicated whenever possible. If the ventricular rate is rapid, the patient is hemodynamically unstable, or underlying disease such as angina or CHF is exacerbated, immediate DC cardioversion under controlled circumstances is indicated. In patients with severe underlying cardiac disease or on potentially arrhythmogenic medications such as digoxin, rapid atrial pacing in a cardiac laboratory setting may be a safer alternative for conversion to sinus rhythm. For more stable patients, reversible underlying conditions or precipitating factors can be corrected before conversion is attempted. Cardioversion is successful in restoring sinus rhythm in more than 95% of cases.[14] Although DC cardioversion and atrial pacing have been considered the preferred treatments, medical cardioversion with ibutilide is emerging as an acceptable alternative.[66] Class IA, IC, or III antiarrhythmics can be effective as pretreatment before DC cardioversion or atrial pacing to increase the likelihood of sustaining sinus rhythm. Beta-blockers, calcium channel blockers, or digoxin may slow a rapid ventricular rate but are not considered effective for conversion to sinus rhythm.

Drug therapy has been shown to be of limited effectiveness in preventing recurrent atrial flutter.[14] In the absence of underlying heart disease, class IC agents flecainide and propafenone may be effective in reducing the number of recurrences, but class IA and IC agents have been associated with serious side effects in patients with underlying heart disease. With improved atrial mapping techniques, RFA of the reentrant circuit has emerged as an effective and potentially curative treatment option; in patients with highly symptomatic atrial flutter unresponsive to other treatments, RFA of the AV junction followed by permanent pacemaker insertion should be considered.[14] The association between stroke and atrial flutter is unclear at present, with conflicting reports regarding risk of stroke after conversion to SR and with drug therapy. Current opinion supports the use of warfarin for cardioversion, but no standard has emerged for long-term anticoagulation.

Other AV Conduction Abnormalities

Conduction disturbances in the AV node–His–Purkinje pathway are a relatively common occurrence, ranging from asymptomatic first-degree AV block to potentially lethal third-degree AV block. A full description of the pathophysiology and electrophysiology of AV block is beyond the scope of this chapter, so a summary of the most common types follows.

First-degree block (Fig. 3.3a) is commonly caused by increased vagal tone or as a drug side effect (digoxin). It is characterized by a prolonged PR interval of more than 0.2 second with an otherwise normal ECG. Unless it is accompanied by significant bradycardia, treatment is not necessary.

There are two varieties of second-degree AV block. Mobitz type I (Wenckebach block) (Fig. 3.3b) is often transient, occurring after cardiac surgery, during an acute MI, or with digoxin toxicity. It is characterized by a constant PP interval, progressive prolongation of the PR interval, and shortening of the RR interval followed by complete block of an atrial impulse and a dropped beat. This rhythm may be perceived on cardiac auscultation as grouped beats followed by a missed beat in a regular pattern. Treatment is generally not necessary. If significant bradycardia and hypoperfusion occur, a cardiac pacemaker may be needed. Mobitz type II block (Fig. 3.3c) is associated with damage to the His–Purkinje system, often due to organic heart disease. Its ECG appearance is as a dropped beat after a normal P wave with otherwise constant PR intervals. It is often associated with intraventricular conduction delays and a slightly wide or atypical QRS complex. This pattern is usually not transient, as it is associated with damage to the conduction system, and is likely to progress to complete heart block. Treatment with a cardiac pacemaker is usually indicated.[67]

Third-degree AV block (complete heart block) (Fig. 3.3d) indicates complete absence of AV conduction. It is usually caused by serious organic heart disease. P waves are present but not conducted, and QRS complexes are usually atypical and widened, reflecting their junctional or ventricular origin. The ventricular rate is most often the idioventricular "escape" frequency of 30 to 40 bpm, but faster heart rates or episodes of asystole can occur. Treatment with a cardiac pacemaker is necessary.

Ventricular Arrhythmias

Most ventricular arrhythmias (VAs) arise from a reentry mechanism involving ventricular myocardium or the portion of the cardiac con-

Figure 3a: First-degree atrioventricular block

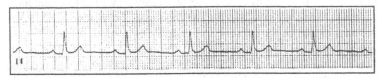

Figure 3b: Second-degree atrioventricular block, Mobitz type I ("Wenckebach" block)

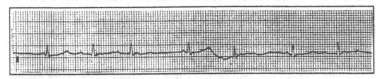

Figure 3c: Second-degree atrioventricular block, Mobitz type II

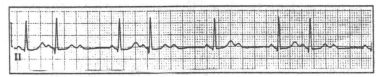

Figure 3d: Third-degree atrioventricular block

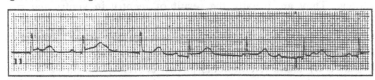

Fig. 3.3. Selected atrioventricular (AV) conduction abnormalities: sample ECG tracings. ECG leads from which tracings were obtained are listed in the lower left corner. Note the progressive prolongation of the PR interval prior to the missed beat in Mobitz type I block (b), the fixed PR interval prior to the missed beat in Mobitz type II block (c), and complete dissociation of atrial and ventricular depolarization in third-degree block (d). See text for discussion of specific ECG features of each arrhythmia.

duction pathway located below the AV node.[68] Predisposing factors include ischemic or valvular heart disease, structural congenital anomalies, cardiomyopathy, CHF, genetic mutations in ion channel proteins (the cause of congenital long QT syndrome), and autonomic hypersensitivity. Their clinical importance lies in their association with SCD, which accounts for over 350,000 deaths in the U.S. annually.[69] In patients without underlying cardiac disease, the risk of

SCD is low and treatment necessary only in special circumstances ["complex" VA such as ventricular tachycardia (VT) or frequent multifocal ventricular premature beats]. However, the risk of SCD in VA is much higher in the presence of underlying cardiac disease, particularly CHF, cardiomyopathy, or in the post-MI setting. The emergence of the ICD as an effective preventive intervention has reduced drug therapy to a secondary and supportive role in treatment of VA. Because most VAs occur outside of the hospital setting, major efforts are now being made to integrate AEDs into out-of-hospital resuscitation protocols.

In general, in the routine office setting family physicians should diagnose this arrhythmia based on ECG, Holter monitoring, or cardiac event monitoring, and search for evidence of underlying cardiac disease or reversible precipitating factors before deciding on therapy. Drug therapy should be initiated with caution and only when clearly indicated.

Ventricular Premature Beats

Ventricular premature beats (VPBs) are the single most common cardiac arrhythmia and perhaps the most overtreated of all cardiac conditions. They are usually the result of reentry in ventricular myocardium or the terminal portion of the Purkinje system; one to several reentry circuits can be present in an individual. They commonly occur in the absence of underlying heart disease and are precipitated by anxiety, emotional stress, exercise, caffeine and other sympathomimetics, electrolyte or acid–base abnormalities, alcohol, and many medications. They also occur in patients with underlying heart disease and in the setting of acute ischemia or MI, acute infection, CHF, chronic ischemia, cardiomyopathy, and some forms of valvular or structural heart disease, including mitral valve prolapse.

The VPBs are most often asymptomatic and are found on routine auscultation or an ECG obtained for other reasons. Patients with frequent VPBs may report palpitations, dizziness, or weakness. On physical examination, VPBs are noted as an early beat with a following compensatory pause. The ECG (Fig. 3.4a) shows baseline sinus rhythm with the VPB seen as an early QRS, which is wide (>0.12 second), notched, and slurred, and not preceded by a P wave. The T wave is often opposite in direction from the QRS due to aberrant repolarization. A P wave following the QRS or embedded in the T wave may be seen, the result of retrograde conduction. The SA node is generally not depolarized by the VPB, creating a "compensatory pause" following the early beat; one sinus beat is suppressed due to a refractory myocardium and conduction system, but the regular SA

Figure 4a: Ventricular premature beats (premature ventricular complexes)

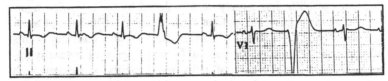

Figure 4b: Nonsustained ventricular tachycardia

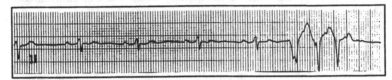

Figure 4c: Sustained ventricular tachycardia

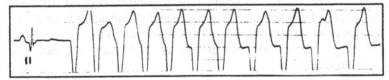

Figure 4d: Ventricular fibrillation

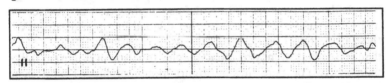

Figure 4e: Torsades de pointes (at initiation)

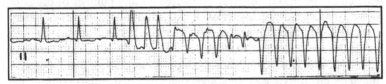

Fig. 3.4. Selected ventricular arrhythmias: sample ECG tracings. ECG leads from which tracings were obtained are listed in the lower left corner. See text for discussion of specific ECG features of each arrhythmia

node pacing is maintained. VPBs can be unifocal or multifocal (the result of more than one reentrant focus), and can occur in patterns such as trigeminy (once every three beats), bigeminy, or couplets (two in a row).

The Lown classification, formerly used to grade the risk of various types of VPB, has largely been replaced by the following treatment "rules." In patients without heart disease, VPBs are not associated with an increased risk of sudden death or other coronary events and generally should not be treated. In the presence of severe symptoms, a careful discussion of risks and benefits of therapy with patients should take place prior to initiating drug therapy. Beta-blockers are the first choice for therapy under most circumstances. The use of class I agents in patients with VPBs has been repeatedly shown to increase the risk of sudden death or coronary events, and these agents should be avoided.[18,19,22] In the post-MI setting, treatment with beta-blockers and angiotensin-converting enzyme inhibitors (ACEIs), preferably in combination, has been shown to have a beneficial effect regarding mortality.[70] Low-dose amiodarone may be helpful in patients who cannot use beta-blockers or ACEIs. Calcium channel blockers are not effective and should not be used. Some experts now recommend that post-MI patients with VPBs undergo EP study so that patients at high risk for SCD (those with inducible VT) can receive an ICD.[71]

Ventricular Tachycardia

Ventricular tachycardia (VT) is defined as the presence of three or more consecutive VPBs; it is further divided into nonsustained VT (NSVT), lasting less than 30 seconds, and sustained, lasting more than 30 seconds. It may be monomorphic (one site of origin) or polymorphic (two or more sites of origin). Monomorphic VT may occur in healthy individuals during exercise, with vagal stimulation, or with excitement or fright, and may be caused by any number of drugs or other substances, notably class I antiarrhythmics, tricyclic antidepressants, and phenothiazines. Polymorphic VT (torsades de pointes being the most familiar example) is associated with congenital long QT syndrome and organophosphate poisoning, and it can be precipitated by electrolyte abnormalities, digoxin, most antiarrhythmic and tricyclic medications, and medication combinations such astemizole and itraconazole. Either type of VT is commonly seen in the setting of acute MI and other serious heart disease.

Nonsustained VT is often asymptomatic but may produce palpitations, weakness, and presyncope; sustained VT is rarely asymptomatic and presents with symptoms ranging from palpitations to sudden death. On auscultation the heart rate may be slightly irregular, with the pulse ranging from 100 to 300 bpm. Other clinical findings vary, as cardiac perfusion changes from beat to beat. With monomorphic VT, the ECG shows a single QRS morphology with the QRS duration more than 0.12 second and the T wave polarity opposite to the QRS polarity. Atrial activity is usually not discernible. Polymorphic VT (Fig. 3.4b) shows several QRS morphologies. Torsades de pointes (Fig. 3.4e) is characterized by alternation of QRS polarity or amplitude (or both) in repeated cycles of 5 to 20 beats.

Most experts do not recommend treatment for NSVT in the absence of underlying heart disease, as there appears to be no increased risk of SCD. If underlying heart disease is present, a careful search to identify those at high risk for SCD is indicated. Various tests have been studied alone or in combination, including echocardiography, Holter monitoring, enhanced ECG-based methods (QT interval dispersion, T-wave alternans, heart rate variability, and signal-averaged ECG), baroreflex sensitivity, and inducibility of VT on EP study, but no standard protocol has yet emerged. Many experts now recommend that patients with underlying heart disease and NSVT undergo an EP study, with the presence of inducible VT identifying high-risk patients who will benefit from ICD placement.[71] The major role for drug therapy is in treatment of underlying cardiac disease: beta-blockers and ACE inhibitors reduce mortality post-MI and in CHF, but it is not clear whether they reduce the rate of SCD. Although amiodarone has been shown to reduce mortality in patients at high risk for SCD,[72] clinical trials directly comparing ICD placement to amiodarone have confirmed the superior effectiveness of ICDs.[73,74] EP studies paired with RFA offer potentially curative therapy for reentrant NSVT and are currently under study.

Sustained VT (Fig. 3.4c) requires emergent treatment guided by current advanced cardiac life support (ACLS) protocols, followed by transfer to an appropriate facility for definitive care.

Ventricular Fibrillation

Ventricular fibrillation (VF) is a state of chaotic ventricular activity caused by the random firing of multiple ectopic foci, probably due to a complex reentry mechanism.[75] It may result from degeneration of VT and most often occurs in the setting of an acute MI. The arrhythmia results in random, ineffective activity in the ventricles, preventing effective blood circulation. Death occurs within minutes if effective resuscitation is not initiated. The ECG (Fig. 3.4d) shows erratic oscillations without any recognizable complexes; an amplitude of more than 1 mm is termed "coarse" VF and is considered to be more amenable to defibrillation than "fine" VF.

Treatment should begin immediately with cardiopulmonary resuscitation efforts as outlined in Basic Life Support (BLS) and ACLS protocols, including the use of AEDs as soon as possible.[44] Transfer to the hospital for definitive care should occur as soon as possible. Patients who survive VF are candidates for ICD placement.

Conclusion

Although diagnostic and treatment options for patients with cardiac arrhythmias are growing rapidly, successful management still rests on a careful and thorough clinical approach to this problem. Family physicians should be able to (1) correctly diagnose common specific arrhythmias, (2) search for and treat underlying or predisposing conditions, (3) determine whether specific treatment is indicated and initiate therapy where possible, and (4) effectively work with consultants when specialized diagnostic or therapeutic approaches are required.

References

1. Priori SG, Barhanin J, Hauer RN, et al. Genetic and molecular basis of cardiac arrhythmias: impact on clinical management parts I and II. Circulation 1999;99:518–28.
2. Bennett PB, Yazawa K, Makita N, George AL Jr. Molecular mechanism for an inherited cardiac arrhythmia. Nature 1995;376:683–5.
3. Splawski I, Timothy KW, Vincent GM, Atkinson DL, Keating MT. Molecular basis of the long-QT syndrome associated with deafness. N Engl J Med 1997;336:1562–7.
4. Zimetbaum PJ, Josephson ME. The evolving role of ambulatory arrhythmia monitoring in general clinical practice. Ann Intern Med 1999;130:848–56.
5. Graboys T. Appropriate indications for ambulatory electrocardiographic monitoring. Cardiol Clin 1992;10:551–4.
6. Weitz HH, Weinstock PJ. Approach to the patient with palpitations. Med Clin North Am 1995;79:449–56.
7. Thamilarasan M, Klein AL. Transesophageal echocardiography (TEE) in atrial fibrillation. Cardiol Clin 2000;18:819–31.
8. Klein AL, Grimm RA, Murray RD, et al. Use of transesophageal echocardiography to guide cardioversion in patients with atrial fibrillation. N Engl J Med 2001;344:1411–20.
9. Grimm RA. Transesophageal echocardiography-guided cardioversion of atrial fibrillation. Echocardiography 2000;17:383–92.
10. Morady F. Radio-frequency ablation as treatment for cardiac arrhythmias. N Engl J Med 1999;340:534–44.
11. Jais P, Shah DC, Haissaguerre M, Hocini M, Peng JT, Clementy J. Catheter ablation for atrial fibrillation. Annu Rev Med 2000;51:431–41.
12. Grubb NR, Furniss S. Science, medicine, and the future: radio-frequency ablation for atrial fibrillation. BMJ 2001;322:777–80.

13. Chauhan VS, Krahn AD, Klein GJ, Skanes AC, Yee R. Supraventricular tachycardia. Med Clin North Am 2001;85:193–223.
14. Waldo AL, Mackall JA, Biblo LA. Mechanisms and medical management of patients with atrial flutter. Cardiol Clin 1997;15:661–76.
15. Vaughan—Williams EM. A classification of antiarrhythmic actions reassessed after a decade of new drugs. J Clin Pharmacol 1984;24:129–47.
16. Morganroth J, Goin JE. Quinidine-related mortality in the short-to-medium-term treatment of ventricular arrhythmias. A meta-analysis. Circulation 1991;84:1977–83.
17. Echt DS, Liebson PR, Mitchell LB, et al. Mortality and morbidity in patients receiving encainide, flecainide, or placebo. The Cardiac Arrhythmia Suppression Trial. N Engl J Med 1991;324:781–8.
18. Epstein AE, Bigger JT Jr, Wyse DG, Romhilt DW, Reynolds-Haertle RA, Hallstrom AP. Events in the Cardiac Arrhythmia Suppression Trial (CAST): mortality in the entire population enrolled. J Am Coll Cardiol 1991;18:14–9.
19. Chaudhry GM, Haffajee CI. Antiarrhythmic agents and proarrhythmia. Crit Care Med 2000;28:N158–64.
20. Boriani G, Biffi M, Capucci A, et al. Oral propafenone to convert recent-onset atrial fibrillation in patients with and without underlying heart disease. A randomized, controlled trial. Ann Intern Med 1997;126:621–5.
21. Chimienti M, Cullen MT, Casadei G. Flecainide and Propa-fenone Italian Study Group. Safety of long-term flecainide and propafenone in the management of symptomatic paroxysmal atrial fibrillation. Am J Cardiol 1996;77:66A–71A.
22. Teo KK, Yusuf S, Furberg CD. Effects of prophylactic antiarrhythmic drug therapy in acute myocardial infarction. An over-view of results from randomized controlled trials. JAMA 1993;270:1589–95.
23. Sim I, McDonald KM, Lavori PW, Norbutas CM, Hlatky MA. Quantitative overview of randomized trials of amiodarone to prevent sudden cardiac death. Circulation 1997;96:2823–9.
24. Peuhkurinen K, Niemela M, Ylitalo A, Linnaluoto M, Lilja M, Juvonen J. Effectiveness of amiodarone as a single oral dose for recent-onset atrial fibrillation. Am J Cardiol 2000;85:462–5.
25. Mason JW. A comparison of seven antiarrhythmic drugs in patients with ventricular tachyarrhythmias. Electrophysiologic Study versus Electrocardiographic Monitoring Investigators. N Engl J Med 1993;329:452–8.
26. Miller MR, McNamara RL, Segal JB, et al. Efficacy of agents for pharmacologic conversion of atrial fibrillation and subsequent maintenance of sinus rhythm: a meta-analysis of clinical trials. J Fam Pract 2000;49:1033–46.
27. Falk RH, Pollak A, Singh SN, et al. Intravenous dofetilide: a class III antiarrhythmic agent, for the termination of sustained atrial fibrillation or flutter. J Am Coll Cardiol 1997;340:385–90.
28. Vukmir RB. Cardiac arrhythmia therapy. Am J Emerg Med 1995;13:459–70.
29. Kerin NZ, Somberg J. Proarrhythmia: definition, risk factors, causes, treatment, and controversies. Am Heart J 1994;128:575–85.

30. Naccarelli GV, Wolbrette DL, Luck JC. Proarrhythmia. Med Clin North Am 2001;85:503–26.
31. Faber TS, Zehender M, Just H. Drug-induced torsade de pointes: incidence, management and prevention. Drug Safety 1994;11:463–76.
32. Trohman RG, Parrillo JE. Direct current cardioversion: indications, techniques, and recent advances. Crit Care Med 2000;28:N170–3.
33. Cox JL, Ferguson TB. Cardiac arrhythmia surgery. Curr Probl Surg 1989;26:193–278.
34. Schaff HV, Dearani JA, Daly RC, Orszulak TA, Danielson GK. Cox-Maze procedure for atrial fibrillation: the Mayo Clinic experience. Semin Thorac Cardiovasc Surg 2000;12:30–7.
35. Hogenhuis W, Stevens SK, Wang P, et al. Cost-effectiveness of radio-frequency ablation compared with other strategies in Wolff-Parkinson-White syndrome. Circulation 1993;88(5 pt 2):II:437–46.
36. Kalbfleisch SJ, Calkins H, Langberg JJ, et al. Comparison of the cost of radiofrequency catheter modification of the atrioventricular node and medical therapy for drug-refractory atrioventricular node reentrant tachycardia. J Am Coll Cardiol 1992;19:1583–7.
37. Fitzpatrick AP, Kourouyan HD, Siu A, et al. Quality of life and outcomes after radiofrequency His-bundle catheter ablation and permanent pacemaker implantation: impact of treatment in paroxysmal and established atrial fibrillation. Am Heart J 1996;131:499–507.
38. Gregoratos G, Cheitlin MD, Conill A, et al. ACC/AHA guidelines for implantation of cardiac pacemakers and antiarrhythmia devices: a report of the American College of Cardiology/American Heart Association Task Force on Practice Guidelines (Committee on Pacemaker Implantation). J Am Coll Cardiol 1998;31:1175–209.
39. The Antiarrhythmics versus Implantable Defibrillators (AVID) Investigators. A comparison of antiarrhythmic-drug therapy with implantable defibrillators in patients resuscitated from near-fatal ventricular arrhythmias. N Engl J Med 1997;337:1576–83.
40. Connolly SJ, Gent M, Roberts RS, et al. Canadian implantable defibrillator study (CIDS): a randomized trial of the implantable cardioverter defibrillator against amiodarone. Circulation 2000;101:1297–302.
41. Buxton AE, Lee KL, Fisher JD, Josephson ME, Prystowsky EN, Hafley G. A randomized study of the prevention of sudden death in patients with coronary artery disease. Multicenter Unsustained Tachycardia Trial Investigators. N Engl J Med 1999;341:1882–90.
42. Gollob MH, Seger JJ. Current status of the implantable cardioverter-defibrillator. Chest 2001;119:1210–21.
43. O'Brien BJ, Yee R. Chapter 10: Current evidence on the cost effectiveness of the implantable cardioverter defibrillator. Can J Cardiol 2000;16(suppl C):45C–7C.
44. Atkins DL, Bossaert LL, Hazinski MF, et al. Automated external defibrillation/public access defibrillation. Ann Emerg Med 2001;37:S60–S67.
45. White RD, Hankins DG, Bugliosi TF, et al. Seven years' experience with early defibrillation by police and paramedics in an emergency medical services system. Resuscitation 1998;39:145–51.

46. Stiell IG, Wells GA, Field BJ, et al. Improved out-of-hospital cardiac arrest survival through the inexpensive optimization of an existing defibrillation program: OPALS Study Phase II. JAMA 1999;281:1175–81.
47. Schwartz M, Rodman D, Lowenstein SR. Recognition and treatment of multifocal atrial tachycardia: a critical review. J Emerg Med 1994;12: 353–60.
48. Camm AJ, Garratt AJ. Adenosine and supraventricular tachycardia. N Engl J Med 1991;32:1621–7.
49. Go AS, Hylek EM, Phillips KA, et al. Prevalence of diagnosed atrial fibrillation in adults: national implications for rhythm management and stroke prevention: the Anticoagulation and Risk Factors in Atrial Fibrillation (ATRIA) Study. JAMA 2001;285:2370–5.
50. Falk RH. Atrial fibrillation. N Engl J Med 2001;344:1067–78.
51. Nattel S, Li D, Yue L. Basic mechanisms of atrial fibrillation—very new insights into very old ideas. Annu Rev Physiol 2000;62:51–77.
52. Danias PG, Caulfield TA, Weigner MJ, Silverman DI, Manning WJ. Likelihood of spontaneous conversion of atrial fibrillation to sinus rhythm. J Am Coll Cardiol 1998;31:588–92.
53. Carlsson J, Neuzner J, Rosenberg YD. Therapy of atrial fibrillation: rhythm control versus rate control. Pacing Clin Electrophysiol 2000;23:891–903.
54. Dries DL, Exner DV, Gersh BJ, Domanski MJ, Waclawiw MA, Stevenson LW. Atrial fibrillation is associated with an increased risk for mortality and heart failure progression in patients with asymptomatic and symptomatic left ventricular systolic dysfunction: a retrospective analysis of the SOLVD trials. J Am Coll Cardiol 1998;32:695–703.
55. Roy D, Talajic M, Dorian P, et al. Amiodarone to prevent recurrence of atrial fibrillation: Canadian Trial of Atrial Fibrillation Investigators. N Engl J Med 2000;342:913–20.
56. Carlson MD. How to manage atrial fibrillation: an update on recent clinical trials. Cardiol Rev 2001;9:60–9.
57. Haissaguerre M, Jais P, Shah DC, et al. Electrophysiological end point for catheter ablation of atrial fibrillation initiated from multiple pulmonary venous foci. Circulation 2000;101:1409–17.
58. Wolf PA, Abbott R, Savage D. Atrial fibrillation as an independent risk factor for stroke: the Framingham Study. Stroke 1991;22:983–8.
59. Petersen P, Boysen G, Godtfredson J, Andersen E, Andersen B. Placebo-controlled, randomized trial of warfarin and aspirin for prevention of thromboembolic complications in chronic atrial fibrillation: the Copenhagen AFASAK study. Lancet 1989;1:175–9.
60. Connolly SJ, Laupacis A, Gent M, Roberts RS, Cairns JA, Joyner C. Canadian Atrial Fibrillation Anticoagulation (CAFA) study. J Am Coll Cardiol 1991;18:349–55.
61. Ezekowitz MD, Bridges SL, James KE, et al. Warfarin in the prevention of stroke associated with nonrheumatic atrial fibrillation. Veterans Affairs Stroke Prevention in Nonrheumatic Atrial Fibrillation Investigators. N Engl J Med 1992;327:1406–12.
62. Boston Area Anticoagualation Trial for Atrial Fibrillation Investigators. The effect of low-dose warfarin on the risk of stroke in patients with nonrheumatic atrial fibrillation. N Engl J Med 1990;323:1505–11.

63. Blackshear JL, Baker VS, Rubino F, et al. Adjusted-dose warfarin versus low-intensity, fixed-dose warfarin plus aspirin for high-risk patients with atrial fibrillation: Stroke Prevention in Atrial Fibrillation III randomized clinical trial. Lancet 1996;348:633–8.
64. Atrial Fibrillation Investigators. Risk factors for stroke and efficacy of antithrombotic therapy in atrial fibrillation: analysis of pooled data from five randomized controlled trials. Arch Intern Med 1994;154:1449–57.
65. Segal JB, McNamara RL, Miller MR, et al. Anticoagulants or antiplatelet therapy for non-rheumatic atrial fibrillation and flutter (Cochrane Review). In: The Cochrane Library, issue 1. Oxford: Update Software, 2001.
66. Stambler BS, Wood MA, Ellenbogen KA, Perry KT, Wakefield LK, VanderLugt JT. Efficacy and safety of repeated intravenous doses of ibutilide for rapid conversion of atrial flutter or fibrillation. Ibutilide Repeat Dose Study Investigators. Circulation 1996;94:1613–21.
67. Barold SS, Hayes DL. Second-degree atrioventricular block: a reappraisal. Mayo Clin Proc 2001;76:44–57.
68. Alpert MA, Mukerji V, Bikkina M, Concannon MD, Hashimi MW. Pathogenesis, recognition, and management of common cardiac arrhythmias. Part I: ventricular premature beats and tachyarrhythmias. South Med J 1995;88:1–21.
69. Myerburg RJ, Kessler KM, Castellanos A. Sudden cardiac death. Structure, function, and time-dependence of risk. Circulation 1992;85:I2–10.
70. Burkart F, Pfisterer M, Kiowski W, Follath F, Burckhardt D. Effect of antiarrhythmic therapy on mortality in survivors of myocardial infarction with asymptomatic complex ventricular arrhythmias: Basel Antiarrhythmic Study of Infarct Survival (BASIS). J Am Coll Cardiol 1990;16:1711–8.
71. Windhagen-Mahnert B, Kadish AH. Application of noninvasive and invasive tests for risk assessment in patients with ventricular arrhythmias. Cardiol Clin 2000;18:243–63.
72. Investigators of Amiodarone Trial Meta-Analyses. Effect of prophylactic amiodarone on mortality after acute myocardial infarction and in congestive heart failure: meta-analysis of individual data from 6500 patients from randomized trials. Lancet 1997;350:1417–24.
73. Moss AJ, Hall WJ, Cannon DS, et al. Improved survival with an implanted defibrillator in patients with coronary disease at high risk for ventricular arrhythmia. Multicenter Automatic Defibrillator Implantation Trial Investigators. N Engl J Med 1996;395:1933–40.
74. Zipes DP, Wyse DG, Friedman PL, et al. A comparison of antiarrhythmic drug therapy with implanatable defibrillators in patients resuscitated from near-fatal ventricular arrhythmias. N Engl J Med 1997;337:1576–83.
75. Jalife J. Ventricular fibrillation: mechanisms of initiation and maintenance. Annu Rev Physiol 2000;62:25–50.

4
Valvular Heart Disease

Eric Walsh

Introduction

Timely and appropriate diagnosis and treatment of valvular heart disease is an important skill for family physicians. Excessive consultation and diagnostic testing of patients who present with murmurs creates unnecessary anxiety and cost. Yet the failure to make a timely diagnosis of valvular heart disease, or to refer when appropriate, can lead to irreversible cardiac damage, decreased functional status, and even death. In making the diagnosis of valvular heart disease, it is important to know the clinical maneuvers that can help refine the bedside diagnosis of murmurs. It is useful to know when third and fourth heart sounds (S_3 and S_4) are abnormal, and how to distinguish innocent and physiologic murmurs from murmurs caused by valvular heart disease.

Third Heart Sound

An S_3 is considered normal in patients under 30 who have no other signs of heart disease. An S_3 heard in patients between ages 30 and 40 is suspicious. In this age group, conditions such as thyrotoxicosis, pregnancy, anxiety, and postexercise states can cause an S_3 not associated with heart disease.

An S_3 heard past age 40 should be considered a likely sign of heart disease. It can be caused by three types of cardiac disease: ventricular diastolic overload, ventricular dysfunction, and constrictive pericarditis. Ventricular diastolic overload is most commonly caused by mitral regurgitation or aortic insufficiency. The S_3 heard with these states of ventricular diastolic overload is almost invariably associated with a murmur. An S_3 not associated with a ventricular diastolic overload state suggests global ventricular dysfunction. Diastolic overload over long periods of time can lead to ventricular dysfunction, which is the most serious and irreversible cause of the S_3. Other non-valvular problems, such as chronic ischemia can also lead to global dysfunction and an S_3. Pericardial disease can cause an S_3. In the case of pericardial disease, it is the sudden deceleration of ventricular relaxation and filling caused by the pericardial pathology that creates the S_3.

Fourth Heart Sound

There is debate about whether an S_4 can be considered normal in the geriatric population, where there is some physiologic loss of ventricular compliance; but as a general rule, an audible S_4 should be considered pathologic. In contrast to an S_3, which gets louder as ventricular compliance decreases, the S_4 becomes softer as the underlying ventricular dysfunction progresses. The underlying cardiac pathology leading to the production of an S_4 is similar to the factors causing an S_3, with two important additions: whereas an S_3 is not heard with hypertrophic cardiomyopathy or left ventricular hypertrophy (LVH) caused by hypertension, an S_4 is common with these conditions.

Innocent and Physiologic Murmurs

Between 90% and 95% of murmurs identified by family physicians are innocent or physiologic murmurs. Innocent murmurs are those present in patients with no cardiac pathology. Murmurs are physiologic when there is an identifiable cause but the heart is normal. Examples of physiologic murmurs include the murmurs heard with anemia, thyrotoxicosis, the increased blood volume of normal pregnancy, and the high output state caused by fever.

Characteristics

Murmurs can be appreciated in 50% to 60% of healthy children, depending on the listening conditions and the cooperation of the child.[1] Soft murmurs can be heard in 30% to 40% of healthy adults.[1] Innocent murmurs are usually best heard along the left sternal border, between the second and the fourth intercostal spaces. Innocent murmurs are always systolic and are rarely louder than grade 2/6. In young patients innocent murmurs are evanescent and usually do not radiate to the carotid area. In older patients it can be more difficult to distinguish pathologic from innocent murmurs. The decreased compliance of the large arteries associated with aging can cause an innocent murmur to be heard in the neck. There are several associated findings that make the diagnosis of an innocent or physiologic murmur less likely. These findings include the presence of more than one sound at S_1, abnormal splitting of S_2, a loud or soft S_1, or a hyperdynamic or sustained ventricular impulse.

Physical Maneuvers

There are a number of simple bedside maneuvers useful for diagnosing an innocent versus a pathologic murmur. These maneuvers increase or decrease preload and increase afterload. The presence of extrasystolic beats, which change the hemodynamics, can affect the quality of murmurs in ways that aid the diagnosis.

Increased Afterload

The best method to increase afterload is the handgrip maneuver. The physician instructs the patient to squeeze the examiner's hand as hard as possible, and the physician returns the pressure. The handgrip should decrease outflow murmurs, including innocent murmurs, physiologic murmurs, and patho-logic aortic outflow murmurs.

Decreased Preload

Decreased preload is created by the Valsalva maneuver or by sudden sitting or standing. Both of these mechanisms cause decreased venous return to the heart. Decreased preload diminishes murmurs that are increased by blood volume, including innocent murmurs, physiologic murmurs, outflow murmurs, and mitral and tricuspid regurgitation. The murmurs of mitral valve prolapse and hypertrophic cardiomyopathy should become louder with a decreased preload.

Increased Preload

Two simple maneuvers can increase preload. The first is lifting the patient's legs while the patient is in the supine position. The second is asking the patient to squat. Increased preload should dilate, to some extent, the left ventricle and thereby decrease the murmurs caused by mitral valve prolapse and hypertrophic cardiomyopathy. The effect of increased preload on other murmurs is variable, but most outflow murmurs become louder with this maneuver.

Ectopic Beats

A premature ventricular beat creates a diagnostic opportunity. If the murmur is an aortic stenosis murmur, it becomes louder after an extrasystolic beat because of the increased pressure gradient across the stenotic valve. The prolonged diastole does not affect most flow murmurs or the murmur caused by mitral regurgitation.

Valvular Heart Disease

Incidence

An important clinical issue is the incidence in the general population of heart murmurs caused by heart disease. If a heart murmur is heard, what is the likelihood that it is caused by heart disease? The incidence of valvular heart disease in the general population is difficult to determine. Murmurs and the pathology that causes them can resolve spontaneously. The loud childhood murmur of a ventricular septal defect can disappear when the defect closes spontaneously. Murmurs can disappear as the pathology worsens; for example, a mitral regurgitant murmur can disappear as the left atrial pressure rises and left ventricular failure occurs. Murmurs that are not pathologic can become so later in life. A bicuspid aortic valve can produce a murmur without a significant gradient early in life, but as valvular calcification develops, significant aortic stenosis can appear. Lastly, the incidence of valvular heart disease depends on the methods by which it is sought: the findings on clinical examination, echocardiography, and autopsy differ.

Good raw data regarding the incidence of valvular heart disease in the general (male) population were obtained in World War I, during which time 2.5 million young men from their late teens to about 30 years old were examined by army doctors.[2] A total of 85,143 men (3.4%) were classified on clinical grounds as having valvular heart disease; 73.4% were diagnosed as having mitral regurgitation, and the remaining 26.6% were about evenly distributed between mitral stenosis, aortic stenosis, and aortic regurgitation, with a small number having right-sided valvular heart disease and nonvalvular heart murmurs such as patent ductus arteriosus (PDA) or ventricular septal defect (VSD). Since World War I the incidence of rheumatic heart disease has declined, making mitral stenosis, which is almost solely caused by rheumatic disease, much rarer.

The use of echocardiography and autopsy increases estimates of the frequency of valvular heart disease. A survey of 18,132 autopsies showed that 6.3% of patients at autopsy had valvular heart disease, 49% involving the mitral valve, 42% the aortic valve, 9% the tricuspid valve, and 0.3% the pulmonic valve.[3] A study of patients over 65 years old found that aortic stenosis was present in 2% overall, with a twofold increase in incidence for each 10 years of life.[4] In 1999, the Framingham Heart Study reported a series of 3,589 color Doppler echocardiograms done on participants between 26 and 83 years old in that ongoing study. The study reported on valvular incompetence, but not valve stenosis.

Using this sophisticated technology, the incidence of valvular incompetence was much higher than previously reported: mitral regurgitation was found in 19.1%, and aortic regurgitation in 10.8%. But when "trivial" and "mild" valvular incompetence are excluded from the analysis, the incidence of "moderate" or "severe" valvular incompetence is reported as 1.9% for the mitral valve, and 0.69% for the aortic valve.[5] Interestingly, a decreased body mass index (BMI) was associated with an increased risk for mitral but not aortic incompetence. A report from the Strong Heart Study, which evaluated echocardiographic data from 3,486 Native Americans, found mitral regurgitation in 21.0% of participants, although regurgitation was moderately severe in only 0.3% and severe in only 0.2%.[6] This study also confirmed the association of lower BMI, as well as female gender, older age, and higher blood pressure with mitral regurgitation.[6]

More recently, the use of anorectic drugs for weight loss, specifically dexfenfluramine, has been associated with an increased risk of the development of valvular regurgitation, most commonly mitral, but also tricuspid and aortic regurgitation (odds ratio 3.1; 95% confidence interval 1.34–7.13).[7] There is reassuring evidence that clinical auscultation is an adequate method of screening for valvular lesions associated with dexfenfluramine, and that discontinuing the drug probably halts progression of the valvular lesions.[7,8]

Mitral Valve Regurgitation

Etiology

There are a large number of causes of mitral regurgitation. Degenerative lesions include the myxomatous change of mitral valve prolapse and the congenital abnormalities of Marfan syndrome, Ehlers-Danlos syndrome, and others. Degenerative changes also include mitral annulus calcification. Inflammatory and infective causes of mitral regurgitation include endocarditis, rheumatic fever, lupus, and scleroderma (see Chapter 11). Ischemia is one of the most important causes of mitral regurgitation. Mitral regurgitation in the setting of ischemia is due to dysfunction of the papillary muscles and/or re-modeling of the ventricle. There is a statistically significant association of mitral regurgitation with increasing age, hypertension, and a lower BMI.[5]

Symptoms

Mitral regurgitation may progress for decades without causing symptoms. Symptoms usually occur insidiously. The first symptom is usually fatigue because of decreased cardiac output. Later dyspnea, orthopnea, and paroxysmal nocturnal dyspnea occur as the left atrial pressure and pulmonary vascular pressure rise. The causes of rapid progression of symptoms with mitral regurgitation include the onset of atrial fibrillation and severe papillary muscle dysfunction or rupture.

Physical Findings

The pulse associated with mitral regurgitation is collapsing in nature. The apical impulse is hyperkinetic and becomes laterally displaced and more diffuse as the disease progresses. The heart sounds are unremarkable. It is unusual to hear an S_4, and the presence of an S_3 indicates advanced disease. The murmur of mitral regurgitation is a holosystolic murmur. It is described as plateau in intensity and blowing in quality. Throughout most of the natural history of mitral regurgitation, the murmur starts at S_1 and ends at S_2. As left atrial pressure and pulmonary pressure rise, the murmur may end before S_2. The murmur of mitral regurgitation becomes softer during the late stages of the disease.

Increasing afterload should increase the intensity of the murmur. Decreasing preload should make the murmur softer, and increasing preload usually makes little or no difference in the murmur. When there is a premature beat and a compensatory pause, the murmur of mitral regurgitation does not change appreciably in the postextrasystolic beat.

Natural History, Complications, Medical Therapy, and Timing of Surgery

As Stapleton[2] suggested, "mitral incompetence is the most benign of left heart valvular lesions. . . . Patients may do well on medical therapy for years after the onset of symptoms." Medical therapy consists of afterload reduction with angiotensin-converting enzyme (ACE) inhibiting agents. As left ventricular function declines, digoxin and diuretics may be added. Atrial fibrillation is a late occurrence and requires rate control. Atrial fibrillation usually denotes marked atrial enlargement, and electrical cardioversion is rarely successful on a long-term basis. The timing of surgery is more controversial for mitral regurgitation than for other valvular heart disease because of the relatively slow course of progression in most cases. Clear indications for valve replacement include left ventricular (LV) failure caused by mitral regurgitation, hemodynamic decompensation with decreased cardiac output (even with normal ejection fraction) at rest or with exercise, and rapid (more than 2 cm per year as measured by echocardiography or chest radiography) increase in ventricular size.[9] More recently, criteria for early replacement of the mitral valve in patients selected as high risk based on low LV ejection fraction (>45%) or low right ventricular (RV) ejection fraction (>30%) have been proposed.[10] Mitral regurgitation that is secondary to ischemia carries a worse prognosis, and mitral valve replacement should be considered earlier than in nonischemic mitral regurgitation. Decisions about valve replacement at the time of coronary artery bypass graft (CABG) surgery should be made on grounds of the severity of heart failure symptoms and LV function, and the clinical severity of regurgitation. Often this is best assessed by intraoperative transesophageal echocardiography (TEE).[11] Mitral regurgitation as a result of myocardial infarction (MI) worsens prognosis independently of other variables, including age and ventricular function. Patients with mitral regurgitation secondary to an MI had a 5-year total mortality of 62% ± 5% vs. total mortality in the control group with MI but no mitral regurgitation of 39% ± 6%. The 5-year cardiac mortality in the group with post-MI mitral regurgitation was 50% ± 6% vs. 30% ± 5% mortality in the control group (both $p < .001$).[11]

Mitral Valve Prolapse

Mitral valve prolapse warrants special mention for a number of reasons. While mitral valve prolapse was previously thought to be common, recent evidence indicates a prevalence of about 2%.[12] There are several unique aspects to the history and physical examination in patients with mitral valve prolapse, and treatment modalities differ in some ways from other causes of mitral regurgitation. In addition, some clinicians have postulated the existence of a mitral valve prolapse syndrome,[13] which involves diffuse autonomic and connective tissue pathology.

Mitral valve prolapse is caused by a combination of factors. There is an abnormality of the connective tissue in the mitral valve, which leads to myxomatous degeneration of the valve and the chordae. Excessive or redundant mitral valve tissue is present and there is often an increased orifice size. Lastly, the length, position, or physiologic function of the papillary muscle and chordae apparatus is abnormal.

Symptoms and Physical Findings

The symptoms of mitral valve prolapse that relate to mitral regurgitation are the same as those seen with other causes of mitral regurgitation. Until recently, it had been reported that palpitations, caused by ventricular ectopy or exaggerated awareness of the heartbeat, and atypical chest pain were more common in patients with mitral valve prolapse. A recent study of mitral valve prolapse, using the Framingham database, has called that association into question.[12]

The mitral valve prolapse syndrome has been defined as mitral valve prolapse associated with increased autonomic tone. Studies have shown increased catecholamine levels and changes in diurnal variation of catecholamine levels in some patients with mitral valve prolapse. In addition, these patients have abnormalities of β-adrenergic receptors and evidence of decreased intravascular volume.[2] Patients with this syndrome may complain of anxiety and show signs of increased adrenergic tone, such as unexplained elevations of the resting pulse. On physical examination S_1 and S_2 are normal, and S_3 and S_4 are usually not present.

Mitral valve prolapse is different from other causes of mitral regurgitation because of the presence of a high-pitched mid-systolic click and the fact that the murmur is not holosystolic. The murmur is mid- to late systolic, follows the click, and often ends before S_2. The findings in mitral valve prolapse are inconstant. There may be no click or murmur one day, but the next day these findings are obvious. An increase in afterload or preload makes the click and murmur occur later, and a decrease in preload makes the click earlier and the murmur louder. The click and murmur of mitral valve prolapse should occur later and may be softer during the beat following the compensatory pause after a premature beat.

Controversies, Complications, Treatment, and Natural History

It is reasonable to wonder when mitral valve prolapse is a disease and when it is a normal variant. Population based studies[12] indicate a low incidence and a benign prognosis. Studies of patients who present with end stage mitral valve regurgitation demonstrate a subgroup of patients with mitral valve prolapse who have serious progressive disease.[14,15] How much workup should be done if an isolated click is heard? What about a click with a murmur? Answering these questions is difficult, particularly when one notes that auscultation may be normal one day and a loud regurgitant murmur may be present the next. The best evidence suggests that the pathology of mitral valve prolapse relates to the degree of mitral regurgitation.[14–16] Risk factors associated with serious mitral valve prolapse requiring valve replacement include increasing age, male sex, increased BMI, and hypertension.

When the severity of mitral valve regurgitation is defined, the medical treatment is the same as for other causes of mitral regurgitation. The adrenergic symptoms, atypical chest pain, and palpitations associated with mitral valve prolapse often respond to beta-blockers.

Mitral Stenosis

Etiology

Mitral stenosis has a single cause: rheumatic heart disease. Although only 50% of patients with mitral stenosis can recall an episode of rheumatic fever, the surgical pathology of stenotic mitral valves virtually always reveals the changes associated with rheumatic heart disease. Congenital mitral stenosis is exceedingly rare.[16] Symptoms can occur as early as 3 years after the episode of rheumatic fever, but most commonly 15 to 25 years elapse between the episode of rheumatic fever and the detection of mitral stenosis. As would be expected, findings and symptoms typically begin during the third to fifth decade of life. The incidence of mitral stenosis has been declining for the last 50 years along with the decline in rheumatic fever.

Symptoms

Symptoms associated with mitral stenosis are directly related to the mitral valve area.[16] With a valve area of more than 2.5 cm^2, assuming a sinus rhythm, no symptoms are present. With a valve area of 1.4 to 2.5 cm^2, there is minimal dyspnea with exertion. With a valve area of 1.0 to 1.3 cm^2, dyspnea on exertion is severe, and orthopnea and paroxysmal nocturnal dyspnea can occur. At valve areas of less than 1 cm^2, resting dyspnea, severe pulmonary edema, and disability occur. The onset of atrial fibrillation, common with advanced mitral stenosis, causes a sudden worsening of symptoms, often frank congestive heart failure (CHF). Pregnancy, infection, and surgery can also cause CHF. Other symptoms associated with mitral stenosis include hemoptysis, which may be the presenting symptom, and frequent bronchitis and wheezing, caused by hyperemia of the bronchi due to increased pulmonary vascular pressure.

Physical Findings and Diagnosis

There are many characteristic physical findings with mitral stenosis, but they are subtle and often overlooked. Ventricular underfilling can cause the carotid pulses to be brisk and brief. The cardiac apex is in the normal location, and the point of maximal impulse (PMI) is small and nonsustained. In fact, the presence of a sustained PMI rules out isolated mitral stenosis. Fine pulmonary crackles may be present, but signs of right heart failure or peripheral edema are typically a sign of end-stage disease.

S_1 is loud with mitral stenosis; in fact, an accentuated S_1, particularly in the setting of atrial fibrillation, should alert the clinician to the possibility of mitral stenosis. As the disease progresses and mitral mobility decreases, S_1 may become softer, but by that time symptoms are usually advanced, and the diagnosis should be obvious. S_2 is either normal or has a loud P2, which can be heard at the apex. S_3 and S_4 are rare because of normal ventricular size, compliance, and slowed diastolic filling.

One of the characteristic heart sounds of mitral stenosis is the opening snap, which occurs after S_2, and is sharper and higher pitched than an S_3. Patients with mitral stenosis usually have a diastolic murmur that is soft, low-pitched (a rumble), and occurs during mid- to late diastole. If the rhythm is sinus, there is presystolic accentuation of the murmur with atrial contraction. Maneuvers that increase or decrease afterload or preload have little effect on the murmur of mitral stenosis.

Natural History, Complications, Medical Therapy, and Timing of Surgery

Mitral stenosis has a more rapid progression and a higher case-fatality rate than mitral regurgitation. Among patients with mild symptoms, 58% are dead in 10 years without surgery; and 85% of patients with mild to moderate symptoms are dead in 10 years without surgery.[16] Rare cases of mitral stenosis remain clinically stable for years, but progression is the rule.

Medical therapy for mitral stenosis is aimed at reducing complications and does not affect the progression of the disease. Diuretics are used to treat pulmonary edema, but digoxin or afterload reduction do not work for this problem. Rate control for atrial fibrillation is essential, and ventricular rates of 50 to 60 beats per minute (bpm) should be the goal of treatment. Digoxin or beta-blockers can be used for rate control. With the onset of atrial fibrillation, electrical cardioversion is attempted and anticoagulation considered, especially if atrial fibrillation persists or recurs.

The assessment of thrombotic risk is an important issue in the diagnosis and treatment of mitral stenosis. Studies have suggested that thrombotic risk is increased with mitral stenosis even with sinus rhythm[17] and with selected echocardiographic findings in atrial fibrillation.[18] Coronary artery disease is rare in the setting of mitral stenosis.

When mitral stenosis is diagnosed, even if symptoms are not present, a workup is initiated to determine left atrial size, valve area, and the atrio-ventricular (AV) pressure gradient. Usually, an echocardiogram is sufficient for this purpose. When moderate symptoms are present or with symptoms such as paroxysmal nocturnal dyspnea or hemoptysis, which suggest significantly elevated pressures, the patient should be referred for surgery. Mitral valve commissurotomy is preferred to mitral valve replacement if possible, although the final decision usually cannot be made until the time of surgery.[18]

Aortic Insufficiency
Etiology
There are multiple etiologies for aortic insufficiency. In an age of a declining incidence of syphilis and rheumatic heart disease, the most common cause is a structural abnormality of the aorta, such as an abnormal valve or aneurysm. In addition to syphilis and rheumatic fever, aortic insufficiency can be caused by subacute bacterial endocarditis, rheumatoid arthritis, ankylosing spondylitis, Reiter's disease, and lupus erythematosus (see Chapter 11). Congenital connective tissue diseases such as Marfan and Ehlers-Danlos syndromes can cause aortic insufficiency, as can severe hypertension.

Symptoms
Patients with aortic insufficiency remain asymptomatic for decades. Early on, patients may complain of palpitations or awareness of heartbeat and mild orthostatic light-headedness. When more severe symptoms occur, they typically begin with fatigue, followed by dyspnea and orthopnea. Later, patients experience angina due to decreased coronary artery flow secondary to the low diastolic pressure in the aorta.

Physical Findings
Patients with aortic insufficiency are often described as flushed and sweaty. Their skin is warm, and until the late stages of the disease

they look healthy. Blood pressure can be normal in aortic insufficiency. With severe regurgitation, there is a wide pulse pressure, and the width of the pulse pressure correlates with the severity of the disease until the left ventricle starts to fail. The fourth Korotkoff sound, muffling, is a more valid indicator of diastolic pressure than the fifth sound, which can sometimes be heard down to 0 mm Hg. The peripheral pulses are bounding and collapsing in nature. The first heart sound is soft with aortic insufficiency. Although S_2 is normal, the aortic component may be lost, so S_2 can sound single. Because of elevated diastolic pressure before the atrial contraction, S_4 is rare until the ventricle is markedly dilated and failing, but an S_3 is common.

The murmur of aortic insufficiency is a high-pitched, soft, blowing diastolic murmur heard best with the diaphragm. It is most audible along the left sternal border with the patient leaning forward and holding expiration. The murmur is sometimes heard at the apex, where it is a lower-pitched rumble (the Austin–Flint murmur) that can be confused with the murmur of mitral stenosis. Because of the greatly elevated stroke volume seen with aortic insufficiency, an outflow murmur mimicking aortic stenosis is common and may be the only murmur appreciated initially. Although one would expect that increasing afterload by the handgrip maneuver would increase the diastolic murmur of aortic insufficiency, it is not always the case. Transient arterial occlusion with two blood pressure cuffs inflated above systolic pressure on the upper extremities often increases the intensity of the murmur. The related outflow murmur usually diminishes with increased afterload. The diastolic murmur does not change appreciably with other maneuvers or after extrasystolic beats.

Natural History, Complications, Medical Therapy, and Timing of Surgery

Stapleton[2] evaluated cases of aortic insufficiency treated medically and noted that among low-risk patients [normal blood pressure, normal electrocardiogram (ECG), no cardiomegaly] 96% were alive 15 years after diagnosis. Among high-risk patients who had two or three ECG abnormalities, cardiomegaly, and an abnormal pulse, 70% were alive at 15 years. Medical therapy consists of providing the kind of follow-up that ensures the appropriate timing of surgical intervention if it becomes necessary. Even before the onset of symptoms, afterload reduction with ACE inhibitors can be done. As symptoms progress, surgery should be strongly considered.

A number of parameters are used as indicators for surgical intervention in patients with asymptomatic or minimally symptomatic aortic insufficiency, but the best combination of these parameters is still a matter of debate. Surgery should be considered if the pulse pressure is more than 100 mm Hg, if there is LVH or ST-T wave abnormalities on the ECG, or if the chest radiograph reveals cardiomegaly, particularly if the cardiothoracic ratio is more than 60%.

Echocardiographic criteria for surgical consultation include an end-diastolic LV diameter of more than 70 mm or an end-systolic diameter of more than 50 mm. An ejection fraction of 40% or less is also an indication for surgical consultation. A decline in ejection fraction during exercise has been shown to identify a cohort of patients at high risk for complications in whom surgery should be considered earlier.[19,20] Because of the embolic and anticoagulation risks of prosthetic aortic valves, the goal of timing surgery is to wait as long as possible, without subjecting the patient to an irreversible loss of LV function.

Aortic Stenosis[21,22]

Etiology

After mitral regurgitation, aortic stenosis is the second most common cause of valvular heart disease in the general population. Male sex predominates by about a 2:1 ratio. Most cases of aortic stenosis are caused by one of three factors: a bicuspid aortic valve, rheumatic fever, or degenerative changes associated with aging (aortic sclerosis). A bicuspid aortic valve is present in 1% to 2% of all births, but it is not known what proportion of these patients progress to having hemodynamically significant aortic stenosis. Isolated cases present with severe symptoms during the teenage years, childhood, or even infancy. Rheumatic fever as a cause of aortic stenosis is declining, whereas age-related aortic stenosis is increasing with increasing life expectancy. An echocardiographic study of patients over 65 found aortic sclerosis in 26% and aortic stenosis in 2%. Risk factors for aortic stenosis include older age, male gender, current smoking, history of hypertension, and elevated low-density lipoprotein and total cholesterol.[4] The risk factors for coronary artery disease are also risk factors for more rapidly progressive aortic stenosis,[21,22] so the index of suspicion for the presence of aortic stenosis or its more rapid progression should be heightened in patients with risk factors for coronary artery disease.

Symptoms

When symptoms due to aortic stenosis develop, they are serious and life-threatening, and the disease is advanced. Angina due to increased LV mass, oxygen consumption, and wall tension can occur even with normal coronary arteries. Medically treated angina due to aortic stenosis is associated with a 5-year life expectancy. Syncope is a frequent presenting symptom of aortic stenosis. Without surgery life expectancy after syncope is 3 years. CHF is also a presenting symptom of aortic stenosis and if not treated surgically carries a 2-year life expectancy. Sudden death is the first symptom of aortic stenosis in 15% of patients with the disease. It is rare for aortic stenosis to present with less serious symptoms.

Physical Findings

Patients with aortic stenosis have normal or low blood pressure. In patients under age 60 an elevated systolic pressure (above 160 to 170 mm Hg) makes severe aortic stenosis unlikely, whereas in elderly patients with diffuse loss of arterial compliance an elevated systolic pressure can be found with moderate to moderately severe aortic stenosis. Low systolic blood pressure and a narrow pulse pressure are ominous signs. Early in the course of aortic stenosis a short, high-pitched opening sound may be heard in the second right intercostal space and may radiate to the neck. As the valvular disease progresses, the opening sound disappears.

The carotid pulse provides the best clue to the presence and severity of aortic stenosis. Called *parvus et tardus* (weak and slow), the carotid pulse rises slowly and often with a shudder. The changes in the carotid pulse are often correlated to the severity of the valvular gradient and the severity of the disease. The cardiac apex is diffuse and often displaced laterally. The PMI is forceful and prolonged. S_1 is usually normal with aortic stenosis. With advanced disease S_2 can be paradoxically split due to prolonged left ventricular systole. An S_3 is rare, but S_4 is common.

The murmur of aortic stenosis is best heard at the second right intercostal space and often radiates to the neck. It is coarse and usually loud. It is described as a crescendo-decrescendo murmur or a diamond-shaped murmur; the later the peak of the crescendo, the more severe is the gradient. The closer to S_2 the murmur ends, the more severe is the disease. The murmur of aortic stenosis is decreased by increased afterload and by decreased preload. The murmur becomes louder with increased preload. The marked accentuation of the murmur after a postextrasystolic beat is one of the most important clues to the presence of aortic stenosis. The physical findings most correlated with severity of disease are a late carotid upstroke; low amplitude of the carotid upstroke; louder, late peaking murmur; and a single second heart sound.[23]

Natural History, Complications, Medical Therapy, and Timing of Surgery

The natural history of aortic stenosis is variable, and the disease can present with clinical symptoms during childhood or during the ninth decade. Once aortic stenosis has been detected, it should be considered a progressive lesion. Presymptomatic medical management should ensure that the rate of progression is well defined. The development of LVH or strain on the ECG and increased cardiac size on the chest radiograph should be followed at least yearly and more often if clinical concern warrants. Serial echocardiography is useful for assessing outflow gradient and LV wall thickness, as the development of a thickened left ventricle can precede the cardiac enlargement seen by radiography.

During the asymptomatic phase of the disease, no medical intervention is indicated. Once symptoms occur, surgery should be considered quickly. Surgery may be considered before symptoms develop if there is ventricular enlargement, segmental wall motion abnormalities suggesting ischemia, severe ECG changes, or frequent ectopy, which might place the patient at risk for sudden death. It has been argued that elderly (older than 75) asymptomatic patients with aortic stenosis who are in sinus rhythm, without bundle branch block and without atrial enlargement, can be followed clinically, no matter what the echocardiographic findings are.[24]

If CHF develops, the use of ACE inhibitors is controversial. Other treatments for complications, pending surgery, consist of accepted medical regimens: digoxin and diuretics for heart failure, cardioversion and chemical stabilization with quinidine for atrial fibrillation (rate control with digoxin or a beta-blocker if cardioversion fails), and nitrates and beta-blockers or calcium channel blockers for angina pectoris.

Hypertrophic Cardiomyopathy

Hypertrophic cardiomyopathy, also known as idiopathic hypertrophic subaortic stenosis (IHSS) and hypertrophic obstructive cardiomyopathy (HOCM), is a hereditary condition causing a murmur that originates in the area below the aortic valve. The murmur is created by thickening of the myocardium with disproportionate septal thickening and subsequent narrowing of the outflow tract. The Venturi effect in the area of subaortic narrowing can cause movement of the anterior mitral valve toward the outflow tract, further worsening the obstruction. The ventricle in patients with hypertrophic cardiomyopathy is hyperkinetic, and systolic emptying of the ventricle is rapid and nearly complete. There is also abnormal relaxation and markedly decreased compliance of the ventricle that causes severe diastolic abnormalities.

The characteristics of this murmur are similar to those of the murmur of aortic stenosis with some key differences. With subaortic stenosis a brisk carotid upstroke is maintained, even in the face of a severe gradient. Contrary to the murmur of aortic stenosis, the murmur of subaortic stenosis becomes softer with increased preload or after a compensatory pause[18] and is louder with decreased preload. Like aortic stenosis, the murmur is softer with increased afterload. The gradient increases with decreased ventricular filling and with lowered systemic resistance. This point is particularly important for athletes, because after exercise both of these conditions are present. Although subvalvular aortic stenosis is an uncommon condition, it causes a disproportionate percentage of unexpected sudden deaths in healthy young people, usually immediately after exercise. Beta-blockers are the medical treatment of choice, but surgery to thin the septum is often necessary.

Right-Sided Heart Murmurs

Right-sided heart murmurs are far less common than left-sided murmurs. The pressures sustained by the valves are lower, which means that valvular dysfunction is less likely to occur. Right-sided murmurs have many of the same characteristics as murmurs involving the analogous left-sided valves with some key differences.

Left-sided murmurs involving the mitral valve cause pulmonary congestion, whereas similar right-sided murmurs involving the tricuspid valve cause central venous congestion and peripheral edema. Whereas left-sided murmurs typically stay the same or diminish slightly with inspiration, right-sided heart murmurs usually become noticeably louder. Increasing afterload by handgrip does not affect right-sided murmurs, nor does the compensatory pause after an extrasystolic beat. Changes in preload, however, affect right-sided murmurs in the same way they affect murmurs originating from the left side of the heart. Lastly, there is no tricuspid analogy to mitral valve prolapse.

Congenital Heart Disease

Murmurs During Infancy

Murmurs are an uncommon finding during infancy. A murmur in an infant should be considered an important finding. A murmur heard

Table 4.1. **Frequency of Congenital Heart Disease (CHD)**

Condition	Percent
Ventricular septal defect (VSD)	32
Pulmonic stenosis	9
Patent ductus arteriosus (PDA)	8
Atrial septal defect (ASD)	7
Coarctation of aorta	7
Aortic stenosis	4
Tetralogy of Fallot	4
Atrioventricular septal defect	4
Hypoplastic left heart	3
D-transposition of vessels	3
Hypoplastic right heart	2
Truncus arteriosus	2
Double outlet right ventricle	1
Single ventricle	1
All other types of CHD	13

during the first 24 hours of life carries a 1 in 12 chance of being caused by congenital heart disease. The most common cause of pathologic murmurs in this age group is patent ductus, which normally resolves spontaneously by 8 weeks of age. A murmur heard at 6 months of age has a one in seven chance of being caused by congenital heart disease, and a murmur heard at 1 year has a 1 in 50 chance of representing congenital heart disease. Table 4.1 lists the frequencies of various types of congenital heart diseases based on a number of epidemiological studies.[25-30]

There are four general findings on physical examination and office laboratory testing that should alert the family physician to pursue the possibility of congenital heart disease in an infant: (1) failure to thrive; (2) abnormal oxygenation, with normal defined as an oxygen saturation of more than 95% in room air (oxygen saturation should not consistently decrease with feeding); (3) signs of CHF, including tachycardia, tachypnea, poor feeding, and sweating; and (4) signs of syndromes (e.g., Down syndrome) or other congenital anomalies.

Maternal risk factors for congenital heart disease in the infant include smoking and gestational diabetes.[31,32] A weak protective effect has been demonstrated for periconceptional multivitamin use (defined as starting at least 3 months before pregnancy and continuing at least 3 months into pregnancy).[33]

The risk of recurrence of congenital heart disease in siblings and offspring is summarized in Table 4.2.

Table 4.2. **Recurrence Risk of Congenital Heart Disease**

Defect	Siblings (%)	Offspring (%)
Ventricular septal defect (VSD)	6	4
Atrial septal defect (ASD)	3	4–10
Atrioventricular (AV) septal defect	2	5–10
Patent ductus arteriosus (PDA)	2.5	3
Valvular aortic stenosis	3	5–10
Valvular pulmonic stenosis	2	6
Coarctation of aorta	2	3
D-transposition of arteries	2	5
Tetralogy of Fallot	2	4
Hypoplastic left heart	1–2	5
Hypoplastic right heart	1	5
Anomalous pulmonary vein	3	5
Truncus arteriosis	8	8
Double outlet ventricle	2	4
Atrial isomerism	5	1
Single ventricle	3	5
Ebstein's malformation	1	5

Ventricular Septal Defect (VSD)

Because VSD is the most common murmur caused by a congenital heart defect, it is important to review its presentation. Newborns and children with a VSD present with a holosystolic murmur similar to the murmur of mitral regurgitation. Murmurs caused by VSDs are typically louder and coarser than the murmur of mitral regurgitation. A VSD is heard best at the left sternal border, and the murmur is often associated with a thrill. About 24% of VSDs close spontaneously by 18 months and 75% by 10 years of age. Those that do not close can cause irreversible pulmonary hypertension, cardiac disability, and early death. If the family physician suspects a VSD, early diagnosis, referral, and close follow-up are critical. Frequent examinations for respiratory status, feeding, and weight gain are mandatory. Any signs of failure to thrive or of RV volume or pressure overload require workup for possible surgical intervention.

Murmurs During Pregnancy

A large percentage of pregnant women develop murmurs because of an increased plasma and blood volume. Studies have shown that most murmurs during pregnancy are benign, and investigations such as echocardiography add little or no benefit to the outcomes of most pregnancies. That is no reason for complacency, however, because certain types of valvular heart disease are likely to become much more serious during pregnancy, even to the point where they threaten the life of the mother or fetus. Pregnant women with known valvular heart disease or in whom there is a diastolic murmur, pansystolic murmur, loud murmur (grade 3 or more), or symptoms of cardiovascular disease must be evaluated for valvular heart disease.

Mitral stenosis, which may be clinically silent prior to conception, can become an important problem during pregnancy. Maternal morbidity and mortality are significantly increased owing to pulmonary edema caused by increased intravascular volume. The fetus suffers from poor growth, and there is increased fetal loss. Mitral regurgitation, on the other hand, is usually well tolerated during pregnancy.

Aortic regurgitation is also well tolerated during pregnancy, except when it is secondary to Marfan syndrome. Increased blood volume can cause dilatation and dissection or rupture of the aortic root. Pregnancy should be avoided in women with Marfan syndrome. Aortic stenosis, although rare in women of childbearing age, causes significant problems during pregnancy. Maternal mortality rates of up to 17% have been reported, and because of sudden depletion of intravascular volume, mortality rates of up to 40% after termination of pregnancy have been reported.[2] Subvalvular aortic stenosis, seen with hypertrophic cardiomyopathy, causes increased maternal morbidity during pregnancy, especially at delivery, when blood loss can worsen outflow obstruction. Any cause of severe left-to-right shunt or pulmonary hypertension creates a contraindication to pregnancy.

Murmurs in the Athlete[34–36]

One of the most important aspects of the physical examination of the athlete is to identify the rare patient in whom risk of sudden death can be avoided. In patients older than 40 years, the most likely cause of sudden death during sports participation is coronary artery disease (see Chapter 2). In the young athlete the most common causes of sudden death are hypertrophic cardiomyopathy,[1,36] and possibly mitral valve prolapse.[34] A 1998 study looked at all sudden deaths in athletes and nonathletes ages 35 or younger in a defined geographical area in Italy with population of 4.4 million people older than 17. This study included 33,735 people who had been screened during that time. The causes of sudden death that would have presented with a murmur, all defined by autopsy, are listed in Table 4.3.[35]

Table 4.3. **Valvular Causes of Sudden Death in 33,735 Athletic Screenings**

Cause of death	Athletes $n = 49$ (%)	Nonathletes $n = 220$ (%)	Total $n = 269$ (%)
Mitral valve prolapse	5 (10.2%)	21 (9.5%)	26 (9.7%)
Hypertrophic cardiomyopathy	1 (2.0%)	16 (7.3%)	17 (6.3%)

The physical findings associated with these problems are covered elsewhere in this chapter. Because hypertrophic cardiomyopathy is a congenital disease, a history of unexplained syncope and a family history of sudden death are key pieces of information. The finding of arrhythmias, a history of syncope, or a family history of sudden death should prompt the family physician to further work up a patient with mitral valve prolapse before sanctioning exercise. Aortic stenosis and other congenital heart conditions associated with pulmonary hypertension are also potential causes of sudden death in young athletes. Current recommendations from the American College of Sports Medicine and the American College of Cardiology for participation in sports by patients with all types of congenital heart disease are found in the Bethesda conference of 1994.[36]

References

1. Harvey WP. Cardiac pearls. Dis Month 1994;40:41–113.
2. Stapleton JF. Natural history of chronic valvular disease. Cardiovasc Clin 1986;16:105–47.
3. Rose AG. Etiology of acquired valvular heart disease in adults. A survey of 18,132 autopsies and 100 consecutive valve replacement operations. Arch Pathol Lab Med 1986;110:385–8.
4. Stewart BF, Siscovick D, Lind BK, et al. Clinical factors associated with aortic valve disease. Cardiovascular health study. J Am Coll Cardiol 1997;29:630–4.
5. Singh JP, Evans JC, Levy D. et al. Prevalence and clinical determinants of mitral, tricuspid and aortic regurgitation (the Framingham Heart Study). Am J Cardiol 1999;83:897–902.
6. Jones EC, Devereux RB, Roman MJ et al. Prevalence and correlates of mitral regurgitation in a population based sample (the Strong Heart Study). Am J Cardiol 2001;87:298–304.
7. Roldan CA, Gill EA, Shivley BK. Prevalence and diagnostic value of precordial murmurs for valvular regurgitation in obese patients treated with dexfenfluramine. Am J Cardiol 2000;86:535–9.

8. Weissman NJ, Panza JA, Tighe JF, Gwynne JT. Natural history of valvular regurgitation 1 year after discontinuation of dexfenfluramine therapy. A randomized double-blind, placebo-controlled trial. Ann Intern Med 2001;134:267–73.
9. Saenz A, Hopkins CB, Humphries JO. Valvular heart disease. In: Chung EK, ed. Quick reference to cardiovascular diseases. Baltimore: Williams & Wilkins, 1987;71–92.
10. Wencker D, Borer JS, Hochreiter C, et al. Preoperative predictors of late postoperative outcome among patients with nonischemic mitral regurgitation with "high risk" descriptors and comparison with non-operated patients. Cardiology 2000;93:37–42.
11. Grigioni F, Enriques-Sarano M, Zehr KJ, et al. Ischemic mitral regurgitation: long term outcome and prognostic implications with quantitative Doppler assessment. Circulation 2001;103:1759–64.
12. Freed LO, Levy D, Levine RA, et al. Prevalence and clinical outcome of mitral valve prolapse. N Engl J Med 1999;339:1–7.
13. Fontana ME, Sparks EA, Harsios B, Wooley CF. Mitral valve prolapse and the mitral valve prolapse syndrome. Curr Probl Cardiol 1991;16: 315–68.
14. Singh RG, Cappucci R, Kramer-Fox R, et al. Severe mitral regurgitation due to mitral valve prolapse: risk factors for development, progression and need for mitral valve surgery. Am J Cardiol 2000;85:193–8.
15. Kolibash AJ, Kilman JW, Bush CA, et al. Evidence of progression from mild to severe mitral regurgitation in mitral valve prolapse. Am J Cardiol 1986;58:762–7.
16. Fukuda M, Oki T, Iuchi A, et al. Predisposing factors for severe mitral regurgitation in idiopathic mitral valve prolapse. Am J Cardiol 1995;76: 503–7.
17. Cheng-Wen C, Sing-Kai L, Yu-Shien K, et al. Predictors of systemic embolism in patients with mitral stenosis: a prospective study. Ann Intern Med 1998;128:885–9.
18. Gonzalez-Torreciella E, Garcia-Fernandez MA, Perez-David E, et al. Predictors of left atrial contrast and thrombi in patients with mitral stenosis and atrial fibrillation. Am J Cardiol 2000;86:529–34.
19. Lindsay J, Silverman A, Van Voorhees LB, Nolan NG. Prognostic implications of left ventricular function during exercise in patients with aortic regurgitation. Angiology 1987;38:386–92.
20. Wahi S, Haluska B, Pasquet A, et al. Exercise echocardiography predicts development of left ventricular dysfunction in medically and surgically treated patients with asymptomatic severe aortic regurgitation. Heart 2000;84:606–14.
21. Palta S, Pai AM, Gill KS, Pai RG. New insights into the progression of aortic stenosis: implications for secondary prevention. Circulation 2000;101:2497–502.
22. Nassimiha D, Aronow WS, Ahn C, Goldman ME. Association of coronary risk factors with progression of aortic valvular stenosis in older persons. Am J Cardiol 2001;87:1313–4.
23. Munt B, Legget ME, Kraft CD et al. Physical examination in valvular aortic stenosis: correlation with stenosis severity and prediction of clinical outcome. Am Heart J 1999;137:298–306.

24. Pierri H, Nussbacher A, Decourt LV, et al. Clinical predictors of prognosis in severe aortic stenosis in unoperated patients > or = to 75 years of age. Am J Cardiol 2000;86:801–4.
25. Samanek N, Voriskova M. Congenital heart disease among 815,569 children born between 1980–1990 and their 15-year survival: a prospective Bohemia survival study. Pediatr Cardiol 1999;20:411–7.
26. Ainsworth S, Wyllie JP, Wren C. Prevalence and significance of cardiac murmurs in neonates. Arch Dis Child (Fetal Neonatal Ed) 1999;80:F43–5.
27. Bosi G, Scorrano M, Tosato G, et al. The Italian Multicentric Study on Epidemiology of Congenital Heart Disease: first step of the analysis. Working Party of the Italian Society of Pediatric Cardiology. Cardiol Young 1999;9:291–9.
28. Wren C, Richmond S, Donaldson L. Presentation of congenital heart disease in infancy: implications for routine examination. Arch Dis Child (Fetal Neonatal Ed) 1999;80:F49–53.
29. Meberg A, Otterstad JE, Froland G, et al. Early clinical screening of neonates for congenital heart defects: the cases we miss. Cardiol Young 1999;9:169–74.
30. Samanek M. Congenital heart malformations: prevalence, severity, survival, and quality of life. Cardiol Young 2000;10:179–85.
31. Kallen K. Maternal smoking and congenital heart defects. Eur J Epidemiol 1999;15:731–7.
32. Aberg A, Westbom L, Kallen B. Congenital malformations among infants whose mothers had gestational diabetes or preexisting diabetes. Early Hum Dev 2001;61:85–95.
33. Botto LD, Mulinare J, Erickson JD. Occurrence of congenital heart defects in relation to maternal multivitamin use. Am J Epidemiol 2000;151:878–84.
34. Maron BJ, Thompson PD, Puffer JC, et al. Cardiovascular preparticipation screening of competitive athletes: a statement for health professionals from the sudden death committee (clinical cardiology) and congenital heart defects committee (cardiovascular disease in the young), American Heart Association. Circulation 1996;94:850–6.
35. Corrado D, Basso C, Schiavon M, Thiene G. Screening for hypertrophic cardiomyopathy in your athletes. N Engl J Med 1998;339:364–5.
36. Graham TP, Bricker JT, James FW, Strong WB. 26th Bethesda Conference: recommendations for determining eligibility for competition in athletes with cardiovascular abnormalities. Task Force 1: congenital heart disease. Med Sci Sports Exerc 1994;26:S46–53.

5
Heart Failure

William A. Norcross and
Denise D. Hermann

Heart failure (HF) is defined as the inability of the heart to generate a cardiac output sufficient to meet the metabolic needs of body tissues at rest or with activity. This definition is sufficiently broad to include systolic and diastolic failure, high-output failure, and cor pulmonale. The adjective "congestive" is appropriate only when there are symptoms or signs of systemic or pulmonary fluid volume overload, typically related to sodium and water retention secondary to activation of the neurohumoral axis (renin-angiotensin-aldosterone system and arginine-vasopressin system) with HF.

Heart failure affects 4.9 million people in the United States and is the only major cardiovascular disorder with increasing incidence and prevalence. Two factors thought to contribute to this phenomenon are increases in average life expectancy and medical advances that have diminished morbidity and mortality from most cardiovascular disorders. The diagnosis of HF accounts for annual health care costs in the United States of more than $18 billion, half of which, it is estimated, could be saved by improvements in outpatient management. Despite modern therapies, however, the morbidity and mortality associated with HF remain high, averaging 10% mortality at 1 year and 50% at 5 years.[1]

The causes of HF are listed in Table 5.1. Coronary artery disease is presently the most common etiology and represents the etiology of HF in nearly 70% of patients with systolic dysfunction in the United States. Idiopathic dilated cardiomyopathy, valvular heart dis-

Table 5.1. **Causes of Heart Failure**

Most common
Coronary artery disease
   Diastolic dysfunction
   Systolic dysfunction
Hypertensive cardiomyopathy
   Diastolic dysfunction
   Systolic dysfunction (late)

Common
   Idiopathic cardiomyopathy
   Alcoholic cardiomyopathy
   Hypertrophic cardiomyopathy
   Diabetic cardiomyopathy
   Valvular heart disease
   Cor pulmonale (right heart failure only)
      Chronic lung disease
      Pulmonary embolic disease
      Primary/secondary pulmonary hypertension

Uncommon
   Infectious cardiomyopathy (viral, bacterial, fungal, parasitic)
   Doxorubicin-induced cardiomyopathy
   Bleomycin-induced cardiomyopathy
   Constrictive pericarditis
   Restrictive cardiomyopathy
      Amyloidosis
      Hemochromatosis
      Sarcoidosis
   Collagen vascular disease-induced cardiomyopathy
   High-output failure
      Anemia
      Arteriovenous shunt
      Paget's disease of bone
      Thyrotoxicosis
   Thiamine deficiency (beriberi) cardiomyopathy
   Radiation-induced cardiomyopathy
   Cardiomyopathy of pregnancy
   Uremic cardiomyopathy
   Endocardial fibroelastosis

ease, and hypertensive cardiomyopathy are also common (see Chapters 1, 4, and 11).

Diastolic (lusitropic) failure occurs when the left ventricle becomes stiff and noncompliant and elevated left ventricular filling pressures develop. Systolic function is generally preserved, and therefore the ejection fraction remains normal to slightly reduced. The cardiac output is preserved at the expense of increased diastolic filling pressure, and is diminished in the setting of hypovolemia and/or excessive systemic afterload. Diastolic failure most commonly results from antecedent hypertension or coronary artery disease. Although the prevalence of chronic diastolic HF in a primary care setting is unknown, studies from tertiary care centers suggest that up to 40% of patients with HF may have primarily diastolic dysfunction.[2] It is important to recognize diastolic dysfunction because certain treatments for systolic dysfunction (diuretics, digoxin) may worsen the patient's hemodynamic profile or clinical condition.

High-output HF is uncommonly encountered in a primary care practice. It is important to recognize because the conditions that cause it (Table 5.1) are often responsive to treatment.

Acute Heart Failure/Cardiogenic Pulmonary Edema

Diagnosis

Although severe acute heart failure (AHF) can manifest in a patient with mild to moderate chronic symptoms, for the purposes of this section the patient with new onset of severe symptoms is described. Air hunger, dyspnea, and anxiety are the most notable symptoms. Classically, the patient expectorates pink, frothy sputum, occasionally blood-streaked due to pulmonary edema and rapid alveolar filling from either pressure or volume overload or both. Physical findings include tachypnea with use of accessory muscles, tachycardia, engorged neck veins, rales, and wheezing (cardiac asthma). The extremities are pale and cool, and peripheral cyanosis may be present. The chest roentgenogram typically shows cardiomegaly (although the heart size and shape may be normal in the setting of acute myocardial infarction, hypertensive crisis, or acute valvular emergency), pulmonary vascular redistribution, Kerley B lines, and perihilar infiltrates with a classic "bat wing" appearance and pleural effusions may be noted (right-sided or bilateral effusions are the rule).

Initial diagnostic testing must include an electrocardiogram (ECG) to rapidly exclude acute myocardial infarction (MI) or a significant arrhythmia, blood chemistries, a complete blood count (CBC), arterial blood gases, and any other tests indicated by the clinical history and examination. Early bedside echocardiography may be helpful, especially for diagnosing acute valvular cardiac disease, helping to differentiate cardiac from noncardiac pulmonary edema, and defining left ventricular (LV) function as preserved or impaired. Severely ill patients (e.g., those with hypotension, oliguria, diminished mentation (cardiogenic shock), or failure to rapidly respond to therapy) require central hemodynamic monitoring by placing an indwelling pulmonary artery catheter (e.g., Swan-Ganz catheter).

Treatment

Acute HF is a medical emergency. Unless severely hypotensive, the patient is placed in a seated position to assist venous pooling and diminish preload. In the absence of chronic obstructive pulmonary disease (COPD) with retention of carbon dioxide, high-flow 100% oxygen is delivered by way of a tight-fitting mask to maintain peripheral oxygen saturation above 94%. Vascular access is established and cardiac monitoring instituted. Rotating tourniquets and phlebotomy are rarely utilized in the modern era, as they have been replaced by aggressive pharmacologic therapy. An acute MI with signs of HF or shock should prompt a rapid evaluation by a cardiologist for percutaneous transluminal coronary angioplasty (PTCA) or administration of thrombolytic agents.

First-Line Agents

Furosemide is generally a first-line agent if the patient is not severely hypotensive. When given intravenously it acts initially as a venodilator and subsequently as a diuretic. The patient is given twice the customary daily oral dose intravenously. If the patient does not take a diuretic, the furosemide dose is 0.5 to 1.0 mg/kg IV slow push. (Rapid, large doses of intravenous furosemide have been associated with permanent ototoxicity.)

Morphine has long had a role in the treatment of cardiogenic pulmonary edema but must be used with caution. It is a potent venodilator and also reduces anxiety. On the other hand, it can cause or worsen hypotension and may mask symptoms and signs that are important for the clinician to observe when sequentially assessing patients with a suspected acute coronary syndrome. The starting dose is 2 to 4 mg IV; subsequent doses can be titrated according to the patient's response. Nitroglycerin, a potent venodilator, may also be considered a first-line drug, especially in patients with concomitant chest pain or ischemia. Because of the peripheral vasoconstriction associated with AHF, topical nitroglycerin is avoided. Nitroglycerin 0.3 mg sublingually or a similar dose of the oral spray may be used and repeated depending on the patient's response. Care is taken to avoid symptomatic hypotension, especially in patients with diastolic

HF, those in whom right ventricular infarction is suspected, and those with an acute coronary syndrome.

Second-Line and Third-Line Agents

The choice of a second-line agent depends on the patient's clinical parameters. It is reasonable to use the guidelines of the American Heart Association adopted from the recommendations made at the International Guidelines Conference on Cardiopulmonary Resuscitation (CPR) and Emergency Cardiac Care (ECC).[3] If systolic blood pressure is below 70 mm Hg, consider norepinephrine 0.5 to 30.0 μg/min IV. If the systolic blood pressure is between 70 and 100 mm Hg, and there are symptoms or signs of shock, consider using dopamine in a range of 2.5 to 15.0 μg/kg/min IV. If the systolic blood pressure is between 70 and 100 mm Hg, and there are no symptoms or signs of shock, use dobutamine 2 to 20 μg/kg/min IV. If the systolic blood pressure is above 100 mm Hg and the patient is not significantly hypertensive, consider nitroglycerin 10 to 20 μg/min IV. If the diastolic blood pressure is above 110 mm Hg, consider nitroglycerin at a starting dose of 10 to 20 μg/min IV and titrate to the desired or optimal effect, or use nitroprusside 0.1 to 5.0 μg/kg/min IV.

By the time third-line agents are required, and possibly before, it is presumed that such a patient would be admitted to a coronary care unit (CCU) and a cardiologist consulted. In patients who do not respond promptly to initial treatment, right heart catheterization (e.g., Swan-Ganz catheter) is desirable to rule out noncardiogenic pulmonary edema and to guide subsequent therapy. Along with drug therapy, it is also reasonable to consider the institution of positive end-expiratory pressure (PEEP), continuous positive airway pressure (CPAP), or intubation with ventilatory support. Third-line agents include amrinone, milrinone, and aminophylline. Other interventions that may be appropriate, depending on the clinical situation, include intraaortic balloon counterpulsation and various surgical procedures such as coronary artery bypass grafting (CABG), valve replacement, and even cardiac transplantation.

Chronic Heart Failure

Clinical Manifestations

The New York Heart Association (NYHA) classification system is widely used to grade heart failure according to symptoms. Unfortunately, it lacks objectivity. NYHA class I patients have no limitation of physical activity. Class II patients are comfortable at rest, but "ordinary" physical activity results in symptoms (e.g., fatigue, dyspnea). Class III patients are comfortable at rest but have symptoms with low levels of activity. Class IV patients experience symptoms at rest. Classes II and III are often difficult to distinguish. Maintaining a frame of reference to the normal activities of an age- and sex-matched normal individual is helpful.

Risk factors for chronic heart failure include aging, coronary heart disease, diabetes, hypertension, and obesity. Unlike the classic presentation of severe AHF, chronic heart failure can be of slow and insidious onset. Patients at risk for the development of heart failure should be screened for symptoms of *f*atigue, *a*ctivity intolerance, *c*ongestive symptoms, *e*dema, and *s*hortness of breath (FACES). Several studies have convincingly demonstrated that the symptoms, signs, and radiographic findings classically associated with chronic HF have poor positive and negative predictive values.[4] Moreover, left ventricular dysfunction can be asymptomatic or symptoms with exercise can be rationalized and attributed to poor physical conditioning or to aging. Although the individual symptoms and signs of HF are often unreliable, diagnostic accuracy is improved directly with the number of symptoms and signs observed and the acuity of the presentation.

The symptoms and signs of chronic HF are shown in Table 5.2. It is critical to note that symptoms cannot distinguish systolic from diastolic ventricular dysfunction. It is helpful therapeutically to distinguish signs of low cardiac output from congestion (left, right, or biventricular volume overload). The former respond favorably to inotropic agents and vasodilators and the latter to diuretics and vasodilators. In the patient with predominant diastolic ventricular dysfunction, dyspnea on exertion may be the primary symptom. In such patients signs often include hypertension and a prominent S_4. The echocardiogram typically shows normal ventricular dimensions and preserved systolic function; Doppler interrogation of mitral valve inflow and pulmonary vein flow demonstrate diastolic filling abnormalities. Left atrial enlargement and left ventricular hypertrophy (LVH) are common. LVH without systemic hypertension (HTN) warrants an evaluation for infiltrative or primary myocardial disease. In the patient with isolated right ventricular (RV) failure, the most likely etiology is primary or secondary pulmonary disease. RV dysplasia and pericardial constriction may be considered as well, but are uncommon.

Diagnosis

Chronic HF is a clinical syndrome whose diagnosis should be confirmed by further evaluation. All patients with symptoms or signs

Table 5.2. **Symptoms and Signs of Chronic Heart Failure**

Parameter	Low cardiac output,	"Left-heart" congestion (pressure or volume overload, or both)	"Right-heart" or biventricular congestion (pressure or volume overload, or both)
Symptoms	Fatigue, anorexia, poor energy, malaise, decreased exercise capacity, weight loss, weakness, impaired concentration or memory	Dyspnea (rest or exertion), orthopnea, paroxysmal nocturnal dyspnea, cough, nocturia	RUQ or epigastric pain or fullness, abdominal bloating, nausea or anorexia, ankle/leg swelling, weight gain
Signs	Resting tachycardia, S_3, low carotid pulse volume, cool or vasoconstricted extremities, cachexia, reduced urine output, altered mentation	Cardiomegaly, abnormal apical impuse, S_3, tachypnea, rales, loud P_2	Jugular distension, hepato-megaly, hepatojugular reflux, pleural effusions or ascites, dependent edema, RV gallop or lift, loud P_2

RUQ = right upper quadrant; RV = right ventricular.

consistent with HF should undergo an assessment of LV function. Specifically, the ejection fraction should be measured by echocardiography or radionuclide ventriculography. These tests also help distinguish systolic from diastolic dysfunction. After confirming the diagnosis, the next step is to determine the etiology of chronic HF. If there are significant risk factors for coronary artery disease (CAD) or if CAD is otherwise suspected, noninvasive testing or direct coronary angiography should be considered (see Chapter 2). Although it is tempting to treat HF patients empirically based on clinical grounds alone, we strongly recommend the use of a confirmatory test for two reasons: (1) the delivery of a diagnosis with such a grave prognosis (50% mortality at 5 years) mandates precision, and reversible or treatable factors must not be overlooked; and (2) useless or inappropriate therapies may be dangerous to the patient and are expensive in their own right.

One study demonstrated the ECG to be a useful screening tool for HF.[5] Of 96 patients with impaired LV systolic function, as determined by two-dimensional, M-mode, and Doppler echocardiography, 90 had major ECG abnormalities (atrial fibrillation, LVH, prior MI, bundle branch block, or left axis deviation) and none had a completely normal ECG. Using major ECG abnormalities as a marker in this study gives a sensitivity of 94% for systolic HF. If these data are borne out by other, similar studies, the ECG may become a useful test when deciding which patients may benefit from assessment of the ejection fraction (EF). Unfortunately, a high sensitivity for major ECG abnormalities has not been demonstrated for diastolic dysfunction, RV failure, or high-output failure. For instance, the sensitivity and specificity of the ECG for detecting LVH vary widely with the grading criteria employed.

Radionuclide ventriculography and echocardiography with Doppler are appropriate tools for the evaluation of the EF. Compared to the EF as measured by cineangiography, the correlation of radionuclide ventriculography ($r = 0.88$) is slightly better than that of echocardiography ($r = 0.78$).[6] However, most clinicians prefer echocardiography with Doppler sonography because of its added ability to quantitate chamber size and detect LVH and valvular dysfunction. The advantages and disadvantages of the two tests are compared in Table 5.3.

Because HF is often asymptomatic or minimally symptomatic, and because early treatment has been documented to diminish mortality and ameliorate the progression of the disease, it would be desirable to have a simple, inexpensive, accurate test for the diagnosis of HF. Natriuretic peptide assays hold promise for this purpose. Natriuretic

Table 5.3. **Echocardiography Versus Radionuclide Ventriculography for Evaluating Left Ventricular Performance**

Test	Advantages	Disadvantages
Echocardiography	Permits concomitant assessment of valvular disease, LV hypertrophy, and LA size	Difficult to perform in patients with lung disease
	Less expensive than radionuclide ventriculography in most cases	Usually only semiquantitative estimate of EF provided
	Able to detect pericardial effusion and ventricular thrombus	Technically inadequate in up to 18% of patients under optimal circumstances
Radionuclide ventriculography	More precise and reliable measurement of EF	Requires venipuncture and radiation exposure
	Better assessment of RV function	Limited assessment of valvular heart disease and LV hypertrophy

Source: Konstam et al.[1]

LV = left ventricular; LA = left atrial; EF = ejection fraction; RV = right ventricular.

peptides are secreted in high levels in systolic HF secondary to atrial and ventricular wall stress. Their properties include natriuresis, vasodilation, and inhibition of the renin-angiotensin-aldosterone axis. The data to date suggest brain natriuretic peptide (BNP, a 32 amino acid peptide originally named because it was thought to be a neurotransmitter in pig brain, but now known to be secreted by the cardiac ventricle) and N-terminal proBNP (NT-proBNP, the circulating amino terminal portion of the BNP prohormone) correlate best with the diagnosis of systolic heart failure. Test characteristics for BNP show sensitivities of 77% to 97%, specificities of 73% to 87%, and positive predictive values of 16% to 70%.[7] For NT-proBNP sensitivities range from 82% to 94%, specificities from 55% to 69%, and positive predictive values from 50% to 58%.[7] As expected, the test characteristics for both tests depend on the assay utilized and the pretest likelihood of HF in the study population (there is improved accuracy in populations at high risk for systolic HF.) These assays have not been well studied in diastolic HF or high-output HF. There is currently no national consensus as to the best test or specific assay to use, but the technology is promising. Such a test may be used in cases where the diagnosis remains uncertain after conventional diagnostic testing has been performed. The assay may be particularly helpful in the emergency department or outpatient clinic.

Once the clinical syndrome of HF is diagnosed, the etiology can often be ascertained by way of a careful history and physical examination, ECG, chest radiography, chemistry panel, thyroid-stimulating hormone (TSH) assay, CBC, and echocardiography. Some would argue the case for serum iron, iron-binding capacity, and ferritin assays to evaluate for the presence of hemochromatosis.

Alcoholic cardiomyopathy, thought to play a role in 20% to 30% of patients with "idiopathic" cardiomyopathy, is probably more commonly encountered than we realize. A sensitive exploration of the issue is necessary for all patients. Also, alcoholic cardiomyopathy seems to correlate well with the presence of the skeletal myopathy of alcoholism[8]; therefore, a careful neurologic examination is important. Similarly, a history of cocaine or amphetamine abuse, which may result in premature large or small vessel CAD and infarct, may be difficult to elicit.

Prognosis

Despite medical and surgical advances in the treatment of HF, the prognosis generally remains grim. Overall mortality for HF optimally treated with angiotensin-converting enzyme (ACE) inhibitors, digoxin, and diuretics is about 10% annually, with a 5-year mortality of 50%. Approximately 30% to 50% of these deaths are sudden. Data from the Framingham study suggest that this 5-year mortality has not changed appreciably since the 1930s. African Americans have about a 1.5-fold higher risk of mortality from HF than whites. The following variables have been found to be independent predictors of a poor prognosis in HF: severely depressed ejection fraction (<30%); LV size and morphology (globular is worse); functional class (NYHA class IV: 30–50% mortality at 1 year); concomitant RV failure or pulmonary hypertension; increased cardiothoracic ratio on chest roentgenogram; older age; reduced exercise capacity; hyponatremia; atrial and ventricular arrhythmias; and neuroendocrine activation [elevated levels of norepinephrine, angiotensin II, aldosterone, atrial natriuretic factor, tumor necrosis factor-α (TNF-α) and other cytokines] (Table 5.4). TNF-α is responsible for inducing "cardiac cachexia," a chronic muscle wasting syndrome seen frequently in advanced heart failure, cancer, and AIDS. At present, the treatment is directed at the underlying disease, although a clinical trial evaluating the effect of a TNF receptor blocker (etanercept) on prognosis in chronic HF is under way, with results expected in 2002.

Management Principles
Patient Counseling
The establishment of a caring, open, compassionate relationship with the patient and the family is necessary for effective treatment of HF. The clinician should not hesitate to enlist the help of dietitians, pharmacists, nurse educators, and community groups. Home health care resources can be especially helpful. It is believed that better patient education and compliance improve morbidity and mortality statistics and save billions of dollars in health care expenditures.

General Counseling
The patient and family should be informed of the pathophysiology of HF, including an explanation of the symptoms observed, the rationale for complying with treatment recommendations, and, if known or suspected, the cause of the HF. The patient and family are told what symptoms or signs suggest a deteriorating course and what to do in the event such symptoms develop. All treatments are explained carefully, and the patient's responsibilities in treatment are reinforced. When family members are involved in the treatment plan, their responsibilities are also clearly delineated. The patient and fam-

Table 5.4. **Prognostic Factors for Chronic Heart Failure**

Etiology of ventricular dysfunction
  Predominant systolic impairment
  Ischemic heart disease
  Idiopathic, hypertensive, or valvular heart disease
  Other
    Myocarditis: infectious, autoimmune, giant cell
    Hypertrophic cardiomyopathy
    Toxin-related cardiomyopathy (e.g., alcohol, anthracyclines)
    Infiltrative diseases (e.g., amyloid, hemochromatosis)
Patient demographics
  Race
  Gender
  Age
Comorbidities
  Diabetes, systemic or pulmonary hypertension, sleep apnea, renal or
    hepatic dysfunction
Easily measured variables
  Symptoms—NYHA classification, specific activity scale
  Ejection fraction in left and right ventricles
  Exercise capacity: VO_2 max, 6-minute walk distance
  Hemodynamics
  Serum sodium
  Thyroid function
  Arrhythmias/ECG (antiarrhythmic therapy)
  Doppler echocardiography (mitral inflow pattern)
  LV size, volumes, shape, and mass
Other markers; research tools
  Neurohormones: plasma norepinephrine, renin activity,
    aldosterone, atrial natriuretic factor
  Markers of autonomic dysfunction (heart rate variability)
  Signal-averaged ECG
  Endomyocardial biopsy

NYHA = New York Heart Association.

ily should be referred to appropriate support groups and community organizations (e.g., American Heart Association).

Patients should weigh themselves daily and record the results. Because a few pounds may be important, it is important to standardize the method of weighing. It is recommended that the patient be weighed in the morning after awakening, after urinating, but before eating. Although the significance of change in weight is related to "baseline" body mass, a change of 3 to 5 pounds is generally sufficient to merit a call to the primary care provider. Well-educated and compliant patients and their families may adjust the diuretic dosage at home based on daily weights. However, frequent adjustments in diuretic dosage require more frequent monitoring of electrolytes, especially potassium and magnesium.

Every effort is made to get smoking patients to stop. There are few things, if any, more dangerous to patients with HF. Community organizations [American Heart Association (AHA), American Cancer Society (ACS), American Lung Association (ALA)] may be helpful in this regard. HF patients are prime targets for pulmonary infections and therefore should receive appropriate immunizations against influenza and pneumococcus.

Sharing the prognosis with the patient and family is a difficult but necessary task of the primary care provider. It is made more difficult by the imprecision inherent in such a process, particularly when the underlying etiology may be unknown or other conditions affect the patient's health. Still, patients and their families deserve this information so they may plan their lives accordingly. Patients should be advised to create advance directives.

Activity/Exercise

Regular moderate, symptom-limited aerobic exercise may be safely recommended to all patients with stable NYHA class I to III HF; it may improve functional capacity and quality of life and diminish symptoms. Concerns about sexual activity must be fully explored, as patients are unlikely to initiate conversation on this matter. Patients with stable NYHA class I to III HF may engage safely in sexual activity, although practices may have to be altered to accommodate patients with diminished exercise tolerance. Although no specific training or cardiac rehabilitation program can be routinely recommended, such programs may be of benefit to certain patients, particularly those with concerns about exercising and those with concomitant CAD. An observed maximal stress test is often useful to objectively document exercise capacity and provide the patient with reassurance that the resulting exercise prescription (roughly to 60% of maximum) is safe.

Diet

All patients should be placed on a 3-g sodium diet, which is palatable, inexpensive, and achievable for most patients. Patients with continued congestive symptoms or fluid retention on high doses of diuretics may require a 2-g or even 1-g sodium diet, though these are much less palatable and compliance is more difficult to obtain. Low-fat diets must be considered with caution, as many patients with HF are elderly and subject to malnutrition. A vitamin supplement may be reasonable, especially if the patient is at risk for loss of water-soluble vitamins because of diuretics. Alcohol, an agent known to be cardiotoxic and capable of acutely depressing myocardial contractility and causing arrhythmias, should be avoided altogether. If the patient is unwilling to stop, ingestion of more than one drink (total of 1 ounce of alcohol) daily should be strongly discouraged. Because of the critical importance of diet in the successful management of HF, it is recommended that the patient and spouse be referred to a health care professional, such as a dietitian for counseling. Nonsteroidal antiinflammatory drugs, both prescription and over the counter (OTC), should be avoided because of the high risk of renal injury (especially in diabetics and those with underlying renal insufficiency) and decompensation of HF.

Compliance with Treatment

Compliance is the cornerstone of treatment of HF. Excellent compliance with the treatment plan should result in improved quality of life, alleviation of symptoms, lower mortality, decreased emergency room visits and hospitalizations, and much lower cost of care. Research shows that patients are noncompliant because of one or more of the following factors: (1) failure to understand the treatment plan, (2) disbelief that the treatment plan can be effective, (3) forgetfulness, and (4) constraints upon following the treatment plan (e.g., financial). During the period following diagnosis, frequent office visits are necessary to titrate medications, reinforce teaching and treatment, and assess side effects.

Patients should know their drug regimen, including drug name, dosage, and method of taking it. Patients should bring all their drugs, including OTC drugs, to the office visit with the primary care provider immediately after hospitalizations, changes in the regimen, and at intervals throughout the year. Patients should also have a written record of their current drug regimen at home and on their person. Home health services or family support may be necessary for patients with memory problems or other intellectual deficits, as well as for those who are blind or frail or have other major physical limitations. A home care evaluation by knowledgeable staff often yields clues to pitfalls to therapy in refractory patients. Compliance has been shown to improve when the patient and family are involved in the development of the treatment plan, feel fully informed about all aspects of the treatment, and experience open, helpful communication with all members of the treatment team.

A nurse-directed, multidisciplinary outpatient intervention in elderly patients with HF has been shown to produce a significant reduction in hospitalizations, improved quality-of-life scores, and savings in health care costs of $460 per patient over 90 days compared to that for patients assigned to conventional care.[9] The intervention consists of intensive education about HF, dietary instruction by a dietitian, analysis and simplification of the drug regimen, and intensive follow-up through home care services and visits and calls from study team members.

Drugs
Vasodilators

Angiotensin-converting enzyme inhibitors (ACEIs) are the cornerstone of the pharmacologic management of systolic HF, and contemporary therapy of systolic HF mandates an ACEI unless contraindicated. Although the reason that ACEIs are more effective than other vasodilators in reducing HF mortality is not fully known, the Survival and Ventricular Enlargement Trial (SAVE),[10] Cooperative North Scandinavian Enalapril Survival Study (CONSENSUS),[11] Vasodilator-Heart Failure Trial-II (V-HeFT II),[12] and Studies of Left Ventricular Dysfunction (SOLVD)[13] trials demonstrated an approximate 20% reduction in mortality compared to placebo. ACEIs reduce afterload, improve neurohumoral abnormalities, improve symptoms and quality of life, and decrease hospitalizations. In the prevention arm of the SOLVD trials, it was further demonstrated that ACEIs delayed the onset of symptoms of HF and first hospitalization for HF in patients with clinically silent LV dysfunction.

The ACEIs are generally well tolerated. Side effects are infrequent and include rash, angioedema, cough, hypotension, hyperkalemia, and impaired renal function. Some of these side effects may be avoided by using specific angiotensin II receptor blockers (ARBs, e.g., losartan). The Evaluation of Losartan in the Elderly-2 (ELITE-2) trial[14] directly compared the use of ACEIs and ARBs on mortality in chronic heart failure in elderly patients with systolic LV dysfunction and found no significant difference. Because of the study population profile, extrapolation of these data to all subsets of patients is not advised. With the exception of patients who develop angioedema or allergic rash, ACEIs remain preferred therapy. Studies of the combined use of both ACEIs and ARBs in systolic HF are now ongoing. Preliminary results are of concern because of an increase in mortality when ACEIs and ARBs are used in combination with beta-blockers (discussed below). It is premature to recommend the combined use of ACEIs and ARBs at present.

Although a survival benefit in regard to HF has been demonstrated in clinical trials of ACEIs, it has not been translated into a survival benefit for the general HF population, largely because these drugs are underused or underdosed by primary care physicians, generally because of unfounded concerns about excessive blood pressure reduction. In the SOLVD trial, systolic blood pressure decreased by only 5 mm Hg, on average, and diastolic blood pressure by 4 mm Hg. Even in the CONSENSUS trial, which enrolled patients with NYHA class IV HF, only 5.5% of patients treated with enalapril were withdrawn because of symptomatic hypotension.

Therefore, all patients with HF should be offered a trial of ACEIs, except those with specific contraindications: (1) a history of allergy or intolerance to ACEIs; (2) a serum potassium level higher than 5.5 mEq/L that cannot be reduced by conventional means; or (3) symptomatic hypotension, even without ACEI treatment. Caution and careful monitoring are used for patients with systolic blood pressures less than 90 mm Hg and patients with a creatinine level above 3.0 mg/dL or a creatinine clearance less than 30 mL/min. Half the usual dosage of ACEI is given to patients with renal insufficiency, and renal function must be monitored frequently.

In stable patients who are not at high risk for symptomatic hypotension, ACEIs may be started as for the treatment of hypertension, with the dosage titrated upward every 2 to 4 weeks to a target dose equivalent to those used in the large-scale clinical trials of ACEIs for HF. Examples of target doses are captopril 50 mg tid and enalapril 10 mg bid. All ACEIs are believed to be equally effective for the treatment of HF, and a corresponding dosage of any other ACEI may be used.

Patients at high risk for symptomatic hypotension should be treated with a low dose of a short-acting ACEI (e.g., captopril 6.25 mg). It is reasonable to consider hospitalizing patients at especially high risk for hypotension, though most patients can be safely monitored in the outpatient setting. If the first dose is tolerated, the patient may be started on captopril 6.25 to 12.5 mg tid. If this dose is tolerated, the patient may be switched to an ACEI with qd or bid dosing intervals and slowly titrated up to the target dose. Patients with renal insufficiency or high risk for hypotension should initially be seen at least weekly and the serum creatinine and potassium levels monitored carefully. In the event of worsening renal function (increased serum creatinine of 0.5 mg/dL or more), hyperkalemia (5.5 mEq/L or higher), or symptomatic hypotension, the patient is reevaluated and the regimen modified. Excessive diuretic administration is a common reason for ACEI intolerance.

Beta-Blockers

Beta-blocker therapy should be added to standard therapy in all patients with NYHA class II or III systolic HF. There are insufficient data to make firm recommendations regarding the efficacy and risk/benefit ratio of treatment of patients with NYHA class I or IV HF with beta-blockers. There is strong evidence to support a mortality benefit and reduced hospitalizations with the use of carvedilol,[15] bisoprolol,[16] and metoprolol CR/XL[17] in patients with NYHA class II or III systolic HF. Unlike ACEIs and ARBs, beta-blockers do not exhibit a "class effect," so that the administration of such agents to patients with HF should be limited to the agents studied in clinical trials. Studies comparing the agents mentioned above are ongoing, but at presently convincing data do not support the use of one drug over another. Regardless of the choice of agent, similar recommendations can be made for the addition of beta-blockers to standard therapy. First, patients should be carefully assessed for clinical stability. Patients with worsening edema, dyspnea, or other manifestations of decompensating HF should be stabilized and should be stable for at least 1 week before beta-blockers are started. The dosage of beta-blockers should be individualized and patients must be closely monitored. Beta-blockers should be started at low dose and titrated upward no more frequently than every 2 weeks. When increasing the dosage, it is wise to give the new dose in the office and to observe the patient for at least 1 hour afterward for symptoms of dizziness or light-headedness or marked changes in vital signs. Patients who do manifest worsening HF should first have their other drugs (diuretics, ACEIs, etc.) adjusted to try to compensate, or the dose of beta-blocker decreased or discontinued. With careful management, most patients can tolerate beta-blocker therapy, even those whose HF may transiently decompensate while titrating therapy. The starting dose of carvedilol (Coreg) is 3.125 mg orally twice daily. If tolerated, the dose can be doubled every 2 weeks to a maximum of 25 mg twice daily for patients weighing less than 85 kg and 50 mg twice daily for those weighing 85 kg or more. The starting dose of metoprolol CR/XL is 25 mg orally daily for patients with NYHA class II and 12.5 mg daily for those with NYHA Class III. The dose is titrated upward every 2 weeks to a target dose of 200 mg daily. The starting dose of bisoprolol is 1.25 mg orally daily titrated upward in a similar manner to a maximum dose of 10 mg daily.

For patients unable to take ACEIs or ARBs, the currently accepted alternate regimen, for which a mortality benefit has been demonstrated at 1 and 3 years,[18] is the combination of hydralazine and isosorbide dinitrate. However, compared to ACEIs, this combination has a worse side-effect profile, and in clinical trials 18% to 33% of patients discontinued one or both agents. Headaches, palpitations, nasal congestion, and hypotension are the most common side effects. The two agents are started concurrently and slowly titrated upward. Isosorbide dinitrate is started at a dose of 10 mg tid and titrated to 40 mg tid. Hydralazine is started at a dose of 10 to 25 mg tid and titrated to 75 mg tid. The drugs are then titrated upward incrementally and no sooner than weekly. In the V-HeFT II trial,[12] which compared the hydralazine–isosorbide dinitrate regimen to enalapril in patients with HF, the average total daily doses were hydralazine 200 mg and isosorbide dinitrate 100 mg. It is unknown if lower dosages would be effective.

Digoxin

A number of studies have found digoxin to improve symptoms and functional status in patients with systolic HF[19]; yet two centuries after its first use in HF by Withering, its effect on mortality has only recently been determined. The National Heart, Lung and Blood Institute: Digitalis Investigation Group (NHLBI-DIG) study found no overall mortality benefit attributable to digoxin in systolic HF; however, a morbidity benefit was observed in that over an average follow-up period of 37 months there were 6% fewer hospitalizations for HF in the digoxin-treated group.[20] It is clear, also, that digoxin withdrawal precipitates clinical worsening and increases hospitalizations.[19]

Even among cardiologists there is debate about when to initiate digoxin in the clinical course of patients with systolic HF. Some clinicians routinely prescribe digoxin for all patients with LV systolic dysfunction (EF <40%). Others institute digoxin only if symptoms and functional status are not satisfactorily improved by ACEIs, beta-blockers, and diuretics. Most agree that digoxin should be prescribed for patients with severe HF and in HF patients with concurrent atrial fibrillation and a rapid ventricular response. The primary mechanism of action of digoxin for symptom alleviation in HF may not be its mild positive inotropic action but rather its vagotonic effects, which antagonize the sympathetic nervous system activation during HF.

Prior to instituting digoxin, the patient's serum electrolytes, blood urea nitrogen (BUN), and creatinine must be tested and a recent ECG reviewed. For stable patients in the outpatient setting, digoxin is started orally and loading doses are almost never required. In younger patients with normal renal function, a dose of 0.25 mg once daily may be prescribed. In elderly, small, or hypothyroid patients, start with 0.125 mg daily. For patients with renal insufficiency, consult one of the widely available nomograms to determine the digoxin dose. When digoxin levels have achieved steady state (approximately 1 week for patients with normal renal function and 3 weeks for those with renal insufficiency), determine the serum digoxin level and repeat the serum BUN, creatinine, and electrolytes. Also obtain and review the ECG.

After steady state has been reached and the patient is stable on a dose of digoxin that results in serum levels within the therapeutic range, it is usually not helpful to determine digoxin levels regularly. Many clinicians recommend checking the digoxin level annually, and it must be obtained if the patient (1) develops symptoms or signs of digoxin toxicity (nausea, mental status change, visual disturbance, ectopy); (2) suffers deterioration of cardiac status; (3) suffers deterioration of renal status; or (4) is prescribed a drug known to interact with digoxin (verapamil, quinidine, amiodarone, antibiotics, and anticholinergic agents).

Diuretics

Diuretic therapy is used only in patients with HF who demonstrate symptoms or signs of fluid volume overload ("congestive" heart failure). Diuretics improve the clinical status of patients with CHF by promoting renal excretion of so-dium and water, but they also activate the renin-angiotensin-aldosterone axis, potentiate the hypotensive effect of ACEIs, and may decrease cardiac output, especially in patients with diastolic dysfunction. While diuretics should not be used routinely in all patients with HF, most patients will require them during their clinical course.

Thiazide diuretics may be useful for mild CHF, but they are ineffective when the glomerular filtration rate (GFR) falls below 30 mL/min. Patients with moderate to severe CHF, a GFR less than 30 mL/min, or marked fluid volume overload should be given a loop diuretic such as furosemide, orally or intravenously, depending on the acuity of the clinical situation. Average oral starting doses of furosemide range from 10 to 40 mg. (Initial, target, and suggested maximal doses for most of the drugs commonly used in HF can be found in Table 5.5.)

Most patients respond to a single daily morning dose of diuretic. If a larger dose of diuretic is needed, increasing the morning dose rather than splitting the dose generally achieves a better diuresis. An alternative to increasing the dose of diuretic, especially when it has superseded the target dose, is to add a diuretic from a different class (e.g., addition of triamterene to the regimen of a patient taking furosemide).

Table 5.5. **Drugs Commonly Used for Chronic Heart Failure**

Drug	Initial dose (mg)	Target dose (mg)	Recommended maximum dose (mg)	Average wholesale price (AWP) for 100 tablets at average or target dose (generic used, when available)
Thiazide diuretics				
Hydrochlorothiazide	25 qd	As needed	50 qd	$7.74
Chlorthalidone	25 qd	As needed	50 qd	$18.40
Loop diuretics				
Furosemide	10–40 qd	As needed	240 bid	$14.30
Bumetanide	0.5–1.0 qd	As needed	10 qd	$75.18
Ethacrynic acid	50 qd	As needed	200 bid	$53.24
Thiazide-related diuretic				
Metolazone	2.5 (test dose)	As needed	10 qd	$93.18
Potassium-sparing diuretic				
Spironolactone	25 qd	As needed	100 bid	$45.94
Triamterene	50 qd	As needed	100 bid	$87.12
Amiloride	5 qd	As needed	40 qd	$47.57

ACE inhibitors				
Enalapril	2.5 bid	10 bid	20 bid	$107.22
Captopril	6.25–12.5 tid	50 tid	100 tid	$131.46
Lisinopril	5 qd	20 qd	40 qd	$108.29
Quinapril	5 bid	20 bid	20 bid	$95.99
Benazepril	10 qd	20 qd	40 qd	$90.01
Ramipril	2.5 qd	10 qd	20 qd	$131.45
Fosinopril	10 qd	20 qd	40 qd	$87.74
Beta blockers				
Bisoprolol	1.25 qd	10 qd		$131.10
Carvedilol	3.125 bid	25 bid		$163.21
Metoprolol succinate	12.5 qd	200 qd		$80.10

Source: Adapted from Konstam et al.[1]

Metolazone is a diuretic commonly reserved for patients with severe or refractory HF because of its potency. It must be used with great caution. A typical starting dose of metolazone is 2.5 mg once daily. The major side effects are similar to those of other diuretic agents: volume depletion, hypotension, hypokalemia, and hypomagnesemia. The combination of furosemide and metolazone is exceptionally potent and necessitates frequent monitoring of fluid status and serum electrolytes. Although there are no set rules for following serum potassium and magnesium levels, it seems reasonable to check levels when starting or changing the regimen of diuretics and ACEIs. Stable patients on diuretics should have the serum potassium measured every 3 to 6 months, but this suggestion is clearly a guideline and should not supplant clinical judgment. It must also be recalled that potassium is a predominantly intracellular cation, and that serum levels do not often accurately reflect intracellular stores. Therefore, clinicians should consider potassium supplementation in patients whose serum potassium falls below 4 mEq/dL. Potassium supplementation is undertaken with great caution in patients with renal insufficiency (including the elderly with a "normal" BUN and creatinine) and those on ACEIs or potassium-conserving diuretics. High-dose diuretic regimens also may cause excessive renal excretion of magnesium and calcium. It may be necessary to replace these nutrients as well.

The Randomized Aldactone Evaluation Study (RALES) Trial[21] demonstrated a mortality benefit in patients in NYHA class III or IV from spironolactone 25 mg orally daily. The study has not been duplicated and its results can be applied only to patients with moderate to severe systolic HF. Although little hyperkalemia was seen in the study, clinicians must be particularly concerned about this risk in general practice because the drug will generally be added to a regimen that already contains potassium-conserving drugs in patients with renal hypoperfusion. Candidates for spironolactone therapy should have NYHA class III or VI systolic HF, be normo-kalemic and have a creatinine less than 2.5 mg/dL. Strong consideration should be given to discontinuing supplemental potassium when spironolactone is added to the regimen. The serum potassium and sodium should be checked at weekly intervals until stable, frequently thereafter, and at any time there is a change in regimen or clinical status.

Anticoagulants

Although some clinicians have suggested the use of warfarin routinely in patients with HF, there is insufficient evidence to support such a recommendation at this time. As 60% to 75% of HF populations have concomitant CAD, antiplatelet therapy may be strongly indicated and empiric use of warfarin increases bleeding risk. HF patients with primary valvular disease, atrial fibrillation, pulmonary embolism or other systemic embolic event, or an LV thrombus should be anticoagulated to an international normalization ratio (INR) in the range of 2.0 to 3.0.

Pacemaker Therapy of Systolic Heart Failure

Increasingly it is becoming recognized that systolic heart failure is characterized by conduction system abnormalities and rhythm disturbances in addition to the well-known problems with myocardial contractility and neurohumoral imbalances. In some HF patients, conduction disturbances diminish cardiac output through reduced diastolic filling, abnormal wall motion and prolonged regurgitation through the mitral and tricuspid valves. Some studies have shown benefit from biventricular pacing in patients with significantly widened QRS complex on quality of life scores, exercise tolerance, and improvement in NYHA functional class.[22] At present, application of this therapy should be individualized. Ongoing studies will define the risks and benefits of this treatment, characterize the survival benefit, and identify those patients most likely to be helped by it.

Drug Management of Diastolic Heart Failure

Although some causes of diastolic dysfunction are irreversible (e.g., myocardial fibrosis), potentially reversible conditions are found in many patients. Therapies that reduce arterial blood pressure, diminish myocardial ischemia, and promote regression of LVH may reverse some of the diastolic abnormalities. Supraventricular arrhythmias are common and poorly tolerated, as tachycardia reduces LV filling time and further increases diastolic pressures.

Because of LV stiffness, patients with diastolic HF are sensitive to changes in LV end-diastolic volume. Diuretics are almost always necessary for congestive symptoms, but overly aggressive diuresis may reduce stroke volume and cardiac output. With hypertrophic cardiomyopathy (HCM), even a mild positive inotrope such as digoxin can worsen outflow tract obstruction. Beta-blockers and calcium channel blockers promote myocardial relaxation and are usually considered first-line agents for the treatment of diastolic HF. ACEIs have not been extensively studied for diastolic HF. However, because tissue-based ACE activity is upregulated in LVH secondary to pressure overload and because it, in turn, leads to reductions in LV relaxation, it is tempting to speculate that ACEIs may have a salutary effect on diastolic function at the level of the myocardium.[23]

Revascularization

Despite the widespread use of CABG and PTCA, few data exist on the efficacy of aggressive treatment of asymptomatic coronary arterial lesions in patients with HF; moreover, there are no randomized, controlled clinical trials that have evaluated outcomes of any procedure in patients with systolic LV dysfunction, other than transplantation for end-stage heart failure. Several cohort studies evaluating the effect of CABG have shown a survival benefit from CABG in patients with clinically symptomatic HF or severe systolic dysfunction and severe or activity-limiting angina.[24-26] Neither CABG nor PTCA has been proved to improve survival in HF patients without angina. Nonetheless, because of the high prevalence of CAD in patients with HF, the suspected high prevalence of "silent" ischemia in this population, and our increasing understanding of "hibernating" myocardium (nonfunctioning or hypofunctioning heart wall that is underperfused but viable), it is conceivable that detection and revascularization of stenotic coronary arteries may improve prognosis via the prevention of future MIs and the diminishing mortality due to HF (see Chapter 2).

Because of the uncertainty surrounding this issue and the high stakes involved, the Heart Failure Guideline Panel of the Agency for Health Care Policy and Research (AHCPR) has developed an algorithm to help patients and providers deal with this clinical situation.[1] These guidelines were devised in 1994, and updated recommendations are expected in 2001–2002 from the combined American College of Cardiology/American Heart Association Task Force and the Heart Failure Society of America. PTCA has not been shown to improve survival in patients with HF of any type, so CABG is considered the procedure of choice. The clinician and patient, though, must also use judgment when choosing a revascularization procedure. A patient may not be a candidate for revascularization if CABG or PTCA is not an acceptable procedure to the patient, anatomic or technical factors (e.g., prior chest irradiation, severe distal disease) jeopardize the likelihood of a successful result, severe comorbid diseases exist, or the ejection fraction is low (<20%).

Once a patient has been determined to be a candidate for revascularization, the HF guideline panel recommended that HF patients be categorized and offered evaluation and treatment as follows:

1. Heart failure patients with severe or activity-limiting angina, frequent episodes of pulmonary edema, or angina decubitus should be advised to undergo coronary arteriography as the first diagnostic modality, to be followed by CABG, if operable lesions are found (see Chapter 2). This group of patients is at greatest risk, has the highest likelihood of having treatable CAD, and is likely to receive the greatest benefit from revascularization.

2. Heart failure patients with mild angina or a history of MI should be advised to undergo a noninvasive test for myocardial ischemia as the first diagnostic modality. Appropriate tests include exercise or pharmacologic stress myocardial perfusion scintigraphy (e.g., thallium scanning), exercise or pharmacologic stress (dobutamine) echocardiography, or stress radionuclide angiocardiography. Patients with evidence of ischemic myocardium should be advised to undergo coronary angiography with revascularization to follow if operable lesions are discovered.

3. Heart failure patients without angina or a history of any manifestation of CAD are, along with their physicians, in a quandary. There are no data to support routine evaluation of this group for myocardial ischemia. The patient and physician should discuss this issue thoroughly and consider the presence of risk factors that make CAD likely or those that explain the patient's HF (e.g., alcoholism) by way of another etiology. If the patient and physician agree that it would be appropriate to screen for myocardial ischemia, the evaluation should begin with one of the noninvasive tests.

Patient Monitoring

Office Visit

The family physician inquires about changes in chronic symptoms or the development of new symptoms. Special attention is given to inquiring about dyspnea or fatigue on exertion, orthopnea, edema, and paroxysmal nocturnal dyspnea. At selected intervals the physician reviews all of the areas covered in the section on patient counseling, especially activity and functional ability, diet, medication regimen, and mental health issues. Patients should bring a record of daily weights to the office visit, and, if requested by the physician, all of their medications (prescription and OTC). Evidence of snoring, episodes of apnea or hypopnea, or other signs of sleep disturbance is sought from the patient and sleep partner.

In a study of 42 patients with stable, "optimally treated" HF, 45% were found to have a moderate to severe degree of sleep-disordered breathing, often associated with prolonged and severe hypoxemia.[27] Patients in whom sleep apnea-hypopnea is suspected are referred to a sleep disorder specialist.

The physical examination includes weight, vital signs, and assessment for edema, rales, or findings suggestive of pleural effusion, jugular venous distention, hepatomegaly, and hepatojugular reflux. A careful cardiac examination is performed with attention to changes in heart rate, cardiac impulse, murmurs and gallops, and especially a third heart sound (S_3). The use of the echocardiogram or any other noninvasive or invasive testing for the purposes of routinely monitoring a patient with HF is not recommended.

All of the data obtained from the history and physical examination at the time of the office visit are carefully considered and used to make appropriate changes, when necessary, in the patient's therapeutic regimen. It is believed that this careful outpatient clinical assessment and subsequent adjustment of therapy is critical for improving quality of life, decreasing mortality, maintaining functional status, and decreasing the frequency of hospital admissions for HF patients.

Exacerbations

Although HF patients and their physicians are disappointed and sometimes alarmed when an episode of clinical deterioration occurs, the occasion can also be used for education that may prevent future decompensations. The physician must search for intercurrent or comorbid diseases that may have caused the deterioration (e.g., thyroid disease, anemia, infection, sleep apnea, arrhythmias, MI, pulmonary embolism, cardiac valvular disease, renal insufficiency, hepatic dysfunction, diabetes, uncontrolled hypertension). The physician must also search for etiologies related to patient noncompliance (e.g., not taking medications or following diet, alcohol or illicit drug abuse) or iatrogenic or OTC drugs that either conserve sodium (nonsteroidal antiinflammatory drugs) or have negative cardiac inotropic effects (e.g., diltiazem, verapamil, beta-blockers, quinidine, disopyramide). Episodes of clinical deterioration in HF patients should not be accepted as part of the natural history of HF. Rather, a careful, thoughtful search for the etiology is almost always fruitful and provides important information that can be used to educate patient and physician alike and prevent future incidents of decompensation.

Prevention of HF

Primary Prevention

Family physicians practicing good preventive medicine and health promotion are already preventing HF. Hypertension and CAD are the two most commonly encountered antecedents of HF, and aggressive detection and treatment of hypertension and other treatable risk factors for CAD (smoking, dyslipidemia, obesity, inactivity, diabetes) can do much to prevent HF. Additionally, physicians must counsel their patients to drink alcohol in moderation (≤2 oz daily) or not at all and to abstain completely from the use of cocaine and other illicit drugs.

Some have made a strong case for routine screening for hemochromatosis,[28] but this recommendation has not been met with widespread enthusiasm. The issue is not addressed by the U.S. Preventive Services Task Force in the second edition of the *Guide to Clinical Preventive Services*.

Secondary Prevention

All patients found to have an EF of less than 40% should be treated with a "target dose" of an ACEI, unless contraindications exist. All patients who suffer a nonfatal MI (except those with small, uncomplicated, non–Q-wave inferior MIs and who have not previously had an MI) should have their EF measured noninvasively prior to discharge and within 6 to 12 months thereafter. If an ACEI was not initiated during periinfarction management, all those with an EF of less than 40% should be treated with target doses of an ACEI.

Future Therapy for Heart Failure

The morbidity and mortality related to the diagnosis of heart failure averages 10% annually despite treatment with ACE inhibitors. It approaches 40% to 50% annually for the most symptomatic patients. Surgical procedures such as cardio-myoplasty, implantation of ventricular assist devices, and cardiac transplantation are viable options for a few such patients. Pharmaceutical agents with additive survival benefit have been sought with great interest. Despite exhibiting great promise in early trials, a number of agents have been demonstrated to be ineffective or actually increase the mortality rate compared to placebo. The latter group includes oral milrinone, flosequinan, and vesnarinone, suggesting that chronic inotropic stimulation is disadvantageous in heart failure.

Refractory Chronic Heart Failure and the Heart Failure Specialist

Primary care providers should consider referral to a heart failure specialist or cardiologist to assist in case management when patients remain symptomatic (NYHA class III or IV) despite (or are intolerant of) "standard therapy." There are other specific indications for referral: when the presence or severity of heart failure is uncertain; patients with two or more hospitalizations or emergency room visits for heart failure within 6 months; patients with suspected acute myocarditis; heart failure with moderate to severe aortic or mitral regurgitation; patients with evidence of myocardial ischemia or potentially reversible myocardial dysfunction; and consideration of clinical trial participation.

Patients in whom cardiac transplantation might be considered during the next 1 or 2 years should be referred early, as serial assessment is invaluable to the transplant team for determining the tempo of disease progression. An "elective" transplant evaluation and the concomitant educational process typically is conducted over several weeks. Once the patient has been listed for transplantation, the wait for an appropriate donor organ may exceed 10 to 14 months, depending on the patient's blood type, body habitus, and other conditions. Urgent transplantation places the patient at increased risk of morbidity from renal or hepatic damage, a prolonged hospitalization and recovery phase, or death while awaiting surgery. Valuable relationships with members of the transplant team are also more difficult to develop in emergent situations.

References

1. Konstam M, Dracup K, Baker D, et al. Heart failure: evaluation and care of patients with left-ventricular systolic dysfunction. Clinical practice guideline no. 11. AHCPR publication no. 94-0612. Rockville, MD: Agency for Health Care Policy and Research, Public Health Service, U.S. Department of Health and Human Services, 1994.
2. Bonow RO, Udelson JE. Left ventricular diastolic dysfunction as a cause of congestive heart failure. Ann Intern Med 1992;117:502–10.
3. International Guidelines on CPR and ECC. Circulation 2000;102(suppl): 1–384.

4. Chakko CS, Woska D, Martinez H, et al. Clinical, radiographic, and hemodynamic correlations in chronic congestive heart failure: conflicting
results may lead to inappropriate care. Am J Med 1991;90:353–9.

5. Davie AP, Francis CM, Love MP, et al. Value of the electrocardiogram
in identifying heart failure due to left ventricular systolic dysfunction.
BMJ 1996;312:222–6.

6. Folland ED, Parisi AF, Moynihan PF, et al. Assessment of left-
ventricular ejection fraction and volumes by real-time, two-dimensional
echocardiography: a comparison of cineangiographic and radionuclide
techniques. Circulation 1979;60:760–6.

7. Talwar S, Downie PF, Ng LL, et al. Towards a blood test for heart failure: the potential use of circulating natriuretic peptides. Br J Clin Pharmacol 2000;50:15–20.

8. Urbano-Marquez A, Estruch R, Navarro-Lopez F, et al. The effects of
alcoholism on skeletal and cardiac muscle. N Engl J Med 1989;320:
409–15.

9. Rich MW, Beckham V, Wittenberg C, et al. A multidisciplinary intervention to prevent the readmission of elderly patients with congestive
heart failure. N Engl J Med 1995;333:1190–5.

10. Pfeffer MA, Braunwald E, Moyé LA, et al. Effect of captopril on mortality and morbidity in patients with left-ventricular dysfunction after
myocardial infarction: results of the survival and ventricular enlargement trial. N Engl J Med 1992;327:669–77.

11. CONSENSUS Trial Study Group. Effects of enalapril on mortality in
severe congestive heart failure. N Engl J Med 1987;316:1429–35.

12. Cohn JN, Johnson G, Ziesche S, et al. A comparison of enalapril with
hydralazine-isosorbide dinitrate in the treatment of chronic congestive
heart failure. N Engl J Med 1991;325:303–10.

13. SOLVD Investigators. Effect of enalapril on mortality and the development of heart failure in asymptomatic patients with reduced left-
ventricular ejection fractions. N Engl J Med 1992;327:685–91.

14. Pitt B, Poole-Wilson PA, Segal R, et al. Effect of losartan compared
with captopril on mortality in patients with symptomatic heart failure:
randomized trial—the Losartan Heart Failure Survival Study ELITE II.
Lancet 2000;355:1582–87.

15. Packer M, Bristow MR, Cohn JN, et al. The effect of carvedilol on morbidity and mortality in patients with chronic heart failure. N Engl J Med
1996;334:1349–55.

16. CIBIS-II Investigators and Committees. The Cardiac Insufficiency Bisoprolol Study II: a randomised trial. Lancet 1999;353:9–13.

17. Hjalmarson A, Goldstein S, Fagerberg B, et al. Effects of controlled-
release metoprolol on total mortality, hospitalizations, and well-being in
patients with heart failure. JAMA 2000;283:1295–302.

18. Cohn JN, Archibald DG, Ziesche S, et al. Effect of vasodilator therapy
on mortality in chronic congestive heart failure: results of a Veteran's
Administration Cooperative Study. N Engl J Med 1986;314:1547–52.

19. Packer M, Gheorghiade M, Young D, et al. Withdrawal of digoxin from
patients with chronic heart failure treated with angiotensin-converting-
enzyme inhibitors. N Engl J Med 1993;329:1–7.

20. The Digitalis Investigation Group. The effect of digoxin on mortality and morbidity in patients with heart failure. N Engl J Med 1997;336: 525–33.
21. Pitt B, Zannad F, Remme WJ, et al. The effect of spironolactone on morbidity and mortality in patients with severe heart failure. N Engl J Med 1999;341:709–17.
22. Bryce M, Spielman SR, Greenspan AM, et al. Evolving indications for permanent pacemakers. Ann Intern Med 2001;134:1130–41.
23. Katz AM. The cardiomyopathy of overload: an unnatural growth response in the hypertrophied heart. Ann Intern Med 1994;121:363–71.
24. Bounous EP, Mark DB, Pollock BG, et al. Surgical survival benefits for coronary disease patients with left-ventricular dysfunction. Circulation 1988;78(suppl I):151–7.
25. Coronary Artery Surgery Study (CASS) Principal Investigators and Associates. Coronary artery surgery study: a randomized trial of coronary artery bypass surgery: survival data. Circulation 1983;68:939–50.
26. Califf RM, Harrell FE Jr, Lee KL, et al. The evolution of medical and surgical therapy for coronary artery disease: a 15-year perspective. JAMA 1989;261:2077–86.
27. Javaheri S, Parker TJ, Wexler L, et al. Occult sleep-disordered breathing in stable congestive heart failure. Ann Intern Med 1995;122:487–92.
28. Edwards CQ, Kushner JP. Screening for hemochromatosis. N Engl J Med 1993;328:1616–20.

6
Dyslipidemias

Patrick E. McBride, Gail Underbakke, and James H. Stein

Dyslipidemias, which include lipoprotein overproduction or deficiencies, are primary disorders of lipoprotein metabolism or secondary disorders induced by behavioral or other metabolic causes. These disorders are a common clinical problem, with 25% to 30% of adults in the United States having total cholesterol (TChol) levels of 240 mg/dL or higher and over half having TChol levels exceeding 200 mg/dL.[1] The four major classes of lipoproteins include the triglyceride-rich particles—chylomicrons and very low density lipoprotein (VLDL)—and the cholesterol-rich particles—low-density lipoprotein (LDL) and high-density lipoprotein (HDL). Evidence from epidemiologic, pathologic, animal, genetic, and metabolic studies strongly support a causal relation between serum lipoprotein concentrations and atherosclerosis.[2]

Optimum and at-risk lipoprotein levels are shown in Table 6.1. These levels are based on population percentiles and a vast research base, but are still arbitrary because the associated risk is linear. Lipoproteins act synergistically with environmental and metabolic factors, e.g., smoking, diabetes mellitus (DM), obesity, and high blood pressure, to promote atherosclerosis and thrombosis.[1,3]

Treatment of dyslipidemias has been proven to reduce coronary heart disease (CHD) morbidity and mortality, and total mortality, in many primary and secondary prevention trials.[3-8] These studies and others have demonstrated that treatment of lipoprotein disorders leads to plaque stabilization, improved endothelial function, prevention of atherosclerotic lesion formation, and regression of existing plaques, reducing CHD symptoms and adverse clinical events.[5,7-10] The pa-

Table 6.1. **National Cholesterol Education Program Adult Treatment Panel III (ATP III) Classification of LDL, Total, and HDL Cholesterol, and Triglycerides (mg/dL)**

LDL-cholesterol—primary target of therapy	
<100	Optimal
100–129	Near optimal/above optimal
130–159	Borderline high
160–189	High
≥190	Very high
Total cholesterol	
<200	Desirable
200–239	Borderline high
≥240	High
HDL cholesterol	
<40	Low
≥60	High
Triglycerides	
<150	Normal
150–199	Borderline high
200–499	High
>499	Very high

HDL = high-density lipoprotein; LDL = low-density lipoprotein.

tients who benefit most from lipid treatment are those who have CHD or noncoronary atherosclerosis, genetic dyslipidemias, diabetes mellitus, or multiple risk factors, including multiple lipoprotein abnormalities.[3] The benefits of lipid therapy have been demonstrated in men and women, and in older patients.[4,5,11]

The National Cholesterol Education Program Adult Treatment Panel III (NCEP ATP III) guidelines recommend evaluation for underlying atherosclerosis and comprehensive risk assessment for all patients prior to determining lipoprotein goals.[3] LDL cholesterol (LDL-C) treatment goals are risk-stratified, using 10-year risk estimates derived from Framingham Heart Study data. CHD risk can be estimated using downloadable risk calculators (for desktop or handheld computers) and paper handouts available at *http://www.nhlbi.nih.gov/guidelines/cholesterol/index.htm*. A 10-year CHD risk >20% is termed a "CHD-risk equivalent," as this is the same CHD event risk as a person with known CHD. High-risk primary prevention patients, including those with diabetes mellitus or noncoronary atherosclerosis, and individuals with a 10-year CHD risk >20%, have the same lipoprotein goals as a person with CHD. Patients with a 10-year risk of 10% to 20% or <10% have higher LDL-C goals and are therefore not treated as aggressively (Table 6.2).

Table 6.2. LDL-Cholesterol Goals Plus Cutpoints for Initiating Lifestyle Changes or Medical Therapy

Patient risk group	LDL-C goal (mg/dL)	LDL-C level at which to start lifestyle changes (mg/dL)	LDL-C level at which to consider starting medical therapy (mg/dL)
CHD or CHD risk equivalent[a] (10-year risk >20%)	<100	≥100	≥130 (100–129; medical therapy optional)[b]
2+ risk factors (10-year risk ≤20%)	<130	≥130	≥130 (if 10-yr risk = 10–20%) ≥160 (if 10-yr risk = <10%)
0–1 risk factors[c]	<160	≥160	≥190 (160–189: medical therapy optional)

[a]A CHD risk equivalent is a condition that carries an absolute risk for developing new CHD equal to the risk for having recurrent CHD events in persons with established CHD.

[b]Some authorities recommend the use of LDL-lowering medications in this category if levels of <100 mg/dL cannot be achieved by lifestyle changes alone. Others prefer use of medications that primarily modify TGs and HDL, e.g., nicotinic acid or fibrate. Clinical judgment also may call for deferring medications for some patients in this subcategory.

[c]Almost all people with 0–1 risk factor have a 10-year risk <10%; thus, 10-year risk assessment in people with 0–1 risk factor is not necessary.

Note: Risk calculators can be downloaded for the office at www.nhlbi.nih.gov/guidelines/cholesterol/profmats.htm.

CHD = coronary heart disease; LDL-C = low-density lipoprotein cholesterol; TG = triglyceride.

The presence of multiple risk factors exponentially increases overall atherosclerotic risk. A clinical evaluation, including a personal and family history, nutritional evaluation, focused physical examination, assessment of potential secondary causes of the dyslipidemia, and confirmation of lipoprotein abnormalities, is essential to characterize overall risk, identify genetic and environmental influences on dyslipidemias, and to determine treatment.

Screening

Current recommendations are that all adults age 20 years and older and children from high-risk families have a fasting lipoprotein profile every 5 years.[3] If a patient presents to the clinic in nonfasting state, an acceptable alternative is to measure TChol and HDL cholesterol (HDL-C) levels, since these measures are reliable in nonfasting individuals and provide important information for an initial risk assessment. A fasting lipoprotein profile should be obtained if the patient has a TChol >200 or HDL-C <40 mg/dL, or a family history of premature CHD or dyslipidemia. Because people who have TChol less than 200 mg/dL may develop atherosclerosis due to low HDL-C, abnormalities of other lipoproteins, or multiple risk factors, a lipoprotein profile is necessary for a thorough risk evaluation for patients with atherosclerosis or risk factors.[1,3] Lipoprotein profile evaluation is especially important for individuals with a personal history of atherosclerosis, two or more CHD risk factors, a family history of dyslipidemia, or premature CHD in a first-degree relative (grandparent, parent, sibling, or child), or a TChol averaging greater than 200 mg/dL on two occasions. It is important to note that approximately 50% of CHD events occur in individuals with no family history of CHD,[12] so the entire risk factor history and laboratory profile should guide assessment and treatment.

Evidence indicates that HDL-C and LDL-C remain important risk factors past age 65, particularly in the presence of atherosclerosis.[11,13] Evaluation of older adults for dyslipidemia treatment is based on the individual's motivation, prognosis, comorbidities, and potential improvement in quality and quantity of life.[11,13]

Dyslipidemias include a variety of common primarily autosomal-dominant genetic disorders that are influenced by both genetic and environmental factors (e.g., lifestyle) and may affect multiple members of high-risk families.[12,14] The presence of a family history of premature atherosclerosis (prior to age 55–65 years old) requires a thorough screening evaluation of the patient and first-degree relatives due to the high incidence of dyslipidemias and other risk factors in these families. Children or adolescents in families with premature atherosclerosis or with dyslipidemias in parents, grandparents, and siblings should be screened in childhood for lipid disorders and other risk factors. Detailed guidelines are available for screening and treatment in children and adolescents.[15] Routine screening of all children remains controversial, but measurement and treatment is recommended for children from families with premature atherosclerosis or genetic cholesterol disorders.

Office cholesterol testing is practical and reliable owing to the availability of advanced testing equipment and national standardization programs. Patients who are acutely or chronically ill, including a recent myocardial infarction, surgery, a mild viral illness, and even those who are pregnant or have had significant weight loss, will have fluctuating lipoprotein levels and should not be tested until they are stabilized.[3] It takes approximately 3 months for cholesterol levels to return to baseline levels after a major illness. Proper phlebotomy technique, such as avoiding prolonged tourniquet time (>1 min), or "milking" the finger for a fingerstick, may also influence cholesterol measures. Biologic variation and standard measurement errors produce a 6% to 9% daily variance for TChol, making it important to average at least two cholesterol measures from different days prior to management decisions.

A TChol higher than 240 mg/dL, if LDL-C is higher than 160 mg/dL, is associated with a marked increase in atherosclerotic risk and is called "high blood cholesterol" for adults[1,3] (Table 6.1). A TChol of 200 to 239 mg/dL, with LDL-C 130 to 159 mg/dL, is considered "borderline" due to increasing risk in this range, particularly in the presence of other risk factors. A TChol of 200 mg/dL or more (with LDL-C >130 mg/dL) in children and adolescents (ages 2–19 years) is higher than the 90th percentile and is considered "high blood cholesterol," whereas a TChol of 170 to 199 mg/dL is considered a borderline elevation for children.[15]

Lipoprotein profiles must be done after a 12- to 14-hour fast because triglyceride (TG) measurements are variable in the nonfasting state. When TChol, TG, and HDL-C are measured, LDL-C can be estimated using the formula:

$$LDL\text{-}C = TChol - HDL\text{-}C - TG/5$$

Dividing clinical TG levels by 5 provides an estimate of VLDL-C cholesterol. These LDL-C calculations are not accurate if the TG exceeds 400 mg/dL.

A lipoprotein profile usually is sufficient to develop a clinical classification and treatment approach for dyslipidemias. Lipoprotein phenotyping to determine the specific biochemical abnormality, using the Fredrickson-Levy classification, may be useful to direct treatment when the TG level is more than 400 mg/dL. It is important to recognize that when TG is >400 mg/dL, the TChol, HDL-C, and LDL-C are much less accurate in most clinical laboratories, and should not be relied on for clinical decisions.

Secondary Causes of Abnormal Cholesterol Levels

The following secondary causes of dyslipidemias should be considered prior to extensive testing or treatment:

Uncontrolled diabetes mellitus
Obesity and the metabolic syndrome
Medications (steroids including estrogen, progesterone, prednisone, anabolic steroids, and others; beta-blockers, or *cis*-retinoic acid)
Obstructive liver disease
Nephrotic syndrome
Multiple myeloma
Hypothyroidism
Excess dietary alcohol, fat, or caloric intake

A directed medical history, nutrition history, thyroid-stimulating hormone (TSH) assay, and fasting chemistry survey (including glucose, liver enzymes, and creatinine) can rule out most of the common secondary causes of dyslipidemias. Hypothyroidism should be considered especially in an older patient or a patient with previously normal lipid levels who develops a sudden elevation of LDL-C or TG. Treatment of secondary causes usually results in a marked improvement, or normalization, of abnormal lipoprotein levels.

Dyslipidemia Classification

A practical system of dyslipidemia classification yields four categories based on clinical, genetic, and biochemical parameters, as listed in Table 6.3 and discussed below. This approach uses screening lipoprotein results and is compatible with the more complex Fredrickson-Levy system. Each of the four dyslipidemia categories has a specific therapeutic approach.

Table 6.3. **Classifications of Dyslipidemias**

Lipoprotein levels (mg/dL)	Fredrickson-Levy class	Genetic disorder
LDL-C elevated	IIA	Familial hypercholesterolemia (LDL >200)
LDL-C >130		Primary hypercholesterolemia (LDL 130–199)
TG <150		
HDL-C >40		
Triglycerides elevated	I, V	LPL deficiency
TG >500[a]		Apo C-III deficiency
LDL-C NA		Familial hypertriglyceridemia
HDL-C NA		
HDL-C decreased	—	Hypo-α-lipoproteinemia
HDL-C <40		
TG <150		
LDL-C <130		
Combined dyslipidemias	IIB, IV, III	Familial combined hyperlipidemia
LDL-C >130		Familial dysbetalipoproteinemia
TG >150		
HDL-C <40		

[a]LDL-C, HDL-C and Total cholesterol levels are not accurate when TG >500 mg/dL.

NA = not applicable.

Elevated LDL-C Cholesterol (LDL-C >130 mg/dL, TG <150 mg/dL)

Elevation of LDL-C, without an elevation of TG, is considered either primary or familial hypercholesterolemia. Familial hypercholesterolemia (FH) is a relatively common disorder caused by defects in the LDL receptor gene, with the heterozygous form affecting approximately 1 in 500 Americans and 1 in 200 French Canadians. FH is expressed during childhood and is autosomal dominant, with selective elevation of LDL-C (usually >220 mg/dL), and often extensor tendon thickening (primarily the Achilles tenderness) or xanthomas. Most individuals with isolated LDL-C elevations <200 mg/dL do not have FH and are considered to have primary hypercholesterolemia, likely due to multiple factors, including nutrition, obesity, and genetic factors.

Very High Triglyceride (TG >500 mg/dL)

Hypertriglyceridemias are elevations of either chylomicrons, intermediate-density lipoproteins (IDL), or VLDL. Because all of these forms of dyslipidemia result in elevated TG, lipoprotein electrophoresis (phenotyping) may be useful for distinguishing among these disorders (Table 6.3). Fasting TG levels over 1000 mg/dL can be due to genetic influences, or a combination of genetic predisposition and secondary causes, such as alcohol abuse, poorly controlled diabetes, obesity, renal disease, or corticosteroids in patients with an underlying moderate hypertriglyceridemia.[14,16]

Patients with TG levels over 1000 mg/dL have a relatively low risk of CHD, but have a high risk of associated pancreatitis (10–15% annually), most likely due to lipemia and subsequent hyperviscosity, which results in obstruction of the microvasculature in the pancreas.[17] The priority of medical therapy in these patients is the prevention of pancreatitis. It is important to note that TG levels drop precipitously during acute attacks, which may mask the etiology of this life-threatening condition. A careful family history, family lipid screening, and remeasurement of TG levels after recovery can identify hypertriglyceridemia as the cause of pancreatitis.

Combined Dyslipidemias (LDL-C >130 mg/dL, TG >150 mg/dL, HDL-C <40 mg/dL)

Combined dyslipidemia, a very common and important disorder, is found in a high percentage of patients who survive myocardial infarction or have coronary revascularization.[18] Combined dyslipidemias include abnormalities of several lipoproteins, usually elevated LDL-C and TG with low HDL-C. Family history will often include the presence of multiple first-degree family members with CHD. As these disorders may be polygenic, affected patients and family members often present with a variety of dyslipidemias, including approximately one third with elevated TG, one third with elevated LDL-C alone, and the rest with a combined dyslipidemia.[14] This disorder is not usually expressed until adulthood, although it is now identified in children due to the recent increase in childhood obesity in the U.S.

Although TG is not metabolically independent of other lipoproteins, research documenting increased atherosclero-sis risk while accounting for the interaction of TG, LDL-C, HDL-C, and other risk factors has led to the designation of TG as an independent CHD risk factor.[3,10] Moderate-range hypertriglyceridemia (TG 200–499 mg/dL) is usually associated with alteration of LDL and VLDL into highly atherogenic forms (small, dense particles), low HDL-C due to reduced HDL production, and altered HDL effectiveness in reverse cholesterol transport.[3,10]

Non-HDL cholesterol, equal to TChol − (HDL-C), can be used to monitor treatment of patients who have had an initial TG measurement of 200 to 499 mg/dL. The non–HDL-C estimate includes all of the atherogenic lipoproteins, and should be <30 points higher than the LDL-C goals. Therefore, for a patient with CHD or DM or for a patient with a 10-year risk greater than 20%, the non–HDL-C cholesterol goal is <130 mg/dL, and for a patient with a 10-year CHD risk of 10% to 20%, the non–HDL-C cholesterol goal is <160 mg/dL. Because only TChol and HDL-C are necessary, the non–HDL-C calculation does not require a fasting blood test, and the non–HDL-C value more accurately assesses risk in patients with TG of 200 to 499 mg/dL.[3]

The metabolic syndrome is a high-risk, common syndrome that resembles familial combined hyperlipidemia and frequently results in premature clinical manifestations. Previously called syndrome X or the insulin-resistance syndrome, this syndrome includes a combined dyslipidemia and metabolic abnormalities associated with central obesity and insulin resistance (glucose intolerance or type II DM, hypertension, and hyperuricemia). Specific measures that identify this syndrome are listed in Table 6.4. Patients with metabolic syndrome can be effectively detected in the office by measuring the waist circumference at the iliac crest (on exhalation). The lipoprotein profile common to the metabolic syndrome includes small, dense LDL particles, which are more easily oxidized and recognized by scavenger

Table 6.4. **Clinical Identification of the Metabolic Syndrome—Any Three of the Following:**

Risk factor	Defining level
Abdominal obesity[a]	Waist circumference
Men	>102 cm (>40 in)
Women	>88 cm (>35 in)
Triglycerides	≥150 mg/dL
HDL cholesterol	
Men	<40 mg/dL
Women	<50 mg/dL
Blood pressure	≥130/≥85 mm Hg
Fasting glucose	≥110 mg/dL

[a]Overweight and obesity are associated with insulin resistance and the metabolic syndrome. However, the presence of abdominal obesity is more highly correlated with the metabolic risk factors than is an elevated body mass index (BMI). Therefore, the simple measure of waist circumference is recommended to identify the body weight component of the metabolic syndrome.

macrophages, rather than the usual lipoprotein receptors, and therefore are more likely to cause atherosclerosis.[18]

In addition to the metabolic syndrome, other causes of combined dyslipidemias are a lack of physical activity, hypothyroidism, DM, alcohol abuse, nephrotic syndrome, and use of glucocorticoids. A rare subtype of the combined dyslipidemias, associated with premature CHD and peripheral arterial disease, is familial dysbetalipoproteinemia (type III). The type III disorder is characterized by elevations of both fasting TChol and TG levels (exceeding 300 mg/dL) and the presence of xanthomas. Lipoprotein electrophoresis is recommended when levels of both LDL-C and TG are very high because treatment recommendations differ from those for other combined dyslipidemias (see below).

Low HDL Cholesterol (HDL-C <40 mg/dL, TG <150 mg/dL)

HDL-C is an independent risk factor and is the most powerful predictor of premature CHD.[19] Low HDL-C is associated with genetic factors, male sex, hypertriglyceridemias, smoking, obesity, and a sedentary lifestyle. Familial hypoalphalipoproteinemia (low HDL-C) is a syndrome found in 7% to 10% of CHD patients less than age 60. This disorder is characterized by an HDL-C level of less than 40 mg/dL, a TG level less than 200 mg/dL, and an autosomal-dominant inheritance.[18] Many other genetic forms of HDL-C deficiency exist but are far less common. Medications, including beta-blockers (non-sympathomimetic), retinoids, progestins, and anabolic steroids can significantly lower HDL-C.

Nonpharmacologic Management of Dyslipidemias

Nutrition and Weight Management

Lifestyle changes are the cornerstone of any treatment program to modify serum lipids. The U.S. Dietary Guidelines and the Food Pyramid recommend food choices that will reduce the risk of heart disease in the general population, and form the foundation for diet guidelines to treat dyslipidemias.[20] Patients with dyslipidemias or a diagnosis of CHD should use the Food Pyramid as a guide, but further limit saturated fat to <7% of calories, and dietary cholesterol to <200 mg/day. See Table 6.5 for a summary of diet recommendations. Trans fat, created during hydrogenation of vegetable oils, raises LDL-C and may reduce HDL-C, so it should be limited by considering it part of the daily saturated fat intake. The major sources of trans fats in the American diet are commercial baked goods, fried foods, and stick margarines.[21] Weight management through caloric reduction and increased activity is encouraged if needed to achieve a body mass index (BMI) of <25. The addition of water-soluble (viscous) fibers and plant stanols/sterols (usually found in margarines) is encouraged if lipids are not normalized by a reduction of saturated fat and cholesterol. Because omega-3 fat found in fish lowers TG levels and is associated with a lower risk for CHD, consumption of two to three fish meals per week is recommended. Inclusion of soy protein is encouraged because it helps reduce LDL-C levels and has other health benefits.[22]

There is debate about the optimal fat content of the diet for the treatment of dyslipidemia. A diet very low in fat (<10% of calories) can reduce LDL-C, but may also reduce HDL-C and increase TG due to a higher carbohydrate content.[23] A Mediterranean-type diet (30–40% of calories as total fat, an emphasis on monounsaturated fat, and saturated fat limited to <7% of calories) can reduce LDL-C without decreasing HDL-C and increasing TG, but the higher fat intake may make calorie control and weight loss more difficult. Medical nutrition therapy in consultation with a registered dietitian is rec-

Table 6.5. Nutritional Recommendations

	AHA/NCEP general population[a]	AHA/NCEP dyslipidemia or CHD[b]	Very low fat diet	Mediterranean dietary pattern
Total fat (% of calories)	<30%	<30%	10%	30–40%
Saturated fat	<10%	<7%	—	7–10%
Monounsaturated fat	10–15%	10–15%	—	15–30%
Polyunsaturated fat	≤10%	≤10%	—	<10%
Carbohydrate	50–60%	50–60%	70–75%	40–55%
Protein	10–20%	10–20%	15–20%	15–20%
Cholesterol	<300 mg/day	<200 mg/day	5 mg/day	<200 mg/day

[a]American Heart Association/National Cholesterol Education Program guidelines for the general, healthy American population.

[b]AHA/NCEP guidelines for anyone with CHD, CHD risk equivalent, or dyslipidemia.

ommended to tailor guidelines and maximize the lipid response to diet.

Serum cholesterol reduction from diet modification varies significantly between individuals, but averages 10% to 15%.[3] Triglycerides are very responsive to diet change, weight loss, and exercise, while the main dietary influences on HDL-C are weight loss and the balance of fat and carbohydrate in the diet. Diet recommendations for dyslipidemia should be individualized based on the patient's lipid pattern, body weight, food preferences, and level of motivation.

Elevated LDL-C

Patients with familial hypercholesterolemia are less responsive to diet changes than those with other forms of hyper-cholesterolemia, but all patients with elevated TChol should reduce their intake of saturated fat, trans fat, and cholesterol, as they are the primary dietary elements that raise LDL-C.

Increased consumption of foods high in soluble (viscous) fiber may be beneficial for some patients with LDL-C elevations. The primary sources of water-soluble fiber are oats, barley, legumes (dried beans and peas), fruits, and some vegetables. Including 20 to 30 g of dietary fiber per day, of which 10 to 25 g is soluble, could result in an additional 5% to 15% reduction in TChol and LDL-C.[24] Fiber supplements (psyllium) may be recommended for patients who are not able to consume adequate fiber through their diet, but it is preferable to obtain fiber from food because of the additional nutrients provided by high-fiber foods. Plant stanols and sterols reduce the absorption of dietary cholesterol, and can reduce LDL-C by up to 15% when used in a dose of 2 to 3 g/day.[21] Stanols and sterols are currently marketed in margarines. To prevent weight gain, patients should take care to compensate for the extra calories that these products contain. Soy protein can reduce LDL-C levels in some people, especially when soy is substituted for foods higher in saturated fat and cholesterol. Studies indicate that 25 g of soy protein per day can reduce LDL-C by 5%.[24]

Very High Triglycerides

TG levels are influenced by the total amount of fat and carbohydrate consumed, but not by the type of fat. For patients with triglycerides between 150 and 500 mg/dL, emphasis is on weight reduction. Very low fat (and consequently higher carbohydrate) diets can lead to significant increases in serum triglycerides in some patients, usually those with the metabolic syndrome. For these patients, nutritional plans of no more than 30% fat with an emphasis on monounsaturated fat are recommended. Patients who do not experience increased TG with higher carbohydrate intakes achieve the best results on a diet containing 20% of calories as fat. Optimal therapy is determined on an individual basis and requires follow-up to allow adjustment. Limitation or avoidance of alcohol is recommended for patients with high TG, and limitation of concentrated sweets is recommended for patients with glucose intolerance and high TG.

A strict control of total fat to 10% of calories is recommended for the patient with very high TG (TG >500 mg/dL) to prevent pancreatitis. Because medium-chain triglycerides (MCTs) are directly absorbed into the portal vein and do not increase chylomicron production, MCT oil (obtained from a pharmacy) can be used by patients who are not overweight to make food more palatable and to provide adequate calories. Consultation with a registered dietitian is recommended to ensure that the very low fat diet is nutritionally adequate.

Combined Dyslipidemias

Patients with combined dyslipidemia and the metabolic syndrome should make weight control and regular exercise a priority, since these changes will have a favorable impact on all serum lipoproteins and the other risks often noted with this pattern (abdominal obesity, glucose intolerance, and hypertension). Patients do not have to reach goal weight to see benefits, since a 10% reduction in body weight is associated with up to a 30% reduction in abdominal obesity. Patients should attempt to reduce body weight by limiting total fat intake to 25% to 30% of calories and saturated fat to <7% of calories. Total carbohydrate intake should not exceed 60% of calories, with an emphasis on complex carbohydrates (whole grains, vegetables, legumes) rather than simple carbohydrates (sugars, sweetened drinks, desserts). Serving sizes of starchy foods (pasta, bread, rice, potatoes, etc.) should be monitored, since they can often be a source of excess calories and may raise TG due to their refined carbohydrate content. Alcohol restriction or avoidance is recommended for reduction of caloric intake and TG.

Low HDL-C

No specific foods or nutrients increase HDL-C levels, with the exception of ethanol. However, ethanol is addictive, myotoxic, raises blood pressure and TG levels, and has variable effects on subspecies of HDL-C.[25] Alcohol should not be recommended as a treatment for low HDL-C. Because HDL-C levels are reduced in patients who are overweight or who have the metabolic syndrome, the normalization of body weight through calorie restriction and increased exercise is the primary goal for patients with low HDL-C. HDL-C levels may also increase in response to a diet higher in monounsaturated fats (nuts, avocado, canola, or olive oil) or the omega-3 polyunsaturated fats found in fish. If fat intake is increased, the quantity of carbohydrate foods will need to be decreased in order to maintain a consistent calorie intake and prevent weight gain.

Other Nutritional CVD Benefits

Plant foods (fruits, vegetables, whole grains, legumes, nuts) contain nutrients and other chemicals that help reduce the risk of heart disease, stroke, and high blood pressure. Antioxidant nutrients can reduce lipoprotein atherogenicity by protecting LDL-C from oxidation but are best obtained by consuming foods containing these vitamins rather than by taking supplements.[26-28] Flavonoids and fish oils reduce platelet aggregation and may reduce inflammation and CHD events.[29] Adequate intake of folic acid (400 μg/day) can help prevent elevations of serum homocysteine, which increases the risk of CHD and stroke.[30] The identity, function, and safe doses of protective nutrients are not completely understood, so it is not possible to establish appropriate guidelines for supplement use. Until more information is available, reasonable amounts of these and other potentially beneficial nutrients can be obtained by consuming at least five servings of fruits and vegetables per day, at least six servings of grain products (with at least half being whole grain), soy or legumes several times per week, fish two to three times per week, and a handful of nuts several times per week.

The practical application of nutritional guidelines by patients and health care providers requires counseling for behavior change and translation of recommendations based on percentage of calories to actual food choices. Table 6.6 lists the daily total fat and saturated fat gram allowances at different calorie levels and fat recommendations. The five food categories listed in Table 6.7 account for more

Table 6.6. **Percentage of Calories as Fat Translated to Fat Grams**

Calorie intake	30% of calories (g)	10% of calories (g)	7% of calories (g)
1500	50	17	12
1800	60	20	14
2000	67	22	16
2400	80	27	19

Table 6.7. **Major Food Group Sources of Saturated Fat and Cholesterol**

Food group	Suggestions
Meats	Smaller portions (6–8 oz/day) Use lean meats, trim fat Broil, bake, or grill Include fish several times per week Plan some meatless meals using soy, dried beans, or peas
Dairy products	Use skim or low-fat products Use part-skim or low-fat cheeses as a meat substitute Substitute low-fat frozen desserts for ice cream
Eggs	Limit yolks to four per week Use egg whites or egg substitute when baking
Fats/oils	Use smaller amounts of all fats Substitute unsaturated fats like olive oil, canola oil, or soft margarine for butter, stick margarine, or shortening Use reduced-fat mayonnaise/salad dressings
Snacks/desserts	Substitute low-fat snack foods (pretzels, popcorn, fruit) for deep fried snacks Use smaller servings of desserts Substitute fruit for other desserts Eat small amounts of nuts or seeds several times per week

than 90% of the fat, saturated fat, and cholesterol consumed in the typical American diet.[31] Counseling for low-fat and low-cholesterol eating should focus on substitution in these five food categories because of their significant contribution to dietary fat, and on recommendations to increase the consumption of plant-based foods.

Exercise

Physical activity is associated with improvement in the lipoprotein profile, but results depend on baseline lifestyle habits, presence of obesity or diabetes, type of dyslipidemia, and the specific exercise program. Both endurance and resistance exercise are helpful in achieving weight reduction and in reducing triglycerides and raising HDL-C, but have little influence on LDL-C unless there is significant weight loss.[14] Daily physical activity increases the clearance of TG-rich lipoproteins and glucose, and is often moderately effective in treating hypertriglyceridemia and combined dyslipidemia. Exercise of moderate intensity, longer duration, and increased frequency appears to have more benefit for dyslipidemia and weight loss than higher intensity, less frequent activity.[14] However, both resistance and endurance activity will improve dyslipidemias, and any regular activity that the patient enjoys should be encouraged. A clear physician message about the importance of physical activity has a significant impact in increasing patient's physical activity.[32]

Smoking Cessation

Cigarette smoking is associated with a number of metabolic processes that affect lipoproteins, including increasing plasma free fatty acids, glucose, and VLDL-C, and lowering HDL-C. Smoking cessation is associated with an average increase in HDL-C of 6 to 8 mg/dL.[33]

Pharmacologic Management

Indications

The use of medications for cholesterol treatment should follow careful consideration and implementation of the nonphar-macologic methods discussed above. The following guidelines are general recommendations and cannot specifically address every clinical situation. Treatment recommendations do not replace the physician's clinical judgment in dealing with an individual patient. Treatment is individualized based on overall risk, pattern of dyslipidemia, and associated medical conditions. Other important factors include cost, prognosis, and patient motivation. Medication use is recommended for those at highest risk who fail to reach goal cholesterol levels after an adequate trial of lifestyle change (usually 3 to 6 months). Any recommendation for early pharmacologic treatment (with lifestyle changes) is focused on the highest risk individuals: those with prior CHD events or "CHD-risk equivalents" (patients with DM or multiple risk factors and a 10-year risk of CHD events >20%), and those with ge-netic lipid disorders (LDL-C >220, TG >1000, or HDL-C <30 mg/dL).[3]

The new NCEP ATP III guidelines use 10-year CHD risk estimates to stratify risk for primary prevention patients with two or more CHD risk factors into LDL-C treatment goal categories to guide treatment decisions (Table 6.2).[3] The risk estimate tools are simple and risk can be calculated using these tools in a minimal amount of time. Patients with one risk factor, or none, usually have a 10-year CHD risk of <10%, so they usually do not require risk calculations. Patients with a 10-year CHD risk of less than 10% have a recommended goal LDL-C of <160 mg/dL, while those with a 10-year risk of 10% to 20% have a goal LDL-C of <130 mg/dL. For patients with a 10-year CHD risk of greater than 20% ("CHD-risk equivalents") the LDL-C goal is <100 mg/dL, the same as for patients with known CHD, as the risk for future CHD is similar (Table 6.2).

Medications

The cholesterol-lowering medications are listed in Table 6.8. Given the limited choice of medications and their specificity, family physicians must be familiar with all these medication classes to effectively treat dyslipidemias. More detailed prescribing information and management principles are available through many current resources.[3,14,16] Some of the medications are expensive, but cost-effective therapy is possible with good working knowledge of the medications.[34]

Medications within each class listed in Table 6.8 have similar intraclass effects and side effects. However, if side effects occur, medications may be substituted within a class with caution, since pharmacokinetics vary. The statins primarily reduce LDL-C, but also moderately reduce TG and raise HDL. The bile acid resins primarily lower LDL-C, but may exacerbate TG elevations. Plant sterols and psyllium are food derivatives that lower LDL-C modestly, but this effect can be enhanced in combination with other medications. Niacin is effective for elevated TG and low HDL-C, but lowers LDL-C only at higher doses, and is somewhat limited by side effects. Gemfibrozil primarily reduces TG (and subsequently raises HDL-C), but may also raise LDL-C as TG is lowered. Fenofibrate (Tricor) is effective for TG, HDL-C, and LDL-C, but may also elevate LDL-C if the baseline TG is high (>300 mg/dL). Due to safety concerns raised in clinical trials, clofibrate (Atromid-S), also a fibrate, is limited to use for high-risk patients with hypertriglyceridemias who cannot take other fibrates or niacin.[14] Medications such as the statins and niacin have recently been shown to have effects beyond lipid-lowering, including antiinflammatory effects, that appear to contribute to their effectiveness in reducing CHD events.[35]

Medication Use for Specific Dyslipidemia Classification

The pattern of dyslipidemia dictates the appropriate choice of medication as discussed below and presented in Table 6.3 and Fig. 6.1.

Table 6.8. Cholesterol-Lowering Medications

Medication	Dose range	LDL reduction (%)	Cost	Side effects and special considerations
HMG-CoA reductase inhibitors (statins)[a]				
Atorvastatin (Lipitor)	10 mg qd min 80 mg qd max	35–38 50–60	$$$–$$$$	Note: this list is for all statins: Increased hepatic transaminases and other minor GI effects (2–3%) May continue if liver function tests (LFTs) are elevated but <2–3 times normal—remonitor Myalgias/arthralgias (2–3%)[b,c]
Fluvastatin (Lescol)	20 mg qhs min 40 mg bid or 80 mg XL max	20–25 35–38	$$+	[b,c]
Lovastatin	10 mg qhs min	25–30	$$–$$$$	[b,c]Lovastatin is now available as a generic medication
(Mevacor)	80 mg qhs or 40 mg bid max	35–40		
Pravastatin (Pravachol)	10 mg qhs min 40 mg qhs max	25–32 30–35	$$$–$$$$	[b]Note: Only statin without CYP450 metabolism; less interaction with other meds
Simvastatin (Zocor)	10 mg qhs min 80 mg qhs max	35–40% 45–50%	$$$–$$$$	[b,c]

(continued)

Table 6.8 (Continued).

Medication	Dose range	LDL reduction (%)	Cost	Side effects and special considerations
Bile acid sequestrants				Second line for LDL-C disorders Potent combination with statins
Colestipol (Colestid)	4–8 g bid–tid	10–25%	$$$–$$$$	May increase TG Bloating, constipation
Cholestyramine (Questran)	5–10 g bid–tid (start at a low dose)	TG may increase moderately	$$–$$$	Interferes with some medication and fat-soluble vitamin absorption
Colesevelam (Welchol)	6 capsules (3 capsules bid or 6 qd with meal)		$$$$	Colesevelam has less GI toxicity and may interference less with absorption of other medications
Psyllium	5–15 g bid–tid	0–10%	$	Bloating, diarrhea/constipation
Plant stanols or sterols (dietary supplement Benecol Take Control	3 tablespoons of margarine tid or used as salad dressing bid	8–15%	$–$$	Minimal to no side effects Weight gain may occur due to increased calorie intake
Niacin				
Niacin plain	500–1500 bid–tid (starting dose: 100 mg)	20–25%	$	Flushing, dry skin, rash Glucose intolerance Elevated uric acid

Extended release (Niaspan only SR-formulation recommended)	Extended release, 500–2000 mg qhs	Also: 50% TG decrease, 25% HDL-C increase	$$–$$$	Dyspepsia or ulcer; Caution with diabetes, gout, history of gastritis or peptic ulcer
Fibrates				
Gemfibrozil (Lopid)	600 mg bid	TG 50% decrease; HDL-C 5–20% increase; LDL-C 10% increase to 20% decrease	$$–$$$	Nausea; Myositis (2–6%) with statins and cyclosporine
Fenofibrate (Tricor)	67–201 mg qd			

[a] All statins have moderate TG lowering (15–40+%) and HDL raising (5–12%) effects.

[b] Increased myositis with gemfibrozil, and possibly fenofibrate and niacin.

[c] Cytochrome CYP450 metabolism with interaction with other medications that are metabolized there; may result in higher statin levels and possible myositis and/or rhabdomyolysis.

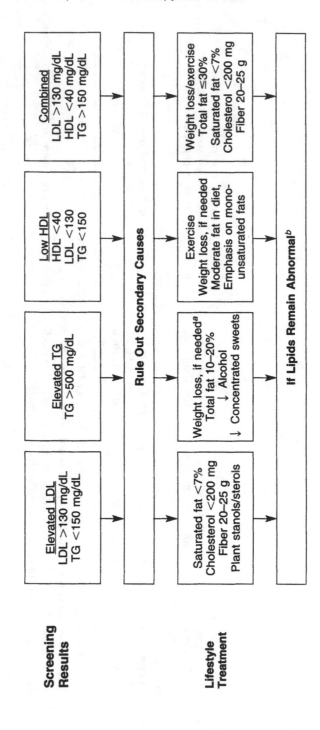

Screening Results

Elevated LDL	Elevated TG	Low HDL	Combined
LDL >130 mg/dL	TG >500 mg/dL	HDL <40	LDL >130 mg/dL
TG <150 mg/dL		LDL <130	HDL <40 mg/dL
		TG <150	TG >150 mg/dL

Rule Out Secondary Causes

Lifestyle Treatment

Saturated fat <7%	Weight loss, if needed[a]	Exercise	Weight loss/exercise
Cholesterol <200 mg	Total fat 10–20%	Weight loss, if needed	Total fat ≤30%
Fiber 20–25 g	↓ Alcohol	Moderate fat in diet,	Saturated fat <7%
Plant stanols/sterols	↓ Concentrated sweets	Emphasis on mono-	Cholesterol <200 mg
		unsaturated fats	Fiber 20–25 g

If Lipids Remain Abnormal[b]

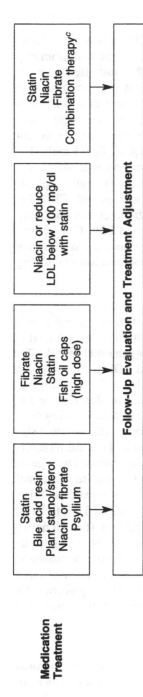

Statin	Fibrate	Niacin or reduce	Statin
Bile acid resin	Niacin	LDL below 100 mg/dl	Niacin
Plant stanol/sterol	Statin	with statin	Fibrate
Niacin or fibrate	Fish oil caps		Combination therapy[c]
Psyllium	(high dose)		

Follow-Up Evaluation and Treatment Adjustment

Medication Treatment

Fig. 6.1. Dyslipidemia treatment summary. [a]Exception: immediate medication (gemfibrozil or niacin) for patients with TG >1000 mg/dL due to high risk of pancreatitis, or LDL-C >220 mg/dL due to genetic basis, and resistance to nonpharmacologic treatment after ruling out secondary causes. [b]Notes: (1) Goal LDL-C <100 with CHD/noncoronary atherosclerosis; diabetes mellitus, 10-yr CHD-risk >20%; (2) goal LDL-C <130 if no known CHD or noncoronary atherosclerosis but high risk (LDL-C >160 mg/dL with two or more risk factors or LDL-C >190 mg/dL in isolation). [c]See text; statins and fibrates and/or niacin may be used in combination with close monitoring for hepatitis or myositis (risk of interaction 2–6%; cerivastatin should not be used in combination with a fibrate).

Elevated LDL-C

For isolated LDL-C elevations, or elevated LDL-C after TG is controlled with combined dyslipidemias, medications that primarily lower LDL-C are recommended. Statins are the most effective treatment. The bile acid resins, plant sterols, and psyllium are modest in efficacy (5–20% mean LDL-C reductions), but side effects are limited to the gastrointestinal tract. Niacin is a potent and inexpensive agent, especially in low-dose combination with bile acid resins, but high doses are generally required to lower LDL-C significantly. Estrogen may effectively reduce LDL-C in postmenopausal women but may also significantly exacerbate TG elevations. Hormone replacement therapy currently is contraindicated in women with CHD due to clinical trial evidence of increased thrombotic events, including CHD events, in three clinical trials.[3,36] Elevated LDL-C in combination with elevated HDL-C in older women is associated with only a modestly increased risk, and nutritional assessment and counseling may be adequate.

Hypertriglyceridemias

After secondary causes are evaluated and treated, niacin and gemfibrozil are the treatments of choice for TG >400 to 500 mg/dL. It is important to realize that when TG is greater than 400 mg/dL, TG usually must be controlled before TChol and LDL-C lowering can be successful. Fibrates are the treatment of choice for hypertriglyceridemia associated with diabetes, gout, gastritis, or ulcer disease due to the potential for niacin to exacerbate these conditions. However, patients with well-controlled diabetes may tolerate niacin without significant worsening of hyperglycemia. Caution and careful monitoring is still advised, however. Note that if TGs are reduced with gemfibrozil, often the LDL-C level rises and may require additional treatment. Fenofibrate will also be effective in these patients, but is more expensive. Omega-3 fish oil capsules (minimum 5.4 g DHA or EPA daily) also can lower TG safely and effectively (though not as effectively as niacin or the fibrates), but may cause abdominal bloating, belching, flatulence, or loose stools. Bile acid resins or estrogens may exacerbate TG elevations, and estrogens, progestins, and other steroids are contraindicated for patients with hypertriglyceridemia (TG >300–400 mg/dL) because they may significantly elevate TG and the high TG may lead to pancreatitis.

Combined Dyslipidemia

This pattern is commonly associated with the metabolic syndrome and premature CHD. The treatments of choice for this disorder are statins, niacin, gemfibrozil, and fenofibrate. Combined dyslipidemias are frequently associated with glucose intolerance and gout, which are relative contraindications to niacin use. Fibrates may be effective but are often limited by a variable response of LDL-C, so treatment may require fibrates in combination with psyllium, a bile acid resin, or a low-dose statin to reduce LDL-C effectively. Statins may be useful if TG levels are moderately elevated but may not be effective if the TG level is over 300 to 400 mg/dL. Patients put on oral contraceptives or hormone replacement therapy should have baseline lipoprotein screening and follow-up testing to ensure that triglycerides are not significantly elevated

Low HDL-C

The only medication that effectively raises isolated low HDL-C (<40 mg/dL) is niacin.[37] Isolated HDL-C deficiencies are slow to respond to treatment, if they respond at all. Patients with documented atherosclerosis or a high-risk family profile with low HDL-C may be candidates for a prolonged trial of low- to moderate-dose niacin (250–500 mg bid) to determine if HDL-C can be increased without significant side effects. Many studies demonstrate CHD event reduction by lowering LDL-C below target levels with statins when HDL-C cannot be raised.[4,5,7]

Combination Therapy

Combining medications to treat cholesterol may be effective when a single agent is insufficient, or to reduce the dosage and side effects of a single medication. Combinations of a statin or other medication that reduces lipoprotein production (i.e., niacin or fibrate) with a medication that reduces bile acid reabsorption (bile acid resin, a plant stanol or sterol, or psyllium) are synergistic in reducing LDL-C levels. Other statins can be combined with niacin or fibrates, but careful education of the patient about identifying and reporting myalgia symptoms is needed, as are more frequent follow-up visits (every 3 to 4 months) to monitor blood chemistry. Combinations of either gemfibrozil or niacin with fluvastatin, prava-statin, or simvastatin increases the risk of myositis to 1% to 2% and combinations with lovastatin increase myositis risk to 5% to 6%.

Monitoring Medications

Patients on medications should be monitored every 4 to 6 weeks to adjust medication doses and evaluate side effects until lipid goals are reached. Evaluations of liver function and the lipoprotein profile are appropriate monitoring tests. Levels of liver function tests such as alanine aminotransferase (ALT) or aspartate aminotransferase (AST) that are less than two to three times normal and that are not progressive can be tolerated with the use of cholesterol medications, especially the statins. More frequent monitoring is recommended for those with severe underlying clinical disease, with liver enzyme elevations or underlying liver disease, on combination cholesterol therapy, or taking other medications that could interact to cause drug-induced hepatitis. Most of the cholesterol medications are metabolized in the liver, with the exception of those that are not absorbed (e.g., resins, stanols, or sterols), and fibrates, which have mixed hepatic and renal metabolism. Due to frequent benign elevations of creatinine kinase (CK) that occur from physical activity, CK levels are only recommended if patients complain of generalized myalgias. When the lipoprotein levels reach treatment goals, monitoring every 4 to 6 months is appropriate to assess side effects and laboratory studies, and to verify diet and medication adherence. Since dyslipidemias are an asymptomatic condition, an initial visit 4 to 6 weeks after initiation of therapy provides an opportunity for valuable patient feedback on medication effectiveness. If patients do not get feedback within that time frame, there is a significant drop in medication adherence.[3]

References

1. American Heart Association. 2001 Heart and Stroke Statistical Update. Dallas, Texas: American Heart Association.
2. LaRosa JC, Hunninghake D, Bush D, et al. The cholesterol facts. A summary of the evidence relating dietary fats, serum cholesterol, and coronary heart disease. A joint statement by the American Heart Association and the National Heart, Lung, and Blood Institute. The Task Force on Cholesterol Issues, American Heart Association. Circulation 1990;81: 1721–33.
3. National Cholesterol Education Program (NCEP) Expert Panel (ATP III). Executive summary of the third report of the National Cholesterol Education Program (NCEP) expert panel on detection, evaluation and treatment of high blood cholesterol in adults (Adult Treatment Panel III). JAMA 2001;285:2486–97.
4. Downs JR, Clearfield M, Weis S. Primary prevention of acute coronary events with lovastatin in men and women with average cholesterol levels: results of AFCAPS/TexCAPS. JAMA 1998;279:1615–22.
5. Scandanavian Simvastatin Survival Study Group. Randomised trial of cholesterol lowering in 4444 patients with coronary heart disease. Lancet 1994;344:1383–9.
6. Shepherd J, Cobbe S, Ford I. Prevention of coronary heart disease with

pravastatin in men with hypercholesterolemia. West of Scotland Coronary Prevention Study Group. N Engl J Med 1995;333:1301–7.
7. Sacks FM, Pfeffer MA, Moye LA, et al. The effect of pravastatin on coronary events after myocardial infarction in patients with average cholesterol levels. Cholesterol and Recurrent Events (CARE) Trial investigators. N Engl J Med 1996;335:1001–9.
8. Lipid Research Clinics Coronary Primary Prevention Trial Results I. Reduction in incidence of coronary heart disease. JAMA 1984;251:351–64.
9. Superko HR, Krauss RM. Coronary artery disease regression. Convincing evidence for the benefit of aggressive lipoprotein management. Circulation 1994;90:1056–69.
10. Ferguson EE. Preventing, stopping, or reversing coronary artery disease—triglyceride-rich lipoproteins and associated lipoprotein and metabolic abnormalities: the need for recognition and treatment. Dis Mon 2000;46:421–503.
11. Carlsson CM, Carnes M, McBride PE, Stein JH. Managing dyslipidemia in older adults. J Am Geriatr Soc 1999;47:1458–65.
12. Williams RR, Hunt SC, Heiss G, et al. Usefulness of cardiovascular family history data for population-based preventive medicine and medical research (the Health Family Tree Study and the NHLBI Family Study). Am J Cardiol 2001;87:129–35.
13. Pacala JT. The relation of serum cholesterol to risk of coronary heart disease: implications for the elderly. J Am Board Fam Pract 1990;3: 271–82.
14. Oberman A, Kreisberg RA, Henkin Y. Principles and management of lipid disorders: a primary care approach. Baltimore: Williams & Wilkins, 1992.
15. National Cholesterol Education Program (NCEP) Expert Panel (ATP II). Highlights of the report of the expert panel on blood cholesterol levels in children and adolescents. Am Fam Physician 1992;45:2127–36.
16. Knopp RH. Drug treatment of lipid disorders. N Engl J Med 1999;341:498–511.
17. Brown WV, Ginsburg H. Classification and diagnosis of the hyperlipidemias. In Steinberg D, Olefsky JM, eds. Hypercholesteremia and atherosclerosis: pathogenesis and prevention. New York: Churchill Livingstone, 1987;143–68.
18. Genest J, Martin-Munley S, McNamara JR, Salem DN, Schaefer EJ. Frequency of genetic dyslipidemias in patients with premature coronary artery disease. Arteriosclerosis 1989;9:701A.
19. Boden WE. High-density lipoprotein cholesterol as an independent risk factor in cardiovascular disease: assessing the data from Framingham to the Veterans Affairs High-Density Lipoprotein Intervention Trial. Am J Cardiol 2000;86:19L–22L.
20. USDA and US Department of Health and Human Services. Dietary guidelines for Americans, 5th ed. Home and Garden bulletin no. 232. Washington, DC: DHHS, 2000.
21. Lichtenstein AH, Deckelbaum RJ. AHA Science Advisory. Stanol/sterol ester-containing foods and blood cholesterol levels. A statement for healthcare professionals from the Nutrition Committee of the Council

on Nutrition, Physical Activity, and Metabolism of the American Heart Association. Circulation 2001;103:1177–9.

22. Krauss RM, Ecked RH, Howard B, et al. AHA Dietary Guidelines: revision 2000: a statement for healthcare professionals from the Nutrition Committee of the American Heart Association. Circulation 2000;102:2284–99.

23. Grundy SM. The optimal ratio of fat-to-carbohydrate in the diet. Annu Rev Nutr 1999;19:325–41.

24. Jenkins DJ, Kendall CW, Vidgen E, et al. The effect on serum lipids and oxidized low-density lipoprotein of supplementing self-selected low-fat diets with soluble-fiber, soy, and vegetable protein foods. Metab Clin Exp 2000;49:67–72.

25. Pearson TA. Alcohol and heart disease. Circulation 1996;94:3023–5.

26. Tribble DL. Antioxidant consumption and risk of coronary heart disease: emphasis on vitamin C, vitamin E, and β-carotene. Circulation 1999;99:591–5.

27. Adams AK, Wermuth EO, McBride PE. Antioxidant vitamins and the prevention of coronary heart disease. Am Fam Physician 1999;60:895–904.

28. Jialal I, Abate N. Therapy and clinical trials. Curr Opin Lipidol 2000;11:93–7.

29. Stone NJ. The Gruppo Italiano per lo Studio della Sopravvivenza nel-l'Infarto Miocardio (GISSI)-Prevenzione Trial on fish oil and vitamin E supplementation in myocardial infarction survivors. Curr Cardiol Rep 2001;2:445–51.

30. Stein JH, McBride PE. Hyperhomocysteinemia and atherosclerotic vascular disease: pathophysiology, screening and treatment. Arch Intern Med 1998;158:1301–6.

31. Subar AF, Krebs-Smith SM, Cook A. Kahle LL. Dietary sources of nutrients among US adults, 1989 to 1991. J Am Diet Assoc 1998;98:537–47.

32. Ockene IS, Hebert JR, Ockene JK, Merriam PA, Hurley TG, Saperia GM. Effect of training and a structured office practice on physician-delivered nutrition counseling: the Worcester-Area Trial for Counseling in Hyperlipidemia (WATCH). Am J Prev Med 1996;12:252–8.

33. McBride PE. The health consequences of smoking. Cardiovascular diseases. Med Clin North Am 1992;76:333–53.

34. Jacobsen TA, Schein JR, Williamson A, Ballantyne CM. Maximizing the cost-effectiveness of lipid-lowering therapy. Arch Intern Med 1998;158:1977–89.

35. Ridker PM, Rifai N, Clearfield M. Measurement of C-reactive protein for the targeting of statin therapy in the primary prevention of acute coronary events. N Engl J Med 2001;344:1959–65.

36. Hulley S, Grady D, Bush T, et al. Randomized trial of estrogen plus progestin for secondary prevention of coronary heart disease in postmenopausal women. Heart and Estrogen/progestin Replacement Study (HERS) Research Group. JAMA 1998;280:605–13.

37. Martin-Jadraque R, Tato F, Mostaza JM, Vega GL, Grundy SM. Effectiveness of low-dose crystalline nicotinic acid in men with low high-density lipoprotein cholesterol levels. Arch Intern Med 1996;156:1081–8.

7
Venous Thromboembolism

*Glenn S. Rodriguez and
Thomas M. Schwartz*

Venous thromboembolism causes substantial disability and death. The incidence of deep venous thrombosis (DVT) is about 1 per 1000 person years. The most serious and potentially preventable complication, pulmonary embolus, kills an estimated 50,000 Americans each year.[1] Venous stasis secondary to chronic valvular incompetence, often a consequence of venous thrombosis, causes varying degrees of pain, edema, and ulceration. The changing demographic patterns, particularly the aging of society, are increasing the risk of venous thromboembolism and the importance of prevention. Recent identification of inherited defects causing thrombosis (inherited thrombophilias) allows improved prevention through identification of individuals at high risk. The knowledge and tools for effective prevention and treatment are available but currently underused.[2] Early identification, office-based diagnostic tests, safer treatments, and targeted education programs for physicians may offer the chance to reduce the incidence of venous thromboembolism and associated morbidity.

Pathophysiology

Virchow hypothesized three factors that predispose a person to venous thrombosis: a hypercoagulable state, injury to the vascular intima, and venous stasis. A century of research has verified this hypothesis. DVT is now understood to be a multifactorial disorder, involving a combination of genetic risk factors and acquired conditions.[3] Known genetic causes are present in 25% of unselected DVT cases and 63% of familial cases.[4] This percentage will probably increase as research identifies more genetic causes. Some conditions that predispose to thrombosis have both genetic and acquired components. Examples are elevated levels of factor VIII[5] and high plasma homocysteine levels. Stasis is the most common precipitating factor. Vascular injury is often the result of surgery or trauma.

A hypercoagulable state results from a disruption of the normal balance between the procoagulant system and the anticoagulant system. The natural anticoagulant system works to confine a beneficial thrombosis to the site of injury and prevent propagation. Major components of this system include antithrombin III, protein C, and protein S. Protein C is activated to the enzyme APC, which functions as a natural anticoagulant by inactivating procoagulant factors Va and VIIIa in the presence of protein S. Antithrombin III directly inhibits thrombin.

Modern molecular genetics is rapidly elucidating the prothrombotic mutations that contribute to hypercoagulable states. The anticoagulant system is impaired by the factor V Leiden mutation, and by deficiencies of proteins C and S and antithrombin. Raised plasma levels of prothrombin 20210A and factor VIII increase risk by accelerating the procoagulant system.

Epidemiology

Reliable incidence data for DVT are not available. Autopsy series show that DVT is often present when not clinically suspected, so hospital discharge diagnosis and death certificate data underestimate the true prevalence. Declining autopsy rates in the United States compound the problem. The best incidence data are from Malmö General Hospital in Sweden, which has maintained an autopsy rate greater than 75% since 1957. The incidence of DVT and fatal pulmonary embolism has been remarkably stable at 35%, representing 9% of all hospital deaths.[6] The Worcester DVT study, a regional survey of hospital discharge diagnoses, reported a diagnosis of DVT in 0.9% of all hospital discharges. The incidence rate increased exponentially with age, rising by a factor of approximately 200 between ages 20 and 80 years.[7] Studies using screening techniques to evaluate hospitalized patients identified surgery of the pelvis or lower extremity and anesthesia lasting more than 30 minutes as the highest risk events (see Chapter 1). More patients hospitalized for medical reasons experience an episode of DVT than did surgical patients because of the greater number of total admissions.

Table 7.1. **Prevalence of Risk Factors for Thrombosis**

Factor	General population[a]	Patients with thrombosis (%)
Genetic		
Factor V Leiden mutation (APC resistance)	~1 in 20	~20[b]
Prothrombin 20210A	~1 in 50	~6
Protein C deficiency	~1 in 300	~3
Protein S deficiency	~1 in 300	~1–2
Antithrombin deficiency	~1 in 3000	~1
Mixed (genetic and acquired components)		
High concentration factor VIII	1 in 10	25
Hyperhomocystinemia	1 in 20	10

[a]Varies significantly in different ethnic populations.

[b]Up to 60% in pregnant patients with deep venous thrombosis (DVT).

Table 7.1 lists the prevalence of risk factors for venous thrombosis.[3] The most common inherited thrombophilia is APC resistance caused by a point mutation producing an abnormal protein known as factor V Leiden. It is present in 5% of Caucasian Americans but has a much lower prevalence in other ethnic groups.[8,9] Women with the factor V Leiden mutation are at increased risk for DVT when taking oral contraceptives. The lifetime risk for DVT in factor V Leiden heterozygotes is approximately 10% and for homozygotes is >80%. Direct molecular genetic testing for the R506Q mutation in the factor V gene is available. Genetic testing can distinguish homozygotes and is the definitive test. The American College of Medical Genetics recommendations for who should be tested for factor V Leiden are listed in Table 7.2.[10] General population screening is not recommended.

Table 7.2. **American College of Medical Genetics (ACMG) Guidelines for Factor V Leiden Testing**

Testing is recommended for individuals who have:
    Any venous thrombosis and are <50 years of age
    Venous thrombosis in unusual sites
    Recurrent venous thrombosis at any age
    Venous thrombosis and a strong family history of thrombotic disease
    Venous thrombosis during pregnancy or in women taking oral contraceptives
    Relatives with venous thrombosis who are under age 50

Clinical Approach

A logical set of principles are basic to the structure of the clinical approach:

1. Venous thrombosis is common. Thrombosis results when an individual with an inherited predisposition to thrombosis suffers venous stasis or vascular injury. Testing to identify the causes of thrombophilia is important.
2. The location of the thrombus is important. The primary source (90%) of pulmonary emboli is the deep veins of the proximal lower extremities. Thrombi limited to the calf pose limited risk (<5%) of pulmonary embolism, but extension to proximal veins occurs.[11] This point is critical to the diagnostic approach outlined in this chapter.
3. Pulmonary embolism is not an independent disease but a complication of DVT. Pulmonary embolism is discussed in Chapter 86.
4. Pulmonary embolism kills quickly; 75% to 90% of those affected die within the first few hours. With limited opportunity for effective diagnosis and treatment, identification of high-risk individuals and primary prevention of DVT is the goal.

Prevention

The key to prevention of thromboembolism is physician recognition of patients at risk, vigorous use of effective treatment, and prophylactic regimens. Selection of appropriate treatments to prevent DVT is imperative whenever a hypercoagulable state is identified or when venous stasis or vascular injury is likely. The 1986 National Institutes of Health (NIH) Consensus Conference outlined such a strategy, and it has been updated.[12] Prophylactic regimens to prevent DVT are discussed in Chapter 57.

Clinical Risk Stratification

Evaluation of the patient with suspected DVT begins with a thorough history and physical examination. DVT occurs predominantly in patients with clinical risk factors. The limitations of physical examination to identify DVT are well known, but physical findings are useful when present. Table 7.3[13,16] lists clinical risk factors and findings that are associated with DVT. Formal clinical risk scoring systems

Table 7.3. **Clinical Risk Factors and Physical Findings Associated with Deep Venous Thrombosis (DVT)**

Risk factors	Physical findings
Active malignancy	Localized tenderness along distribution of deep veins
Recently bedridden	Unilateral pitting edema
Recent paralysis/paresis	Thigh or calf swelling >3 cm compared to the asymptomatic limb
Recent limb immobilization	Dilated superficial (nonvaricose) veins in symptomatic limb only
Trauma	Erythema in symptomatic limb only
Hospital or nursing home confinement	
Pregnancy/puerperium	
Strong family history of DVT	

have been developed to stratify patients with suspected first DVT into low, moderate and high-risk groups. Risk stratification then helps guide evaluation as described below, especially the need for follow-up evaluation if initial studies are negative.[13–16]

Diagnostic Tests

D-Dimer Assay

D-dimer, a degradation product of cross-linked fibrin, is released into the blood during fibrinolysis. D-dimer testing is highly sensitive, but has poor specificity in the diagnosis of DVT because many conditions can lead to elevated serum D-dimer levels.[17] It has been studied as an adjunctive test to help rule out DVT. There are several types of D-dimer assays currently available for clinical use, including enzyme-linked immunosorbent assay (ELISA), latex agglutination, and whole blood agglutination. ELISA testing is very accurate, but the conventional test takes at least several hours and may not be practical for clinical use. Several rapid ELISAs that can be run in less than an hour are now available and have sensitivity that is roughly equivalent to standard ELISA.[18] Latex agglutination assays are inexpensive and rapid, but lack sufficient sensitivity to be useful as screening tests.[19] Whole blood agglutination assays have several advantages. They require only a drop of blood, rather than plasma, and provide results in as little as 2 minutes. Their sensitivity is reported to be similar to that of ELISA.[20] Two studies suggest that DVT can be reliably ruled out in low-risk patients using formal risk stratification in whom whole blood agglutination assay D-dimer testing is negative.[15,16]

Ultrasonography/Duplex Scanning

Real-time compression ultrasonography has been demonstrated to be a reliable technique for noninvasive evaluation of proximal venous thrombosis.[21,22] With this technique the veins under evaluation are visualized and the ability to compress the vein with probe pressure measured. The technique is accurate for thrombi above the knee, with sensitivity and specificity reported to be more than 90% in most series. It is less useful for diagnosing thrombi below the knee. Real-time ultrasonography is widely available, but the reliability of the results may vary with the expertise of the technologist performing the study. Duplex scanning combines real-time ultrasonography with a pulsed Doppler study to diagnose DVT.[23] The reported sensitivity and specificity of this test ranges from 85% to 95%. It also is of limited value for diagnosing calf thrombi.

Duplex scanning should not be confused with a Doppler study. Doppler evaluation of the lower extremity requires only a small hand-held unit and does not use B-mode ultrasonography. It detects only venous occlusion, so significant mural thrombi may be missed. The test has poor sensitivity and no role as a definitive diagnostic test.

Contrast Venography

Contrast venography has long been considered the standard by which all other diagnostic tests for DVT are measured. Performed according to defined techniques, it is highly accurate and has the advantage of reliably diagnosing thrombosis below the knee.[24] Risks include phlebitis, contrast allergy, local extravasation of dye, and discomfort. The overall complication rate is 4%, and the risk of major complications due to a contrast reaction is 1%. Its main use currently is in the evaluation of high-risk patients with a negative compression ultrasound or for diagnosis of recurrent DVT.

Other Diagnostic Tests

Impedance plethysmography and radiofibrinogen scanning are other tests that have been used in the past for diagnosis of DVT. Because of the wide availability of compression ultrasonography, these tests are now rarely used.

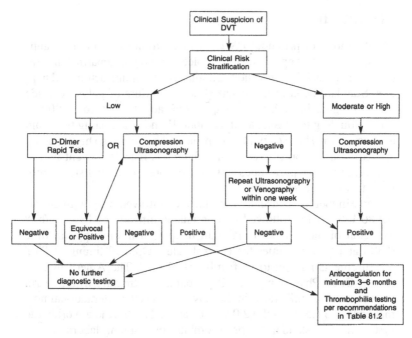

Fig. 7.1. Diagnostic approach to the patient with suspected lower extremity deep venous thrombosis (DVT).

Diagnostic Approach

Many diagnostic strategies for the evaluation of DVT have been proposed,[25] and the preferred strategy will likely change over time. Based on current data we propose the diagnostic approach outlined in Figure 7.1. Using this approach, the evaluation of the patient with suspected DVT should begin with clinical risk stratification. Existing formal scoring systems that allow rapid stratification of patients as low, moderate, or high risk have been clinically validated.[13,16] Moderate- and high-risk patients should promptly undergo compression ultrasound or duplex scanning. A negative study in these patients should be followed by either venography or repeat ultrasound within 1 week. Patients with low clinical risk may undergo D-dimer testing or immediate ultrasound. If D-dimer or ultrasound is negative, then further evaluation is not required. Patients with a positive D-dimer should have ultrasound. Patients with a positive ultrasound or venogram should be treated with anticoagulation.

Treatment

The diagnosis of proximal DVT requires prompt institution of anti-coagulation with heparin or low molecular weight heparin. The traditional approach is intravenous administration of unfractionated heparin. Standard heparin is a heterogeneous mixture of polysaccharide chains ranging in molecular weight from about 3,000 to 30,000. It acts by binding to plasma antithrombin III and inactivating thrombin and factor Xa. These enzymes are protected by fibrin, so higher doses are required to stop extension of a thrombus than to prevent its initial formation. Heparin does not directly prevent embolism or promote thrombus dissolution.

Heparin therapy is usually administered intravenously with an initial 80 U/kg bolus followed by continuous infusion of 18 U/kg/h.[26] The goal of therapy is to maintain the partial thromboplastin time (PTT) at 1.5 to 2.0 times the control value. Optimal timing of PTT measurements has yet to be firmly established. The American College of Chest Physicians (ACCP) recommends treating with heparin for 4 to 5 days, until warfarin therapy increases the international normalized ratio (INR) to the 2.0 to 3.0 range. The INR is a worldwide system used to standardize prothrombin times among laboratories.

The major complications of heparin therapy include hemorrhage, thrombocytopenia, osteoporosis, and anaphylaxis. The risk of hemorrhage increases with age, significant coexistent illness, and the presence of known bleeding sites. Platelet count should be checked daily to monitor for thrombocytopenia during heparin therapy. The effects of heparin can be terminated by intravenous injection of protamine sulfate.

Low molecular weight heparins (LMWHs) are fragments of standard heparin with mean molecular weights of 4000 to 6000. There are three LMWHs available in the United States: dalteparin, enoxaparin, and tinzaparin. LMWHs are theoretically superior to unfractionated heparin because of greater anticoagulant specificity (primary action on factor Xa), a more predictable anticoagulant response, fewer complications, and a longer plasma half-life.[27] Many studies have evaluated specific LMWHs for the treatment of DVT, and a meta-analysis concluded that LMWHs administered subcutaneously in fixed doses, adjusted for body weight, and without laboratory monitoring are more effective and safer than adjusted-dose standard heparin.[28] A Cochrane Database systematic review found LMWH to be at least as effective as heparin in preventing recurrent thromboembolism with lower risk of hemorrhage and lower overall mortality.[29] Although LMWHs are more expensive on a per-unit basis, they may lower the total cost of treatment per episode of DVT. LMWH should be continued for 4 to 5 days until the patient is therapeutic on warfarin with an INR of 2.0 to 3.0.[26]

Two studies have compared the safety and efficacy of subcutaneous LMWH administered at home with intravenous heparin in the hospital.[30,31] These studies demonstrated equivalent safety and efficacy. However, 30% to 60% of potentially eligible patients were excluded from the studies because of additional risk factors. A more recent study compared treatment of DVT with LMWH in hospital for 10 days vs. starting therapy at home.[32] There was no significant difference in outcome between the two groups; however, total costs for the home treatment group were 56% less than the costs for the hospital treatment group. Home-based treatment of DVT with LMWH is becoming more common. Effective protocols for home therapy with LMWH involve a multidisciplinary approach including the physician, pharmacy, and home health nurse. Contraindications to home treatment are listed in Table 7.4.[33]

After treatment with heparin or LMWH, anticoagulation is continued with warfarin. Warfarin should be started concurrently with heparin or LMWH. The duration of warfarin therapy is controversial.[34] The ACCP guideline gives the following recommendations regarding duration of anticoagulation: 3 to 6 months for DVT associated with transient known risk (e.g., surgery), >6 months for idiopathic DVT, and lifelong therapy for recurrent DVT or if associated with a persistent risk factor.[26] The dosage of warfarin is adjusted to maintain a prothrombin time approximately 1.5 times control or an INR of 2.0 to 3.0.[26]

Anticoagulation therapy carries substantial risk of hemorrhage. Warfarin has a narrow therapeutic ratio and is a major cause of pre-

Table 7.4. **Relative and Absolute Contraindications to Home Treatment of DVT**

Concurrent pulmonary embolism
Active bleeding or high clinical risk for bleeding
   Familial bleeding disorder
   Thrombocytopenia
   Severe liver disease
Hemodynamic instability
Limited cardiopulmonary reserve
Significant renal insufficiency
Pregnancy
Severe leg pain and swelling
Uncertain compliance or follow-up

ventable adverse drug reactions. Current recommendations suggest daily measurement of the prothrombin time during initiation of warfarin therapy. Once the INR is in the therapeutic range for two consecutive measurements, weekly monitoring is acceptable. The measurement interval can be extended to 2 to 4 weeks for patients on long-term anticoagulation with stable prothrombin times.[26,33] Optimal management of anticoagulation therapy requires a coordinated program of patient education, drug–drug and drug–food interaction detection, systematic adjustment of warfarin dosage based on prothrombin times, fail-safe systems to communicate the recommendations to patients, and implementation of a patient registry. Organized anticoagulation clinics are cost-effective and demonstrate superior outcomes.[35]

Thrombolytic therapy for DVT has been investigated because it theoretically could prevent postphlebitic syndrome by lysing the clot. It may be appropriate for selected patients with massive iliofemoral DVT. Unfortunately, studies of this therapy have shown a significant increase in major hemorrhage and it is not generally recommended for uncomplicated DVT.[33,36]

References

1. Silverstein MD, Heit JA, Mohr DN, Petterson TM, O'Fallon WM, Melton LJ. Trends in the incidence of deep vein thrombosis and pulmonary embolism: a 25-year population-based cohort study. Arch Intern Med 1998;158:585–93.
2. Anderson FA, Wheeler HB, Goldberg RJ, et al. Physician practices in the prevention of venous thromboembolism. Ann Intern Med 1991;115:591–5.
3. Rosendaal FR. Venous thrombosis: prevalence and interaction of risk factors. Haemostasis 1999;29(suppl S1):1–9.
4. Heijboer H, Brandjes DPM, Buller HR, Sturk A, ten Cate JW. Deficiencies of coagulation-inhibiting and fibrinolytic proteins in outpatients with deep-vein thrombosis. N Engl J Med 1990;323:1512–16.
5. Kyrle P, Minar E, Hirschl M, et al. High plasma levels of factor VIII and the risk of recurrent venous thromboembolism. N Engl J Med 2000;343:457–62.
6. Lindblad B, Sernby NH, Bergqvist D. Incidence of venous thromboembolism verified by necropsy over 30 years. BMJ 1991;302:709–11.
7. Anderson FA, Wheeler HB, Goldberg RJ, et al. A population-based perspective of the hospital incidence and case-fatality rates of deep vein thrombosis and pulmonary embolism. Arch Intern Med 1991;1512:933–8.
8. Ridker PM, Miletich UP, Hennekens CH, Buring JE. Ethnic distribution of factor V Leiden in 4047 men and women: implications for venous thromboembolism screening. JAMA 1997;227:1305–7.

9. Gregg JP, Yamane A, Grody WW. The prevalence of the factor V Leiden mutation in four distinct American ethnic populations. Am J Med Genet 1997;73:334–6.
10. Grody W, Griffen J, Taylor A, Korf B, Heit J. American college of medical genetics consensus statement on factor V Leiden mutation testing. Genet Med 2001;3(2)139–48.
11. Philbrick JT, Becker DM. Calf deep venous thrombosis: a wolf in sheep's clothing? Arch Intern Med 1988;148:2131–8.
12. Clagett GP, Anderson FA, Heit J, et al. Prevention of venous thromboembolism. Chest 1995;108:321S–34S.
13. Wells PS, Anderson DR, Bormanis J, et al. Value of assessment of pretest probability of deep-vein thrombosis in clinical management. Lancet 1997;350:1795–8.
14. Miron MJ, Perrier A, Bounameaux H. Clinical assessment of suspected deep vein thrombosis: comparison between a score and empirical assessment. J Intern Med 2000;247(2):249–54.
15. Kearon C, Ginsberg JS, Douketis J, et al. Management of suspected deep venous thrombosis in outpatients by using clinical assessment and D-dimer testing. Ann Intern Med 2001;135:108–11.
16. Lennox AF, Delis KT, Serunkuma S, et al. Combination of a clinical risk assessment score and rapid whole blood D-dimer testing in the diagnosis of deep vein thrombosis in symptomatic patients. J Vasc Surg 1999;30:794–804.
17. Brill-Edwards B, Lee A. D-dimer testing in the diagnosis of acute venous thromboembolism. Thromb Haemost 1999;82(2):688–94.
18. Lee AY, Ginsberg JS. Laboratory diagnosis of venous thromboembolism. Baillieres Clin Haematol 1998;11:1–18.
19. Becker DM, Philbrick JT, Bachhuber TL, Humphries JE. D-dimer testing and acute venous thromboembolism. A shortcut to accurate diagnosis? Arch Intern Med 1996;156:939–46.
20. Wells PS, Brill-Edwards P, Stevens P, et al. A novel and rapid whole-blood assay for D-dimer in patients with clinically suspected deep vein thrombosis. Circulation 1995;91:2184–7.
21. Perrier A, Desmarais S, Miron M, et al. Non-invasive diagnosis of venous thromboembolism in outpatients. Lancet 1999;353:190–5.
22. Cogo A, Lensing A, Koopman M, et al. Compression ultrasonography for diagnostic management of patients with clinically suspected deep vein thrombosis: prospective cohort study. BMJ 1998;316:17–20.
23. Langsfeld M, Hershey FB, Thorpe L, et al. Duplex B-mode imaging for the diagnosis of deep venous thrombosis. Arch Surg 1987;122:587–91.
24. Hull R, Hirsh J, Sackett DL, et al. Clinical validity of a negative venogram in patients with clinically suspected venous thrombosis. Circulation 1981;64:622–5.
25. Kearon C, Julian J, Math M, Newman T, Ginsberg J. Noninvasive diagnosis for deep venous thrombosis. Ann Intern Med 1998;128:663–77.
26. Hirsch J, Dalen J, Guyatt G. The sixth (2000) ACCP guideline for antithrombotic therapy for prevention and treatment of thrombosis. Chest 2001;119(suppl 1):1S–2S.
27. Schafer AI. Low-molecular-weight heparin—an opportunity for home treatment of venous thrombosis. N Engl J Med 1996;334:724–5.

28. Lensing AW, Prins MH, Davidson BL, et al. Treatment of deep venous thrombosis with low-molecular-weight heparins. Arch Intern Med 1995;155:601–7.
29. Schraibman IG, Milne AA, Royle EM. Home versus in-patient treatment for deep vein thrombosis. Cochrane Database of Systematic Reviews 2001;issue 2.
30. Levin M, Gent M, Hirsh J, et al. A comparison of low-molecular-weight heparin administered primarily at home with unfractionated heparin administered in the hospital for proximal deep-vein thrombosis. N Engl J Med 1996;334:677–81.
31. Koopman MMW, Prandoni P, Piovella F, et al. Treatment of venous thrombosis with intravenous unfractionated heparin administered in the hospital as compared with subcutaneous low-molecular-weight heparin administered at home. N Engl J Med 1996;334:682–7.
32. Boccalon H, Elias A, Chale J-J, Cadene A, Gabriel S. Clinical outcome and cost of hospital vs. home treatment of proximal deep vein thrombosis with a low-molecular-weight heparin. Arch Intern Med 2000;160: 1769–73.
33. Yacovella T, Alter M. Anticoagulation for venous thromboembolism. Postgrad Med 2000;108:43–54.
34. Hutten BA, Prins MH. Duration of treatment with vitamin K antagonists in symptomatic venous thromboembolism. Cochrane Database of Systematic Reviews 2001;issue 2.
35. Asell JE. The value of an anticoagulation management service. In: Managing oral anticoagulation therapy. Gaithersburg, MD: Aspen, 2000;1–6.
36. Sanson B-J, Buller H. Is there a role for thrombolytic therapy in venous thromboembolism? Haemostasis 1999;29(suppl 1):81–3.

8
Cerebrovascular Disease

Michael H. Bross and
David C. Campbell

Strokes are the third leading cause of death in the United States, claiming about 160,000 Americans yearly. Each year over 730,000 Americans have a new or recurrent stroke.[1] Two thirds of stroke survivors are impaired neurologically, with over four million Americans suffering from stroke impairments. These stroke survivors have a high risk of subsequent stroke, with about one third having another stroke within 5 years. The costs of strokes, including both medical care and lost productivity, have been estimated to be $30 billion annually.[2]

With the aging of our population, diseases that disproportionately affect the elderly will assume increasing importance. The incidence rate of first-ever stroke rises sharply with age, from 8.72 per 1000 person-years for individuals age 65 to 84 to 17.31 per 1000 person-years for persons 75 years and older.[3] Since women as a group live longer than men, it is not surprising that over 60% of the stroke deaths involve women.

African Americans have higher rates of both stroke incidence and stroke death, nearly double that for whites. African Americans also suffer from more severe impairments after strokes than other racial groups in the United States.[2] This high rate of strokes among African Americans has led to the southeastern United States being referred to as the "stroke belt."

Pathogenesis

Stroke occurs when there is disrupted blood flow to an area of the brain. The brain is perfused by anterior and posterior circulations. The anterior circulation begins with the carotid arteries and perfuses the anterior four fifths of the brain. The internal carotid arteries give off the ophthalmic branch before terminating at the circle of Willis, branching into the anterior and middle cerebral arteries. The posterior circulation supplies only one fifth of the brain and is derived from the vertebral arteries. The vertebral arteries first supply the cerebellum via the posterior inferior cerebellar arteries. The vertebral arteries then join to form the basilar artery. The basilar artery branches to form the posterior cerebral arteries that supply the occipital lobes.

Arterial and cardiac abnormalities[4] (Fig. 8.1) often develop and lead to ischemic stroke. The most common cause of ischemic stroke is atherosclerosis of large and small arteries. When atherosclerois of an arterial wall leads to thrombus formation, there is partial or com-

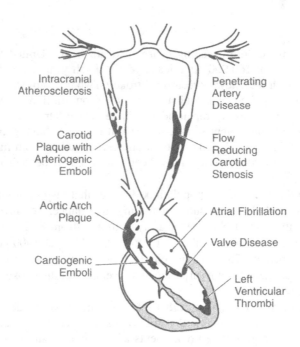

Intracranial
Atherosclerosis

Penetrating
Artery
Disease

Carotid
Plaque with
Arteriogenic
Emboli

Flow
Reducing
Carotid
Stenosis

Aortic Arch
Plaque

Atrial Fibrillation

Valve Disease

Cardiogenic
Emboli

Left
Ventricular
Thrombi

Fig. 8.1. The most frequent sites of arterial and cardiac abnormalities causing ischemic stroke. (From Albers GW, et al,[4] with permission.)

plete disruption of blood flow (thrombotic stroke). The thrombus may also dislodge and occlude a more distal artery (embolic stroke). Large artery pathology commonly occurs in the aortic arch, carotids, and major cerebral vessels. Small vessel atherosclerosis may involve intracranial or penetrating arteries, with more focal or limited brain injury occurring (lacunar stroke). The most common cardiac abnormalities leading to stroke are atrial fibrillation, valvular disease (especially mitral stenosis), and poor ejection fraction. These cardiac problems predispose to thrombus formation, with dislodged thrombi (emboli) occluding cerebral vessels. Less common causes of ischemic stroke include drug use, arterial dissection, fibromuscular dysplasia, arteritis, hypercoagulable states, and migraines.

Hemorrhagic strokes comprise approximately 20% of total strokes and are divided into intracerebral and subarachnoid types. Intracerebral hemorrhage is usually caused by hypertensive vascular disease, with bleeding most often into the putamen, thalamus, pons, or cerebellum. Subarachnoid hemorrhage (SAH) is typically the result of leaking from a saccular aneurysm, but may be secondary to an arteriovenous malformation or other vascular abnormality.

Risk Factors

Stroke risk factors[5] (Table 8.1) have tremendous impact and are often additive in any given patient. Although several risk factors cannot be modified, many of the risks are potentially controllable. Recognition of risk factors and implementing effective interventions will lessen the impact of strokes.

Age, gender, race, and family history as risk factors cannot be modified but are important to consider as the individual patient is treated. A patient at high risk for a potentially devastating disease (as a stroke) will warrant more aggressive preventive treatments. The risk of stroke doubles every 10 years after age 55, with the net result of eight times the risk of stroke by age 85. For similar age groupings, men have a 30% greater incidence of stroke than women. The high rate of strokes in African Americans may be secondary to higher rates of several risk factors, including hypertension, diabetes, smoking, poverty, and sickle cell anemia. A family history of stroke or transient ischemic attack (TIA) also increases stroke risk.

Several additional risk factors for stroke can be lessened with appropriate interventions. Smoking more than doubles the stroke risk as the result of accelerating atherosclerosis, raising blood pressure, and lowering arterial oxygen. In women, smoking cessation for 2 to

Table 8.1. **The Impact of Stroke Risk Factors**

Male gender	1.3× greater
African-American race	2× greater
Age 65 (vs. 55)	2× greater
Smoking	2× greater
Diabetes	3× greater
Carotid artery disease	3× greater
Peripheral vascular disease	3× greater
Age 75 (vs. 55)	4× greater
Left ventricular hypertrophy	4× greater
Previous heart surgery	4× greater
Atrial fibrillation	6× greater
Other heart disease	6× greater
Blood pressure >140/90	6× greater
Age 85 (vs. 55)	8× greater
Previous transient ischemic attack (TIA)	10× greater
Previous stroke	10× greater

Source: National Stroke Association. Stroke risk factors and their impact, 2001, with permission. Available at *www.stroke.org.*

4 years largely decreases the risk of stroke to that of nonsmokers.[6] In men, smoking cessation for 5 years markedly decreases the risk of stroke, but former heavy smokers remain at significant risk for stroke.[7] Cholesterol reduction with the statin drugs reduces stroke rate by almost 30%.[8] Diabetes triples the stroke risk, with accelerated atherosclerosis, hypertension, thrombosis, and hyperlipidemia. For the diabetic patient, tight control of diabetes and lowering low-density lipoprotein (LDL) cholesterol to <100 mg/dL are recommended.[9] In addition, diabetic patients have been found to have a 44% decrease in strokes with tight blood pressure control averaging 144/82.[10]

Carotid artery disease and peripheral vascular disease each triple the stroke risk. With known vascular disease, antiplatelet therapy with aspirin or ticlodipine (Ticlid) has been found to decrease nonfatal strokes by about one third.[11] A newer agent, clopidogrel (Plavix), has been shown to be slightly more effective than aspirin for stroke prevention in patients with vascular disease.[12] In addition, the combination of low-dose aspirin and sustained release dipyridamole (Aggrenox) has been found more effective than aspirin or dipyridamole alone.[13] The surgical treatment of asymptomatic carotid artery disease remains controversial. The Asymptomatic Carotid Atheroslerosis Study compared medical treatment to carotid endarterectomy for the treatment of patients with carotid artery stenosis of 60% or greater.

High-risk patients, with respect to surgical risk and projected 5-year survival, were excluded. The study found surgery patients have 5-year risk reduction for ipsilateral stroke of 66% for men and 7% for women. Women suffer higher perioperative complications than men. For surgical benefit to occur, the carotid endarterectomy must be performed with less than 3% perioperative morbidity and mortality.[14] A subsequent analysis of carotid endarterectomy surgery in Ohio found that higher-volume hospitals have a 71% reduction in risk for 30-day stroke or death compared to lower-volume hospitals.[15] The physician must therefore carefully present the risks and benefits of asymptomatic carotid artery surgery to each affected patient.

Hypertension affects over 50 million Americans and is recognized as the most important controllable risk factor. Since hypertension rarely causes symptoms, it is often untreated. Less than 30% of treated hypertensive patients have blood pressure less than 140/90.[16] A prolonged decrease in diastolic blood pressure of only 5 mm Hg has been found to decrease stroke risk by one third.[17] Treatment of isolated systolic blood pressure, 160 mm Hg or more, has been found to decrease nonfatal stroke by 44% in persons 60 and older.[18]

Cardiac disease increases the risk of stroke by several potential mechanisms. Although the direct effect of emboli from the heart is the most recognized risk, the coexistence of atherosclerosis in the heart and cerebral vasculature needs to be recognized. After myocardial infarction, the risk of stroke is estimated to be 8.1% over the following 5 years. Increasing age, lower ejection fraction, and absence of aspirin or anticoagulant treatment are risk factors for stroke. For every 5% decrease in ejection fraction, there is an 18% increase in the risk of stroke.[19] Atrial fibrillation markedly increases stroke risk, with the incidence of stroke averaging about 5% per year. Stroke risk with atrial fibrillation increases with the coexisting risk factors of increasing age, hypertension, diabetes, impaired left ventricular function, mitral stenosis, and a large left atrium. If feasible, cardioversion to a sinus rhythm is recommended. Oral anticoagulation with adjusted-dose warfarin (Coumadin) to achieve a target international normalized ratio (INR) of 2.0 to 3.0 reduces the stroke rate by two thirds for persistent atrial fibrillation.[20,21] It has been found that a combination of low-dose warfarin plus aspirin is not nearly as effective as adjusted-dose warfarin for the prevention of stroke.[22] In summary, atrial fibrillation patients over age 65 and atrial fibrillation patients with one or more additional risk factors (hypertension, diabetes, prior stroke or TIA, mitral stenosis, or impaired left ventricular function) should strongly be considered for warfarin therapy to achieve a target INR of 2.0 to 3.0. Aspirin or other antiplatelet therapy can be substituted for atrial fibrillation patients who cannot tolerate warfarin or are at low risk for stroke.[23]

Previous TIA and previous stroke confer very high risk for future stroke, and is discussed in the following sections.

Cerebrovascular Ischemia

Cerebrovascular ischemia leads to specific signs and symptoms that can help localize the site of brain involvement (Table 8.2). One of the most important factors is to determine whether the anterior or posterior circulation of the brain is involved. Compromise of the anterior cerebral artery leads to contralateral weakness and sensory loss, with the leg more involved. Since the frontal lobe is injured, judgment and insight are often impaired. Middle cerebral artery lesion

Table 8.2. **Common Clinical Findings with Vascular Lesions**

Anterior cerebral artery
  Contralateral paresis/paralysis/sensory deficits of leg greater than arm
  Confusion, impaired judgment and insight
  Primitive grasp and suck reflexes
  Gait disturbance
  Bowel/bladder incontinence

Middle cerebral artery
  Contralateral paresis/paralysis/sensory deficits of arm and face greater than leg
  Contralateral homonymous hemianopsia
  Speech and language disorder (aphasia) with dominant hemisphere involvement
  Contralateral visual neglect, contralateral sensory neglect, confusion, denial of deficit with nondominant hemisphere involvement

Posterior cerebral artery
  Contralateral homonymous hemianopsia
  Visual hallucinations and trouble recognizing objects (visual agnosia)

Vertebrobasilar artery system
  Diplopia, visual field deficits (homonymous and bilateral)
  Vertigo, syncope
  Dysarthria, dysphagia
  Ataxic gait/limbs
  Bilateral or alternating deficits (sensory and motor)

leads to contralateral weakness and sensory loss, with greater arm and facial involvement. Speech and language are commonly involved with the dominant hemisphere (usually the left hemisphere for right-handed persons). Nondominant hemisphere injuries from the middle cerebral artery commonly lead to symptoms of neglect (the patient does not recognize stimuli to one side of the body). Injury to the posterior circulation of the brain, or vertebrobasilar system, usually affects the brainstem, cerebellum, and occipital lobe. A combination of symptoms usually occurs, including diplopia, vertigo, dysarthria, dysphagia, ataxic gait/limbs, and bilateral or alternating deficits.

Transient Ischemic Attack

Transient ischemic attack is defined as a focal cerebral ischemic event that lasts less than 24 hours and leaves no residual neurologic deficit. The annual incidence rate of TIA, a key predictor of future stroke, rises sharply with age and is 41% of the annual stroke incidence rate.[24] The neurologic symptoms of a TIA usually occur suddenly, without warning, and peak within minutes. Most TIAs last less than 6 hours. A full range of neurologic symptoms (Table 8.2) can occur with TIAs, with common symptoms being unilateral weakness, aphasia, unilateral paresthesias, and partial or complete unilateral loss of vision. Vertebrobasilar symptoms include dysarthria, diplopia, ataxia, and vertigo. Hallucinations, tingling, scintillations, and rhythmic shaking of an extremity may occasionally occur and make the diagnosis more difficult. Extremely brief neurologic symptoms that last a few seconds and a sudden loss of consciousness without additional neurologic symptoms are seldom due to a TIA. The light-headedness associated with sudden change in position is most often due to postural hypotension.

If symptoms suggest a TIA, the physical examination and testing are focused to identify an etiology. Embolic fragments from diseased arteries or the heart are the most common etiologies. Arterial auscultation may reveal bruits in the carotid, aorta, renal, and iliac arteries. Other signs of advanced atherosclerosis may be found with arterial narrowing by funduscopic exam and loss of peripheral pulses. Duplex carotid ultrasound testing is a cost-effective way to screen for significant carotid artery disease, whether or not a carotid bruit is present.[25] Cardiac disease can be detected by listening for the murmur of mitral stenosis or aortic stenosis and the irregularly irregular rhythm of atrial fibrillation. Electrocardiogram readily confirms atrial fibrillation. Transthoracic two-dimensional echocardiography helps to reveal valvular disease and thrombi. Transesophageal echocardiography may be needed to detect small left atrial thrombi, a right to left shunt, and ascending aorta atherosclerosis.

Endarterectomy for symptomatic carotid stenosis is beneficial for patients with ipsilateral high-grade stenosis. The Medical Research Council (MRC) European Carotid Surgery Trial recommends surgery for stenosis 80% or greater.[26] The North American Symptomatic Carotid Endarterectomy Trial found definite benefit with surgery for 70% stenosis or greater and recommended consideration of surgery for 50% to 69% stenosis. To achieve operative benefit with 50% to 69% stenosis, very low endarterectomy risks of <3% for disabling stroke or death must be present.[27]

Chronic atrial fibrillation, mitral stenosis, and thrombi from myocardial injury are best managed with anticoagulation. Warfarin is used to achieve an INR of 2.0 to 3.0.

Ischemic Stroke

Initial Assessment

Symptoms that suggest stroke must be recognized quickly for effective treatment to occur. When blood supply to part of the brain is compromised, the brain tissue that is most directly affected will begin to die within minutes. The brain tissue surrounding the injured area will be hypoperfused. This area of poor perfusion has been termed "ischemic penumbra" and is at high risk for subsequent cellular death. If the stroke is allowed to progress without timely intervention, much of this ischemic penumbra will die and greatly increase the impact of the stroke.

The clinical presentation of a stroke depends on the site of vascular occlusion (Table 8.2). Sudden weakness, confusion, trouble speaking or understanding speech, trouble walking, and vision disturbances are common symptoms. In addition, a severe headache and a sudden decline in consciousness can also indicate stroke. It is important to teach potential patients and their family members to recognize these symptoms and immediately call 911 for timely intervention. Older patients, the highest risk group, are the least knowledgeable about stroke signs.[28]

The prehospital treatment of stroke is first focused on stabilizing airway, breathing, and circulation. Oxygen is administered and an intravenous saline infusion started. Since hypoglycemia can produce many neurologic symptoms, blood glucose is quickly checked. Glucose is given intravenously if hypoglycemia is confirmed. The emergency medical services system should be aware of which local hospitals are equipped to best handle acute stroke and transport to a well-prepared hospital if possible.

Once the patient arrives in the emergency department, pertinent history needs to be obtained. Discerning the time of stroke onset is crucial; information might be provided by any eyewitnesses as well as the patient. If the patient awakens with the symptoms of a stroke, it must be inferred that the symptoms began when the patient fell asleep. Additional key history items include recent trauma, recent signs of illness (temperature, pain, chills, etc.), drug use (alcohol, illicit), medical history, and medications.

Vital signs are checked repeatedly to detect any instability. Elevated blood pressure commonly occurs with an ischemic stroke and may be partially protective, helping perfuse borderline areas. Unless blood pressure consistently exceeds 220 mm Hg systolic or 120 mm Hg diastolic, it should not routinely be treated. Coexisting illnesses, such as myocardial infarction and heart failure, will require more aggressive treatment of blood pressure. In addition, blood pressure should be kept below 180 systolic and 110 diastolic if a thrombolytic agent has been given. Elevation of temperature has been found to be associated with more severe strokes and worse outcomes.[29] Although hypothermic treatment remains controversial, it is prudent to control temperature elevation if possible. The neurologic exam seeks to uncover the most likely site of brain injury, with brief repeated exams to detect changing neurologic status. Cardiovascular exam will detect atrial fibrillation, aortic and mitral murmurs, carotid bruits, and decreased or absent peripheral pulses. If a carotid bruit is heard on the side corresponding to the symptoms, moderate or severe stenosis is more than twice as likely to be present.[25] Ophthalmoscopy will detect signs of long-standing hypertension, chronic diabetes, increased intracranial pressure, and retinal emboli.

Initial diagnostic testing includes an electrocardiogram, pulse oximeter monitoring, complete blood count, prothrombin time (PT) with INR, partial thromboplastin time (PTT), serum electrolytes, glucose, blood urea nitrogen (BUN), and creatinine. Preparations are immediately begun for a non-contrast computed tomography (CT) of the brain. This emergent CT scan is primarily helpful in detecting any bleeding. In addition, local mass effect and ischemia may be seen and help determine the site of injury.

Thrombolytic Treatment

Rapid diagnosis and assessment of stroke is crucial to allow for timely thrombolytic treatment. If thrombolytic treatment with tissue-type plasminogen activator (t-PA) (Activase) is given within 3 hours of symptom onset, it has been shown that partial or total stroke recovery is 1.7 times more likely than in a placebo group.[30] Outcome measures at 3 and 12 months are significantly better.[30,31] In addition to treatment within 3 hours, other inclusion and exclusion criteria must be carefully noted[32] (Table 8.3). It is especially important to exclude bleeding with a CT scan before giving thrombolytic treatment. Since the majority of physicians have difficulty consistently identifying hemorrhage on a CT scan, enhanced training or telemedicine systems may be necessary to widely implement stroke thrombolysis.[33]

Thrombolytic therapy is given at a dose of 0.9 mg/kg, with a 10% bolus and the remainder over 1 hour. Aspirin and anticoagulants are not given for the first 24 hours. If the repeat CT scan at 24 hours shows no evidence of hemorrhage, aspirin or anticoagulants may be started. Blood pressure should be maintained below 180 mm Hg systolic and 110 diastolic. Even with these precautions, intracranial hemorrhage occurs in over 6% of patients with thrombolytic treatment.[30] If the patient exhibits any signs of hemorrhage, such as vomiting or intense headache, thrombolytics/anticoagulants should be held and a CT repeated immediately.

Treatment with intravenous thrombolysis should be limited to within 3 hours of symptom onset, since treatment at from 3 to 5 hours of symptom onset results in increased symptomatic intracranial hemorrhage and mortality.[34] Intraarterial thrombolysis may become more widely used in the future, as one study has found benefit with treatment up to 6 hours after symptom onset with intraarterial prourokinase for middle cerebral artery (MCA) occlusion.[35]

Additional Considerations

Most patients present with stroke after the therapeutic window for thrombolysis has passed. Close monitoring reveals any signs of deterioration. It is important to correct electrolyte disturbances, hypoglycemia and hyperglycemia, hypoxia, and volume disturbances. Patients need to be kept NPO until good swallowing reflexes can be demonstrated. A radiologic swallowing study is often necessary before oral feeding is resumed. The complications of immobility can be minimized with appropriate bedding, frequent turning, good nutrition, and early rehabilitation. Deep vein thrombosis (DVT) prophylaxis and aspiration precautions should be used.

Further evaluation is often necessary to determine the likely cause of the stroke and exclude other diagnoses. A magnetic resonance imaging (MRI) head scan with diffusion weighted imaging is very sensitive for ischemia and may demonstrate stroke even when conventional MRI and CT are negative. Carotid duplex ultrasonography

Table 8.3. **Inclusion and Exclusion Criteria for Intravenous Thrombolytic Therapy**

Inclusion criteria
  Ischemic stroke by clinical assessment
  Persistent neurologic deficit beyond an isolated sensory deficit or
    ataxia
  Cranial computed tomography (CT) negative for hemorrhage
  Initiation of treatment within 3 hours after symptom onset

Exclusion criteria
  Treatment initiated >3 hours after symptoms' onset
  Neurologic deficit is found to be rapidly improving, based on
    history or observation
  A patient whose CT scan shows hemorrhage or hemorrhagic
    transformation of an infarct; exercise caution because the risks
    associated with tissue-type plasminogen activator (t-PA) therapy
    increase in patients with major early infarct signs revealed by CT
    (e.g., substantial edema, mass effect, or midline shift); its use
    should be weighted against the anticipated benefit
  A patient taking oral anticoagulants or with prothrombin time (PT)
    >15 seconds
  A patient receiving heparin within the preceding 48 hours who has
    a prolonged partial thromboplastin time (PTT)
  A patient with platelet counts <100,000 per mm^3
  A patient with a pretreatment systolic blood pressure >184 mm Hg
    or diastolic pressure >110 mm Hg or if aggressive treatment is
    required to reduce blood pressure to the specified limits prior to
    thrombolytic therapy
  A patient who has had prior stroke or any serious head trauma in
    the preceding 3 months
  A patient who has had major surgery within the preceding 14 days
  A patient with prior intracranial hemorrhage
  A patient with gastrointestinal tract or urinary tract hemorrhage
    within the preceding 14 days
  A patient with seizure at the onset of the stroke
  A patient with symptoms suggestive of subarachnoid hemorrhage
  A patient with arterial puncture at a noncompressible site within
    the previous 7 days

Source: National Stroke Association. Stroke the first hours: guidelines for acute treatment, 2000, with permission. Available at *www.stroke. org.*

will reveal extracranial disease up to the angle of the jaw. MRI angiography may be used in conjunction with ultrasound studies to improve diagnostic sensitivity and specificity.[36] CT and MRI angiography are both effective for evaluation of intracranial vasculature.[37] Cerebral angiography and digital subtraction angiography (angiography using less contrast material) are invasive tests that may be indicated if surgery is being considered. A repeat CT scan with intravenous contrast is often necessary to exclude a tumor or abscess. If the posterior fossa portion of the brain is damaged, MRI provides better visualization than a CT scanning. Suspected central nervous system infection will require a lumbar puncture (after CT scanning). An electroencephalogram (EEG) is indicated if seizures are a consideration. Echocardiography is indicated if heart disease is present or suspected. Transesophageal echocardiography is often helpful to further clarify cardiac abnormalities, such as vegetations and thrombi.

A worsening clinical condition often prompts consideration of heparin therapy. Unfortunately, both intravenous low molecular weight heparin and subcutaneous heparin have failed to reduce recurrent strokes and increase hemorrhagic strokes.[38,39] If the stroke is the result of suspected emboli from atrial fibrillation or a poor ejection fraction, warfarin is recommended but only after the stroke has stabilized.

Early therapy with aspirin after an acute stroke has been shown to decrease future strokes and mortality, with no significant increase in hemorrhagic strokes.[39,40] Since aspirin dosing at 81 or 325 mg daily is more effective than higher doses, a practical approach is to administer one adult aspirin (325 mg) daily.[41]

Hemorrhagic Stroke

Subarachnoid Hemorrhage

A subarachnoid hemorrhage is usually the result of leaking from a ruptured saccular or "berry" aneurysm. An aneurysm forms when there is a weakness, either congenitally or acquired, at an arterial bifurcation. The classic location of these aneurysms is in the circle of Willis. Arteriovenous malformations (AVMs) account for most of the remaining cases of SAH.

Clinically the patient has sudden onset of a severe headache, often described as "the worst headache of my life" or a "thunderclap headache." Nausea, vomiting, photophobia, and meningismus are characteristic. Focal neurologic symptoms, such as ptosis or diplopia, may result from cranial nerve compression. The patient will often lapse into a coma as intracranial pressure rises abruptly.

In some patients, a small leaking from the aneurysm may occur before a catastrophic rupture. This "sentinel leak" characteristically causes severe headache, nausea, and vomiting, and may be mistaken for a migraine headache. Nuccal rigidity may or may not be present. The physician is cautioned to consider a sentinel leak whenever a patient develops a new headache that is excruciating or a different type of headache than ever before.

Diagnosis of SAH can be made by CT scan in about 90% of patients by finding blood in the basal cisterns. If the CT scan does not show blood and there is no impending herniation, a lumbar puncture should be performed to reveal cerebrospinal fluid (CSF) blood. A traumatic tap can usually be separated from a SAH, since the blood clears from a traumatic tap by the third tube of CSF. A tube of CSF should be centrifuged immediately to detect xanthochromia (from an earlier bleed).

Once SAH is diagnosed, immediate neurosurgical consultation is recommended. For surgical candidates, cerebral angiography is used to determine the site and size of the bleeding. The timing of angiography and surgery are best determined by the neurosurgeon. Early clipping of a ruptured aneurysm prevents further bleeding but has high mortality if vasospasm has begun. Vasospasm occurs in most SAH patients and produces strokelike symptoms. Nimodipine, a calcium channel blocker, decreases morbidity and mortality from SAH.[42]

Intracerebral Hemorrhage

Intracerebral hemorrhage typically occurs with activity. There is a sudden onset of severe headache, nausea, and vomiting. Focal neurologic deficits, seizures, and mental status changes are common. Blood may extend into the ventricles and subarachnoid space, causing nuccal rigidity. With extensive hemorrhage, patients will lapse into coma. Unfortunately, most patients do not have warning signs. There is usually a history of long-standing hypertension with vascular disease. Other causes of intracranial hemorrhage include trauma, tumor, arteriovenous malformation, and amyloid angiopathy.

Hemorrhage location is categorized as lobar or nonlobar, with nonlobar hemorrhage usually originating in the putamen, thalamus, pons, or cerebellum. Surgical interventions have been disappointing with supratentorial hemorrhage.[43] With large cerebellar hemorrhage or an infarction, rapid brainstem compression can occur. Surgery has been successfully utilized with these cerebellar injuries.[44]

The long-term prognosis of hypertensive intracerebral hemorrhage is reasonably good if the patient survives the acute hospitalization, with a study finding over 90% of survivors ambulatory after an average of 2.5 years.[45] Surviving patients are at increased risk for both ischemic and hemorrhagic stroke, with a slightly higher rate of ischemic stroke than recurrent hemorrhagic stroke.[46] Although antiplatelet therapy remains controversial, additional stroke prevention measures appear warranted.

Strokes in Children and Young Adults

Strokes in children and young adults have some important differences from strokes in older adults. Newborn strokes often present with seizures as the sole manifestation. Perinatal asphyxia and meningitis must be considered. Strokes in children age 1 to 15 are often due to cyanotic heart disease, moyamoya, or a prothrombotic state. The most common prothombotic condition is sickle cell hemoglobinopathy.[47] Young-adult strokes are often the result of a right-to-left atrial shunt, carotid or vertebrobasilar dissection, a hypercoagulable state.[47] A patent foramen ovale (PFO) can be revealed by a transesophageal echocardiogram with a "bubble test." Hypercoagulation can be revealed by testing for protein S deficiency, protein C deficiency, antithrombin III deficiency, and antiphospholipid antibodies. In addition, toxicology studies for drugs of abuse are often warranted.

Recovery and Rehabilitation

The most dramatic improvement following stroke occurs in the first few weeks, and most measurable neurologic recovery occurs in the first 3 months. Reduction of edema, re-covery of local circulation, and resolution of metabolic factors are thought to account for the early recovery, while functional reorganization (plasticity) of the central nervous system is responsible for continuing recovery.

An understanding of the anticipated stages of recovery of motor function is important in accessing the progress of an individual patient. Brunnstrom[48] described six sequential stages of recovery in hemiplegia. The clinician may observe some variability at each stage, and must remember that some patients will plateau short of full recovery. Immediately following the acute episode there is a period of flaccidity, and no movement of the limb can be elicited (stage 1). As recovery begins, minimal voluntary movement responses may be present and spasticity begins to develop (stage 2). During this stage, basic limb synergy patterns may be appear as associated reactions. Synergy patterns are primitive movement patterns associated with spasticity. The synergy patterns include both flexion and extension components, and can be seen in both the upper and lower extremities. Typically the strongest components of these patterns include elbow flexion, shoulder adduction, and forearm pronation of the upper extremity, and hip flexion and adduction, knee extension, and ankle plantarflexion of the lower extremity.[49] Associated reactions are abnormal, automatic responses in the involved limb resulting from action occurring in some other part of the body, such as yawning, sneezing, or stretching. In stage 3 the patient gains voluntary control of the movement synergies. Spasticity increases and may be severe. Stage 4 is marked by a decline in spasticity and mastery of some movement combinations that do not follow the paths of either flexion or extension synergy. If progress continues, more difficult movement combinations are mastered in stage 5 and the primitive limb synergies lose their dominance over motor acts. For those who progress to the disappearance of spasticity (stage 6), individual joint movements become possible and coordination improves toward normal.

Rehabilitation should be initiated as soon as possible after the stroke has been diagnosed. If the patient is medically stable, rehabilitation can begin in the hospital within 48 to 72 hours after the stroke has occurred. The rehabilitative process should begin in the hospital, but will continue through some combination of specialized rehabilitation units, outpatient or home therapy, or through stays at long-term-care facilities that provide therapy and skilled nursing care.

The Agency for Health Care Policy and Research of the United States Department of Health and Human Services has published clinical practice guidelines for post-stroke rehabilitation that stress four basic principles of stroke rehabilitation.[50] The first principle involves the importance of a multidisciplinary care team approach to rehabilitation. While the specific rehabilitation professions involved will vary according to the needs of the individual patient, the team will typically include the family physician, a physiatrist, a neurologist, and possibly specialty consultants and psychiatry. Other critical team members include the physical therapist, occu-pational therapist, rehabilitation nurse, and possibly a recreational therapist, speech and language therapist, social worker, and dietitian. Effective teamwork is challenging and requires clarity of roles and responsibilities, positive leadership, good communication, and strong commitment to the process.

The second basic principle of rehabilitation requires completion and documentation of thorough and consistent ongoing assessment throughout the rehabilitation process. Repeated clinical examinations and use of standardized instruments are key elements of this assessment process, which should monitor neurologic deficits and medical problems as well as physical, cognitive, psychological, and communication disabilities. The validity, sensitivity, and reliability of the assessment tools are critical so that progress can be measured accurately, and adjustments in the rehabilitation program made appropriately.

Continuity of care is the third basic principle of rehabilitation. As noted above the typical patient's rehabilitation will move from the inpatient setting to either a skilled nursing or rehabilitation facility, and, it is hoped, to home and either home or outpatient therapy. The patient's family physician may be the only member of the rehabilitation team to follow the patient from one setting to another. To reduce the risk of gaps in care when the transition from one facility to another takes place, close communication involving the providers and the family is critical. Transfer of all relevant clinical information including the ongoing patient assessments discussed earlier must occur.

The fourth basic principle of rehabilitation is involvement of the patient and the family in rehabilitation decisions. Throughout the rehabilitation process decisions about the determining rehabilitation goals, selection of a rehabilitation settings and interventions, and ultimately decisions about home care or long-term facility placement should involve the patient and their family whenever possible. Once again, the family physician may be the key individual that the family and patient look to for the information they will need to participate in these decisions.

Once the stroke patient is discharged from the inpatient rehabilitation program, it is recommended that a visit with the primary physician should take place within the first month and at regular intervals during the first year. Continued monitoring of the patient's physical, cognitive, and emotional functioning and integration into the family and social roles is especially important. The family physician should direct the patient toward risk factor reduction. If the patient was on platelet inhibiting therapy with aspirin prior to the stroke, this represents an aspirin failure and use of an alternative agent should be considered.

In addition to working with the rehabilitation team to monitor the patient's physical recovery, the primary physician should also closely monitor the patient's emotional state. Frustration with difficulty in communicating, moving, and functioning will take an emotional toll on the stroke patient. Depression may occur in even mildly impaired patients and is most likely to manifest between 6 months and 2 years after the event. It has been noted that depression is more frequent and more severe in patients with lesions of the left hemisphere compared to patients who had right hemisphere or brainstem lesions, suggesting that the etiology of post-stroke depression may involve more than just the psychological reaction to disability.

References

1. Broderick J, Brott T, Kothari R, et al. The Greater Cincinnati/Northern Kentucky Stroke Study: preliminary first-ever and total incidence rates of stroke among blacks. Stroke 1998;29:415–21.
2. Brain attack statistics, 2000. Available at *www.stroke.org*.
3. Di Carlo A. Frequency of stroke in Europe: a collaborative study of population-based cohorts. ILSA Working Group and the Neurologic Diseases in the Elderly Research Group. Italian Lon-gitudinal Study on Aging. Neurology 2000;54(11 suppl 5):S28–33.
4. Albers GW, Easton JD, Sacco RL, Teal P. Antithrombotic and thrombolytic therapy for ischemic stroke. Chest 1998;114:683S–98S.
5. Stroke risk factors and their impact, 2000. Available at *www.stroke.org*.
6. Kawachi I, Colditz GA, Stampfer MJ, et al. Smoking cessation and decreased risk of stroke in women. JAMA 1993;269:232–6.
7. Wannamethee SG, Shaper AG, Whincup PH, Walker M. Smoking cessation and the risk of stroke in middle-aged men. JAMA 1995;274:155–60.
8. Hebert PR, Gaziano JM, Chan KS, Hennekens CH. Cholesterol lowering with statin drugs, risk of stroke, and total mortality. JAMA 1997;278:313–21.
9. Garber AJ. Attenuating cardiovascular risk factors in patients with type 2 diabetes. Am Fam Physician 2000;62:2633–42.
10. UK Prospective Diabetes Study Group. Tight blood pressure control and risk of macrovascular and microvascular complications in type 2 diabetes: UKPDS 38. BMJ 1998;317:703–13.
11. Antiplatelet Trialists' Collaboration. Collaborative overview of randomized trials of antiplatelet therapy—1: prevention of death, myocardial infarction, and stroke by prolonged anti-platelet therapy in various categories of patients. BMJ 1994;308:81–106.
12. CAPRIE Steering Committee. A randomized, blinded, trial of clopidogrel versus aspirin in patients at risk of ischaemic events (CAPRIE). Lancet 1996;348:1329–39.
13. Diener HC Cunha L, Forbes C, Sivenius J, Smets P, Lowenthal A. European Stroke Prevention Study 2. Dipyridamole and acetylsalicylic acid in the secondary prevention of stroke. J Neurol Sci 1996;143:1–13.
14. Executive Committee for the Asymptomatic Carotid Atherosclerosis Study. Endarterectomy for asymptomatic carotid artery stenosis. JAMA 1995;273;1421–8.

15. Cebul RD. Indications, outcomes, and provider volumes for carotid end-arterectomy. JAMA 1998;279:1282–7.
16. The Sixth Report of the Joint National Committee on Prevention, Detection, Evaluation, and Treatment of High Blood Pressure. Arch Intern Med 1997;157:2413–46.
17. MacMahon S, Rodgers A. Primary and secondary prevention of stroke. Clin Exp Hypertens 1996;18:537–46.
18. Staessen JA, Fagard R, Thijs L, et al. Randomised double-blind comparison of placebo and active treatment for older patients with isolated systolic hypertension. Lancet 1997;350:757–64.
19. Loh E, Sutton MS, Wun CC, et al. Ventricular dysfunction and the risk of stroke after myocardial infarction. N Engl J Med 1997;336:251–7.
20. Hankey GJ. Non-valvular atrial fibrillation and stroke prevention. National Blood Pressure Advisory Committee of the National Heart Foundation. Med J Aust 2001;174:234–9.
21. Atrial Fibrillation Investigators. Risk factors for stroke and efficacy of antithrombotic therapy in atrial fibrillation. Analysis of pooled data from five randomized controlled trials. Arch Intern Med 1994;154:1449–57.
22. Stroke Prevention in Atrial Fibrillation Investigators. Adjusted-dose warfarin versus low-intensity, fixed-dose warfarin plus aspirin for high-risk patients with atrial fibrillation: Stroke Prevention in Atrial fibrillation III randomized clinical trial. Lancet 1996;348:633–8.
23. Singer DE, Go AS. Antithrombotic therapy in atrial fibrillation. Clin Geriatr Med 2001;17:131–47.
24. Brown RD, Petty GW, O'Fallon WM, Wiebers DO, Whisnant JP. Incidence of transient ischemic attack in Rochester, Minnesota, 1985–1989. Stroke 1998;29:2109–13.
25. Hankey GJ, Warlow CP. Symptomatic carotid ischaemic events: safest and most cost effective way of selecting patients for angiography, before carotid endarterectomy. BMJ 1990;300:1485–91.
26. European Carotid Surgery Trialists' Collaborative Group. Randomized trial of endarterectomy for recently symptomatic carotid stenosis: final results of the MRC European Carotid Surgery Trial (ECST). Lancet 1998;351:1379–87.
27. Barnett HJ, Taylor DW, Eliasziw M, et al. Benefit of carotid endarterectomy in patients with symptomatic moderate or severe stenosis. N. Engl J Med 1998;339:1415–25.
28. Pancioli AM, Broderick J, Kothari R, et al. Public perception of stroke warning signs and knowledge of potential risk factors. JAMA 1998;279:1288–92.
29. Reith J, Jorgensen HS, Pedersen PM, et al. Body temperature in acute stroke: relation to stroke severity, infarct size, mortality, and outcome. Lancet 1996;347:422–5.
30. The National Institute of Neurological Disorders and Stroke rt-PA Stroke Study Group. Tissue plasminogen activator for acute ischemic stroke. N Engl J Med 1995;333:1581–7.
31. Kwiatkowski TG, Libman RB, Frankel M, et al. Effects of tissue plasminogen activator for acute ischemic stroke at one year. National Insti-

tute of Neurological Disorders and Stroke Recombinant Tissue Plasminogen Activator Stroke Study Group. N Engl J Med 1999;340:1781–7.
32. Stroke the first hours: Guidelines for Acute Treatment, 2000. Available at *www.stroke.org*.
33. Schriger DL, Kalafut M, Starkman S, Krueger M, Saver JL. Cranial computed tomography interpretation in acute stroke. JAMA 1998;279: 1293–7.
34. Clark WM, Wissman S, Albers GW, Jhamandas JH, Madden KP, Hamilton S. Recombinant tissue-type plasminogen activator (Alteplase) for ischemic stroke 3 to 5 hours after symptom onset. The Atlantis Study: a randomized controlled trial. JAMA 1999;282:2019–26.
35. Furlan A, Higashida R, Wechsler L, et al. Intra-arterial prourokinase for acute ischemic stroke. The PROACT 11 study: a randomized controlled trial. Prolyse in acute cerebral thromboembolism. JAMA 1999;282: 2003–11.
36. Young GR, Humphrey PR, Shaw MD, Nixon TE, Smith ET. Comparison of magnetic resonance angiography, duplex ultrasound, and digital subtraction angiography in assessment extracranial internal carotid stenosis. J Neurol Neurosurg Psychiatry 1994;57:166–78.
37. Shrier DA, Tanaka H, Numaguchi Y, Konno S, Patel U, Shibata D. CT angiography in the evaluation of acute stroke. AJNR 1997;18:1021–3.
38. Publications Committee for the Trial of ORG 10172 in Acute Stroke Treatment (Toast) Investigators. Low molecular weight heparinoid, ORG 10172 (Danaparoid), and outcome after acute ischemic stroke. JAMA 1998;279:1265–72.
39. International Stroke Trial Collaborative Group. The International Stroke Trial (IST): a randomized trial of aspirin, subcutaneous heparin, both, or neither among 19,435 patients with acute ischaemic stroke. Lancet 1997;349:1569–81.
40. CAST (Chinese Acute Stroke Trial) Collaborative Group. CAST: randomized placebo-controlled trial of early aspirin use in 20,000 patients with acute ischaemic stroke. Lancet 1997;349:1641–9.
41. Taylor DW. Low-dose and high-dose acetylsalicylic acid for patients undergoing endarterectomy: a randomized controlled trial. ASA and Carotid Endarterectomy (ACE) Trial Collaborators. Lancet 1999;353: 2179–84.
42. Popovic EA, Danks RA, Siu KH. Experience with nimodipine in aneurysmal subarachnoid haemorrhage. Med J Aust 1993;158:91–3.
43. Juvela S, Heiskanen O, Poranen A, Valtonen S, Kuurne T, Kaste M. The treatment of spontaneous intracerebral hemorrhage. A prospective randomized trial of surgical and conservative treatment. J Neurosurg 1989;70:755–8.
44. Heros RC. Surgical treatment of cerebellar infarction. Stroke 1992;23: 937–8.
45. Douglas MA, Haerer AF. Long-term prognosis of hypertensive intracerebral hemorrhage. Stroke 1982;13:488–91.
46. Hill MD, Silver FL, Austin PC, Tu JV. Rate of stroke recurrence in patients with primary intracerebral hemorrhage. Stroke 2000;31:123–7.

47. Williams LS, Garg BP, Cohen M, Fleck JD, Biller J. Subtypes of ischemic stroke in children and young adults. Neurology 1997;49:1541–5.
48. Brunnstrom S: Movement therapy in hemiplegia. New York: Harper & Row, 1970.
49. O'Sullivan S. Stroke. In: O'Sullivan S, Schmitz TJ, eds. Physical rehab assessment and treatment. Philadelphia: FA Davis, 1994;327–59.
50. Clinical Practice Guideline Number 16: post-stroke rehabilitation. AHCPR publication no. 95-0662. Rockville, MD: U.S. Department of Health and Human Services, Public Health Service, Agency for Health Care Policy and Research, May 1995.

9
Cardiovascular Emergencies

*William J. Hueston and
A. Kesh Hebbar*

Cardiac disease accounts for the largest proportion of deaths in the United States. Many patients with underlying cardiac problems present to family physicians with conditions that can lead to death if not properly evaluated and treated. This chapter examines several cardiac emergencies that may be encountered by patients in a primary care practice.

Syncope

Syncope refers to transient loss of consciousness with loss of motor tone. Near-syncope generally refers to patients who lose some motor activity and have a decreased level of consciousness, but do not completely pass out. These conditions are frightening to patients and their family and usually result in patients' seeking care immediately. In one series, syncope-related problems accounted for 3% of all emergency department visits and 6% of all general medical hospital admissions.

Syncope can be the symptom of many different conditions including multiple noncardiac conditions. However, syncope associated with cardiac problems carries a much higher risk of subsequent death than when caused by other noncardiac diseases. In a prospective study of patients identified with syncope, it was found that patients whose syncope was linked to a cardiac cause had a 1-year mortality of 30% compared to 12% when a neurologic diagnosis was made and 6% with syncope from unknown causes.[1] For this reason, the identification of a cardiac problem contributing to syncope is important.

The causes of syncope can be divided into three broad categories: cardiac, neurologic, and other. A list of causes of syncope is shown in Table 9.1.[1,2] This chapter focuses on cardiac causes of syncope and cardiac medications that can result in syncope.

Pathophysiology and Differential Diagnosis

The symptom of syncope usually develops as a result of transient decreases in oxygen delivery to the neurologic centers that control con-

Table 9.1. **Causes of Syncope**

Cardiac syncope
Dysrhythmias
   Ventricular tachycardia
   Supraventricular tachycardia
   Sick-sinus syndrome
   Sinus pause
   Complete heart block
Cardiac ischemia
   Myocardial infarction
   Aortic stenosis
   Hypertrophic cardiomyopathy
Obstruction of inflow/outflow
   Pulmonary embolism
   Aortic dissection
   Atrial myxoma
   Pericardial tamponade

Neurogenic syncope
Vasovagal syncope
Vascular obstruction
   Subclavian steal syndrome
   Vertebral-basilar transient ischemic attacks
Carotid hypersensitivity
Autonomic neuropathies

Other
Idiopathic orthostatic hypotension
Hypovolemia
Medications
Hyperventilation
Psychiatric syncope/conversion reaction

sciousness. Any cardiac, circulatory, or neurologic condition that reduces perfusion to this area of the brain can cause syncope. In a prospective trial of 204 patients presenting with syncope in the early 1980s, Kapoor and colleagues[1] were able to classify 26% as having cardiac problems and another 26% with noncardiac conditions that caused their symptoms. In the remaining 48%, no cause could be found despite extensive investigation.[2]

Cardiac Syncope

Cardiac causes of syncope lead to a reduction in cardiac output that results in decreased perfusion of the brain. This includes cardiac dysrhythmias, cardiac ischemia, and obstruction to cardiac outflow.

The most common cause of transient reductions in cardiac outflow is an acute dysrhythmia. Of the types of rhythm disturbances, nonsustained ventricular tachycardia is the most common dysrhythmia associated with syncope. Since ventricular tachycardia can occur in association with ischemia, patients may have reduced cardiac output preceding the onset of the rhythm disturbance. The other dysrhythmia frequently resulting in syncope is sick sinus syndrome (tachycardia-bradycardia syndrome). In this instance either the tachycardic phase or the bradycardic phase can result in transitory decreases in cardiac output.

Ischemia also should be considered in the patient presenting with syncope (also see Chapter 2). The ischemic event can result in myocardial infarction or can be transient such as that occurring with aortic stenosis. Both of these possibilities should be entertained especially when the syncope is associated with exercise in a patient with risk factors for valvular or atherosclerotic disease. In younger patients, another potential for ischemic-related syncope is hypertrophic cardiomyopathy. Young individuals with exercise-induced syncope should be carefully evaluated for the possibility of hypertrophic cardiomyopathy before being allowed to participate in sports or other exertional activities.

Obstructive cardiac conditions resulting in syncope are uncommon. The most common obstructive cause of syncope is pulmonary embolism. Another emergent cause of syncope that obstructs cardiac filling is cardiac tamponade. In addition, rare cardiac abnormalities can cause syncope. These include atrial myxomas that may obstruct blood flow through the mitral valve, cardiac tumors that can obstruct valvular flow, and thoracic aortic dissection, which can obstruct blood flow to the cerebral vessels. Finally, cardiac tamponade can restrict cardiac filling and result in decreased cardiac output.

Other Causes of Syncope

A variety of neurologic conditions can cause syncopes. These include posterior circulation transient ischemic attacks, vasopressor/vasovagal syncope, and carotid hypersensitivity. Additionally, seizures can mimic syncope. If the syncopal episode is witnessed, tonic-clonic motor activity can indicate an underlying seizure disorder. If the episode is not witnessed, a generalized seizure should remain in the differential diagnosis until a cause is found.

Other nonneurologic conditions to consider that can be associated with syncope include decreased intravascular fluids that occur with hemorrhage or profound dehydration. In addition, psychiatric conditions also should be considered, especially when the syncope tends to occur in dramatic fashion and always in the presence of onlookers. Psychiatric problems such as hyperventilation also can cause the loss of consciousness.

Some common associated findings with each disorder are shown in Table 9.2.[3]

Evaluation

The most important aspects of the evaluation are the history, physical examination, and electrocardiogram testing. These three techniques have been found to yield the diagnosis in about 50% of cases of syncope.[4]

History

As part of a comprehensive history of the event and general health of the patient, several areas should be emphasized. The occurrence of prodromal symptoms and what these symptoms were like may be useful in suggesting a potential cause for the syncope. Generally, neurologic or neurovascular events occur with little warning. Vasovagal syncope often produces a prodrome that includes flushing, sweating, nausea, and anxiety. Some cardiac dysrhythmias are associated with palpitations, but many, such as ventricular tachycardia, may occur without warning; thus, palpitations can be a specific indicator of a cardiac source, but is not very sensitive.

The specific circumstances surrounding the syncope also should be determined. As indicated earlier, events that occur when the neck is turned or compressed or associated with micturition, cough, or straining may indicate carotid hypersensitivity. Orthostatic hypotension occurs with standing or other sudden position changes. Subclavian steal is associated with upper extremity use.

Table 9.2. **Associated History and Physical Examination Findings for Common Causes of Syncope**

Cause	Onset	Other history	Physical exam
Dysrhythmia	Quick, little warning	Higher risk with CAD; family history of hypertrophic cardiomyopathy	Murmur of aortic stenosis; irregular rhythm or rate disturbance
Ischemic heart disease	With exertion	Risk factors for CAD; previous angina	No specific findings
Aortic stenosis	With exercise	Recurrent syncope; rheumatic heart disease	Systolic murmur
Hypertrophic cardiomyopathy	With exercise	Family history of sudden death	Murmur accentuated by Valsalva maneuver
Seizure disorder	May have aura	History of seizures; drug use that reduces seizure threshold; alcohol or other drug withdrawal	Postictal state; loss of bladder or bowel continence
Vertebrobasilar transient ischemic attack	Sudden onset	Risk factors for vascular disease	May find carotid bruits; usually no specific findings
Subclavian steal syndrome	Onset with exercise using left arm	Recurrent syncope with exercise; higher incidence in women	Decreased pulse and blood pressure in left arm
Orthostatic syncope	Usually gradual onset with episodes of near-syncope	Usually progressive in nature; associated with drugs that can cause orthostasis (alpha-blockers, tricyclic antidepressants); associated with diabetes mellitus	Orthostatic drop in blood pressure with rising; with autonomic neuropathy (associated with diabetes) see drop in blood pressure without an accompanying rise in pulse
Psychogenic syncope	Dramatic event	Occurs in times of stress; patient rarely injured in fall	No specific cardiac or neurologic findings

CAD = coronary artery disease.

The occurrence of syncope with exertion is worrisome and raises the possibility of ischemic heart disease from either fixed vessel obstruction or aortic stenosis. Younger patients with syncope or near-syncope during athletic activities should be evaluated for hypertrophic cardiomyopathy.

Past medical history is important to assess the presence and risk factors for atherosclerotic disease. In addition, a number of drugs are associated with syncope (Table 9.3), so a complete medication history is essential.[1,2] A family history of syncope, sudden death (especially at a young age, as frequently occurs in hypertrophic cardiomyopathy), and other illnesses might suggest specific conditions.

In addition, information from an onlooker about what happened during the event may be useful. In particular, the presence of tonic-clonic motor activity may differentiate seizure activity from syncope. Furthermore, information about how the individual fell and his or her activity while "passed out" can be useful in identifying patients with psychiatric syncope.

Table 9.3. **Drugs Associated with Syncope**

Vasodilating agents
   Nitrates
   Calcium channel blockers
   ACE inhibitors
   Minoxidil (topical and systemic)
   Alpha-blocking agents
Psychoactive drugs
   Tricyclic antidepressants
   Phenothiazines
   MAO inhibitors
Drugs lengthening the QT interval
   Type I (quinidine, procainamide, disopyramide, flecainide, encainide)
   Sotalol
   Amiodarone
Diuretics
Others
   Alcohol
   Cocaine
   Digitalis
   Vincristine and other neuropathic drugs
   Marijuana

ACE = angiotensin-converting enzyme; MAO = monoamine oxidase.
Source: Kapoor,[2] with permission.

Physical Examination

A careful physical examination can help confirm some of the conditions suspected from the history. Assessment of the blood pressure in both arms while lying, sitting, and standing with simultaneous measure of the pulse is very useful. Blood pressure testing can reveal orthostasis (with or without pulse increases) and may detect differences in left and right arm blood pressures suggestive of subclavian steal.

Attention to the carotid arteries should include listening for bruits and palpating the pulse. In addition, gentle carotid massage can be useful in assessing for carotid hypersensitivity. Carotid pressure should be avoided if bruits are present to reduce the risk of causing a cerebrovascular embolism with massage. In addition, in patients with a high likelihood for carotid hypersensitivity, intravenous access may be warranted to treat the resulting sinus pause or third-degree atrioventricular (AV) block (also see Chapter 3).

The cardiac examination is important as well. Determination of the resting heart rate and any rhythm disturbances can be signs of a rate problem. The presence of murmurs may signal aortic stenosis or other valvular heart disease (see Chapter 4). The emergence of a murmur or accentuation of a soft aortic murmur while the patient does a Valsalva maneuver and the physician listens over the aortic outflow tract may indicate hypertrophic cardiomyopathy. A pericardial rub can indicate restrictive pericarditis.

Other Testing

Evaluation of the patient with syncope can be performed on an outpatient basis if the patient has not suffered any injury from the fall, has not had recurrent episodes, and is at low risk for ischemic cardiac events or malignant dysrhythmias. This description would most often apply to young healthy individuals for whom this is an isolated, brief episode with full recovery and no injury. Young healthy patients with clear antecedents to the event that suggest a clear cause, such as vasovagal syncope, may require no additional workup for a single event.

Initial evaluation of the patient with syncope should include an electrocardiogram (ECG) to establish the cardiac rhythm and assess for signs of cardiac injury or syncope. If the history is suggestive of a cardiac rhythm disturbance and the initial ECG is normal, further evaluation with a Holter monitor is indicated. If patients experience multiple near-syncope episodes, consideration may be given to an event recorder rather than Holter monitoring, especially if the events are not frequent and are likely to be missed over the 24- or 48-hour period that the Holter monitor is in place.[5]

Patients at risk for ischemic events should have cardiac enzymes determined to rule out myocardial infarction. For patients with syncope related to exertion, further evaluation for ischemia is warranted with a cardiac stress test.

An echocardiogram may be useful in patients with a rub or murmur. Echocardiography will allow for visualization of the valves, and Doppler flow can estimate whether significant pressure gradients exist across the heart valves. Additionally, the echocardiogram may detect areas of previous myocardial injury or hypertrophy, and it evaluates the pericardium.

Routine brain imaging is not likely to be useful in patients without carotid bruits, no other neurologic symptoms, and a normal neurologic examination. Without evidence of motor activity during the event, electroencephalograms are not likely to be helpful.[6]

For patients in whom the previous evaluation has been unrevealing, two additional types of evaluations may be indicated. In patients with suspected or known cardiac disease or whose history is suggestive of a cardiac dysrhythmia, further evaluation with electrophysiologic (EPS) testing may be indicated. In several studies of patients with cardiac disease and unexplained syncope, EPS testing uncovered a presumptive cause for the syncope in 18% to 75% of cases.[3] Treatment of syncope in these cases resulted in a cessation of symptoms in 75% to 85% of patients. In contrast, in patients without cardiac disease, response to treatment ranges from 12% to 20% suggesting that EPS abnormalities uncovered in these individuals were not causing the symptoms.

Patients in whom a vagally mediated mechanism is suspected can be evaluated using the head-up tilt test. The tilt test involves positioning of the tilt table at a 60- to 80-degree angle for 10 to 60 minutes supplemented with the infusion of isoproterenol. A recurrence of symptoms in this circumstance is usually indicative of vasovagal syncope. The tilt test is most useful in patients with recurrent symptoms but no evidence of suspected cardiac disease in whom other evaluations have been unfruitful.

In some patients, psychiatric evaluation is indicated. Psychiatric problems can be uncovered in as many as 25% of patients who have recurrent syncope.[4] Patients at higher risk for psychiatric disorders include those in whom syncope is also witnessed and is dramatic, who have had five or more episodes in 1 year, and have other suspected underlying psychiatric disorders.

Management

Because syncope is a symptom, appropriate management includes identifying the underlying cause and providing effective therapy.

The most important types of syncope to treat are those associated with dysrhythmias and with ischemic heart disease. Once a cardiac problem has been established as the cause of the syncopal episodes, further evaluation with EPS testing and evaluation for underlying ischmic heart disease may be warranted. Control of potential malignant dysrhythmias such as ventricular tachycardia or supraventricular tachycardias with ischemia are essential to prevent sudden death.

A second important aspect in managing syncope is to avoid drugs that can exacerbate orthostasis or contribute to depressed sinus or AV nodal function. Patients who are currently taking these medications should be offered trials of alternatives that may not cause as much orthostatic hypotension. Patients who are prone to orthostasis should be advised to remain well hydrated and avoid situations where they may lose excessive fluids without adequate replacement, such as long hikes in hot, dry environments. Wearing elastic hose to prevent venous pooling and intermittently contracting the leg muscles to promote venous return also may be helpful.[7]

Syncope in Children and Adolescents

Syncope also is a common symptom in children and adolescents. Some studies estimate that up to 20% of all children or adolescents will have at least one fainting episode before reaching adulthood.[8] The challenge for the physician is to differentiate when these episodes are due to benign causes such as breath-holding or hyperventilation and when they signal more serious problems.

In one small study of pediatric patients presenting to an emergency department with syncope, over half of all patients with syncope had a vasovagal attack.[9] In all patients except the 9% in which the cause remained unknown, a benign reason was identified for the attack.

While syncope from serious illness is uncommon in children, there are some warning signs of cardiac disease that should prompt a more thorough investigation[8] (Table 9.4). These include syncope that occurs when the patient is lying down or with no forewarning, syncope provoked by exercise, episodes accompanied by chest pain or palpitations, and loss of consciousness for more than 5 minutes. In addition, children or adolescents who have a family history of cardiomyopathies, sudden death, or aortic stenosis should be evaluated more extensively.

Table 9.4. **Factors Associated with Cardiac-Induced Syncope in Children**

Attack when recumbent
Little or no prodrome preceding attack
Attack associated with exercise
Unconsciousness lasting more than 5 minutes
History of cardiac disease in family member
History of sudden death in family member

Cardiogenic Shock

Traditional classification of shock states has been based on broad but discrete hemodynamic defects. These categories include hypovolemic shock (e.g., hemorrhage, gastroenteritis), obstructive shock (acute pulmonary embolism), distributive shock (anaphylactic and septic shock), and cardiogenic shock. Survival from shock states is dependent on the initial resuscitative efforts to establish tissue perfusion and reverse the underlying etiologic process. Table 9.5 lists the major hemodynamic patterns seen in each of these shock states.

The most frequent cause of cardiogenic shock is acute myocardial infarction (AMI). Anterior MI is by far the most common type of infarction precipitating cardiogenic shock. In the case of an acute anterior wall MI, left anterior descending artery occlusion is usually detected. Lateral wall MIs are not often associated with cardiogenic shock. Inferior MI alone infrequently causes shock.

In the past cardiogenic shock was reported to occur in up to 15% to 20% of individuals with AMI, but with the advent of thrombolytic therapy the incidence has decreased to about 7%.[10,11] The majority

Table 9.5. **Classification of Types of Shock**

Type of shock	CI	SVR	PVR	PaOP
Cardiogenic shock, e.g., AMI	↓	↑	N	↑
Hypovolemic shock	↓	↑	N	↓
Distributive shock, e.g., septic shock	↑		N	N–↓
Obstructive shock, e.g. pulmonary embolism	↓	↑–N	↑	N–↓

AMI = acute myocardial infarction; CI = cardiac index; SVR = systemic vascular resistance; PVR = pulmonary vascular resistance; PaOP = pulmonary artery occlusion pressure; N = normal; ↑ = increased; ↓ = decreased.

Table 9.6. **Differential Diagnosis of Cardiogenic Shock**

Acute myocardial infarction
Septal wall rupture
Dilated cardiomyopathy
Myocarditis
Pericardial tamponade
Right ventricular failure
Arrhythmias

of patients do not present initially in shock but develop this state during hospitalization and usually it is due to an infarct extension. The differential diagnosis of cardiogenic shock is summarized in Table 9.6.

Pathophysiology

Obstruction of coronary blood flow produces myocardial ischemia. Ischemia causes myocardial wall dysfunction, which is reversible if blood flow is reestablished. During these brief episodes of wall dysfunction, pulmonary edema may develop. However, wall motion abnormalities abate with restoration of blood flow, so heart failure usually responds to the usual aggressive management.

In acute MI, ischemia is not relieved. This results in cell necrosis. Loss of myocardial muscle results in irreversible impairment in myocardial contractility and ventricular performance. The resulting decline in cardiac output reduces arterial blood pressure and coronary perfusion pressure. This in turn leads to further cardiac ischemia and extension of the necrosis.

Cardiogenic shock often involves multivessel disease with substantial amount of myocardial damage. At autopsy more than two thirds of patients with cardiogenic shock demonstrated stenosis of 75% or more of luminal diameter of all three major coronary vessels and exhibited necrosis of at least 40% of the left ventricle.[12,13]

Diagnosis

The criteria for the diagnosis of cardiogenic shock include evidence of myocardial wall motion abnormalities combined with (1) hypotension with systolic blood pressure less than 90 mm Hg for at least 30 minutes and the need for vasopressors; (2) clinical evidence of end-organ dysfunction, e.g., cool clammy skin, altered mental status, oliguria (less than 20 mL/h); or (3) confirmatory hemodynamic features, i.e., pulmonary capillary wedge pressure (PCWP) >15 mm Hg and cardiac index <2.2 L/min/m^2.

In evaluating patients with cardiogenic shock, it is important to exclude mechanical complications (e.g., septal rupture, papillary muscle rupture, right ventricular infarction) because they may need urgent operative intervention. These complications can be detected quickly by echocardiography or angiography.

Management

When cardiac shock occurs, immediate resuscitative measures should be undertaken. Oxygenation should be optimized with obtaining a PaO_2 over 60 mm Hg as the goal. Noninvasive ventilation with bilevel positive airway pressure (BiPAP) or intubation and mechanical ventilation may be needed to achieve appropriate oxygenation. Fluid management should be carefully titrated to maintain filling pressure of the left ventricle but avoiding fluid overload. The hematocrit should be maintained at or greater than 30% to improve oxygen delivery to the myocardium.

Vasopressors and inotropic therapy are usually used in the management of cardiogenic shock, but should be considered as supportive and not curative. Supportive therapy without attempts to attain reperfusion does not appear to improve prognosis.

Vasoconstricting agents useful in the management of cardiogenic shock include dopamine, dobutamine and norepinephrine. Dopamine can be used at doses ranging between 5 and 20 μg/kg/min. Low doses help in renal and splanchnic blood flow by vasodilation (2–3 μg/kg/min). At doses of 4 to 6 μg/kg/min dopamine increases cardiac contractility and at higher doses (>10 μg/kg/min) increases blood pressure by activation of peripheral α-receptors. Dobutamine is a powerful inotropic agent and also reduces afterload by peripheral vasodilation. The dose of dobutamine is titrated for effect. The usual starting dose is 2 to 5 μg/kg/min and can be increased to 20 μg/kg/min. Norepinephrine also has α- and β-adrenergic activity and a potent vasoconstricting agent. Among these agents, dopamine is usually preferred because of the multiple effects that can be obtained simply by altering the infusion rate.

Intraaortic balloon pump counterpulsation (IABP) is another option to assist ventricular function and usually is performed on patients who do not respond to medical therapy. The balloon is inserted percutaneously via a femoral catheter and floated to the proximal aorta. The balloon then fills during diastole and deflates during systole. The function of the balloon is controlled electronically and is synchronized with the cardiac cycle. IABP is not a permanent solution, but allows for patient transfer to another facility and gives physicians time to initiate revascularization procedures to reverse ischemia. IABP has consistently been shown to lower in-hospital mortality.[14]

The key to treatment is obtaining revascularization of the threatened myocardium so that myocardial wall function is improved. This can be achieved either surgically or, for patients who present early in the process of an infarction, through clot lysis using a thrombolytic agent. Patients receiving either thrombolytic therapy or IABP have lower mortality rates than those not receiving these therapies. Combining the two approaches appears to confer even greater benefit than either alone.[15]

Even with aggressive management, outcomes for cardiogenic shock are poor. The randomized international SHOCK trial (*should* we emergently revascularize *o*ccluded *c*oronaries for cardiogenic shoc*k*) assessed the effects on 30-day mortality of a direct invasive strategy (emergency early revascularization) compared with initial medical stabilization (including thrombolysis and IABP).[16] Overall, the trial enrolled 302 patients and showed no significant difference in the 30-day mortality for patients treated with early intervention compared to those who were treated with initial medical stabilization. However, when the trial looked at the subset of patients under the age of 75, early revascularization did show significant benefits. In this group, early revascularization was calculated to save 13 lives per 100 patients under age 75.

Sudden Cardiac Death (SCD)

According to the most widely used estimates, between 300,000 and 400,000 people die of sudden cardiac death in the United States every year.[17] Two age-related peaks occur: between 5 and 6 months of age and between 45 and 75 years of age.

In adults, coronary heart disease is by far the structural basis for at least 80% of SCD. Consequently, those at highest risk for coronary heart disease, such as men, are at higher risk for SCD. Additionally, poor cardiac function is a risk factor for SCD. In fact, an ejection fraction equal to or less than 30% is the single most powerful predictor for sudden cardiac death.[18]

It is important to have an understanding of the other causes of sudden cardiac death because recognizing them may be lifesaving. Table 9.7 reviews the causes of SCD.

Table 9.7. **Causes of Sudden Cardiac Death**

Coronary artery abnormalities
  Coronary atherosclerosis
  Congenital abnormalities of coronary arteries
  Coronary arteritis
Hypertrophy
  Left ventricular hypertrophy with coronary artery disease
  Hypertensive heart disease
  Valvular heart disease
  Hypertrophic cardiomyopathy (HCM)
  Primary or secondary pulmonary hypertension
Myocardial disease
  Ischemic cardiomyopathy
  Alcoholic cardiomyopathy
  Postpartum cardiomyopathy
  Acute myocarditis
Congenital heart disease
Electrical abnormalities
  Fibrosis of conduction system
  Prolonged QT syndrome
  Drug effect
Miscellaneous
  Acute cardiac tamponade
  Massive pulmonary embolism
  Dissecting aneurysm of aorta
  Sudden infant death syndrome (SIDS)

Sudden Cardiac Death in Infants, Children, and Adolescents

An estimated 5,000 to 7,000 children die suddenly in the United States annually; this does not include the 5,000 to 7,000 deaths from sudden infant death syndrome (SIDS).[19] Those at highest risk are patients with congenital heart disease who have structural abnormalities that cannot be fully corrected. The development of severe pulmonary hypertension (Eisenmenger syndrome) confers the highest risk. A history of early or sudden unexplained death in other family members should raise the index of suspicion for congenital diseases that increase the risk of SCD such as hypertrophic cardiomyopathy, long QT syndrome, congenital coronary abnormalities, and Marfan syndrome. In children with family members with these disorders, symptoms of chest pain, palpitations, exertional dizziness or syncope may need to be investigated thoroughly before a benign cause is assigned for the symptoms.

In contrast to adults, coronary artery disease is rare in childhood and is usually associated with other disorders such as lipid abnormalities or infectious diseases like Kawasaki syndrome. Kawasaki syndrome is the most common cause of acquired coronary artery disease in infants and young children. SCD occurs in 1% to 2% of patients with untreated Kawasaki syndrome.

Unfortunately for most patients, SCD may be the presenting symptom in many cases, and the underlying condition(s) may be discovered only at the time of autopsy. Although SCD is relatively uncommon, its psychosocial impact is devastating.

Sudden infant death syndrome is defined as sudden death of an apparently healthy infant whose death remains unexplained even after autopsy. Risk factors for SIDS are prematurity, infants of teenage mothers, and exposure to tobacco and cocaine. Apnea is considered to be the main etiology but occlusive lesions of the cardiac conduction tissue arteries have been demonstrated in some children.[20] An observational study by Schwartz et al[21] suggested that abnormal prolongation of QT interval may be the cause of SIDS.

Sudden Death in Young and Middle-Aged Athletes

The incidence of sudden cardiac death in athletes is low and the cause varies with the age of the population studied. In young competitive athletes hypertrophic cardiomyopathy (HCM) is the most frequent cause followed by aberrant coronary arteries. For individuals older than 35 years, coronary artery atherosclerosis is by far the most common cause of sudden cardiac death. These individuals tend to start running at an older age and usually have a strong family history of heart disease or have other recognized risk factors.

Some studies estimate that up to 50% of sudden death in young athletes are due to HCM.[22] Some of the older terms used to describe the condition were *idiopathic hypertrophic subaortic stenosis* (IHSS), *hypertrophic obstructive cardiomyopathy* (HOCM), and *muscular subaortic stenosis*. The characteristic physiologic abnormality is diastolic dysfunction and increased left end-diastolic pressure, which results in pulmonary congestion and dyspnea.

HCM is an autosomal-dominant disease and is identified most often in adults in their 30s and 40s. The majority of the patients are asymptomatic. If patients do experience problems, the most common complaint is dyspnea. Other less common symptoms include angina, fatigue, dizziness on exertion, presyncope, and syncope. On physical examination of patients with HCM the apical impulse is often displaced laterally and forceful. A systolic murmur is sometimes present that resembles aortic stenosis but usually does not radiate to the neck vessels and increases in intensity with Valsalva maneuver and

Table 9.8. **Causes of Sudden Cardiac Death in Athletes**

Coronary atherosclerosis
Hypertrophic cardiomyopathy
Idiopathic left ventricular hypertrophy
Right ventricular hypertrophy
Coronary artery anomalies
Long QT syndrome
Myocarditis

standing. The ECG is usually abnormal in symptomatic patients with evidence of left ventricular hypertrophy (LVH) and ST segment and T wave abnormalities. Prominent Q waves in leads II and III, AVF, and sometimes in the precordial leads can also be seen. Echocardiogram shows the characteristic features of the hypertrophied septum, outflow tract obstruction, and diastolic dysfunction. Screening asymptomatic athletes with echocardiogram is not cost-effective because of the low prevalence of the disease.

The mechanisms of sudden death in HCM include tachyarrhythmias or ischemia from small vessel disease.[23] Beta-blockers remain the mainstay of medical therapy, and dual-chamber pacemakers and surgery are options for the high-risk patient.[24,25]

Causes of sudden death in athletes are summarized in Table 9.8.

Sudden Death in Dilated Cardiomyopathy and Heart Failure

Patients with coronary heart disease are living longer with the aggressive therapeutic interventions over the last two decades. However, while people live longer the proportion of patients with stable heart failure who die suddenly has increased.[26] The primary mechanism of death appears to be due to an acute arrhythmia. In particular, a high incidence of ventricular arrhythmias has been observed during follow-up of patients with aortic valve surgery, multiple valve surgery or cardiomegaly.[27]

For patients who have experienced an acute arrhythmia or who are found to be at high risk for sudden cardiac death, an implantable cardiac defibrillator (ICD) may be lifesaving. ICDs are multiprogrammable devices capable of delivering high-energy defibrillation shocks, antitachycardia pacing, and pacing for bradyarrhythmias. The unit runs on a battery that has a charge capacity that varies from 5 to 9 years.

Two recent major trials have shown convincingly that ICD is superior to antiarrhythmic drugs in certain situations. The Antiarrhyth-

Table 9.9. **Potential Problems Associated with an Implantable Cardiac Defibrillator (ICD)**

Potential problems with insertion or maintenance
  Frequent shocks
  Infection or hematoma at time of insertion
  Pacing malfunction
  Lead dislodgment
Special precautions for patients with ICD
  Procedures needing electrocautery
  Magnetic resonance imaging (MRI) is contraindicated
  ICD may continue to function after death (need to disconnect)

mics Versus Implantable Defibrillators (AVID) trial showed significantly better survival rate over a 3-year follow-up in patients who had survived a near-fatal ventricular fibrillation or had sustained ventricular tachycardia.[28] The Multicenter Automatic Defibrillator Implantation Trial (MADIT) included patients with low ejection fraction and episodes of unsustained ventricular tachycardia, and compared ICD with no therapy.[29] The trial was terminated prematurely because of a marked survival benefit with ICDs. After ICD placement, routine visits at 3- to 6-month intervals are arranged for pacing malfunction and battery failure. Some of the emergencies for patients with ICD are highlighted in Table 9.9.

In patients with an ICD, antibiotic prophylaxis is not recommended for procedures that may induce bacteremia.[30] However, an ICD should be disabled during electrocautery use. An ICD constitutes a strong contraindication to magnetic resonance imaging (MRI). ICD system infection is an uncommon problem but will need removal of the system and IV antibiotics to eradicate infection.[31]

ICDs may have to be inactivated in terminally ill patients when frequent arrhythmias triggers ICD shocks. Consent to inactivate the ICD should be specifically obtained even in a patient with a do-not-resuscitate order.[32] In a patient who is pacemaker dependent, inactivating the ICD bradycardia pacing is not recommended as this may be mistakenly interpreted as physician-assisted suicide. Careful counseling and an informed consent should be in place before deactivating ICD devices.

Cardiopulmonary Resuscitation

More than 200,000 people in the United States die suddenly each year from coronary artery disease before they reach the hospital. An estimated 500,000 patients also will experience a cardiac arrest during their hospitalization.[33] Cardiopulmonary resuscitation (CPR) was designed to intervene in these circumstances and restore a normal cardiac rhythm so that the underlying disease can be addressed and normal health restored.

CPR is guided by protocols approved by the American Heart Association. These protocols are reviewed and updated periodically. The last review was completed in 2000. The published Guidelines 2000 for CPR and Emergency Cardiovascular Care[34] is the first attempt to base recommendation on evidence and make them adaptable to the resources available in different countries.

The fundamentals of CPR have remained the same for the past several decades and continue to include four basic sequential steps: (1) the call for help, (2) chest compression and mouth-to-mouth resuscitation, (3) rapid defibrillation, and (4) medical management of specific cardiac arrhythmias. An algorithm for progressing through CPR is shown in Table 9.10. The prognosis for patients with pulse-

Table 9.10. **Algorithm for Recent Cardiopulmonary Resuscitation (CPR) Protocols**

Primary ABCD survey
(airway, breathing, circulation, defibrillate)
↓
Assess rhythm after first three shocks
↓
If persistent or recurrent ventricular fibrillation/tachycardia
↓
Secondary ABCD survey
Place airway device, confirm breathing, establish
circulation by inserting intravenous line, and
differential diagnosis for reversible causes
↓
1 mg epinephrine intravenously and repeat every 3–5 min
or
40 units of vasopressin intravenous, one time dose
↓
Resume attempt to defibrillate
↓
Consider antiarrhythmics
Amiodarone for persistent or recurrent ventricular
fibrillation/tachycardia
Lidocaine for persistent of recurrent ventricular fibrillation/tachycardia
Magnesium for hypomagnesemic patient
Procainamide
↓
Resume attempts to defibrillate

less electrical activity and asystole is very poor. Potentially treatable conditions should be addressed first. The failure to identify a treatable condition signals poor likelihood to respond to resuscitation efforts.

Common rhythm disturbances encountered in cardiac arrest include ventricular fibrillation, pulseless ventricular tachycardia, pulseless electrical activity, and asystole. Medications useful in cardiac resuscitation are listed in Table 9.11.[35]

Two changes in the CPR protocols should be highlighted. First is the addition of vasopressin for use in patients with shock-resistance ventricular fibrillation. There are no data on the performance of vasopressin in cardiac arrest, but the consensus conference adopting current recommendations believed that this drug would be more effective than epinephrine in shock-resistant ventricular fibrillation.

Table 9.11. **Some Medications Useful in CPR**

Medication	Indication	Adult dose
Amiodarone	VF or pulseless V-tach	300 mg initial followed by 150 mg repeated doses
	Stable V-tach	150 mg over 10 min followed by 1 mg/min infusion for 6 hours, then 0.5 mg/min
	Supraventricular tachycardia	Same as stable V-tach
Atropine	Bradycardia	0.5–1.0 mg IV every 3–5 minutes
	Asystole	1 mg IV repeated every 3–5 minutes
Epinephrine	VF or pulseless V-tach	1 mg IV repeated every 3–5 minutes
	Pulseless electrical activity	As above
	Asystole	As above
	Bradycardia unresponsive to atropine	1–10 μg/min IV titrated to heart rate
Lidocaine	VF or pulseless V-tach	1–1.5 mg/kg IV may repeat in 3–5 minutes
Vasopressin	VF or pulseless V-tach	40 units single dose

V-tach = ventricular tachycardia; VF = ventricular fibrillation.

Source: Adapted with permission from Eisenberg and Mengert.[35] Copyright© 2001 Massachusetts Medical Society. All rights reserved.

Second is the addition of amiodarone as the antiarrhythmic of choice for most ventricular arrhythmias. The substitution of amiodarone for other antiarrhythmics is based on evidence from the Amiodarone for Resuscitation After Out-of-Hospital Cardiac Arrest Due to Ventricular Fibrillation (ARREST) trial. In this study, patients who received amiodarone had improved survival in shock-resistant ventricular fibrillation. No other antiarrhythmics, including lidocaine, has demonstrated any effectiveness in this situation.

A number of controversies persist in the use of CPR. These include issues such as when CPR should be terminated for patients who are not responding, and when CPR is not appropriate. These issues require further clarification and at the present time are left to the best judgment of the clinician caring for the patient and to the family.

References

1. Kapoor WN, Karpf M, Wieland S, et al. A prospective evaluation and follow-up of patients with syncope. N Engl J Med 1983;309;197–204.
2. Kapoor WN. Evaluation and management of the patient with syncope. JAMA 1992;268:2553–60.
3. Manolis AS, Linzer M, Salem D, Estes NAM. Syncope: current diagnostic evaluation and management. Ann Intern Med 1990;112:850–63.
4. Linzer M, Yang EH, Estes M, et al. Diagnosing syncope: part 1: value of history, physical examination, and electrocardiography. Ann Intern Med 1997;126:989–96.
5. Linzer M, Prystowsky EN, Brunetti LL, et al. Recurrent syncope of unknown origin diagnosed by ambulatory continuous loop ECG recording. Am Heart J 1988;116:1632–4.
6. Davis TL, Freeman FR. Electroencephalography should not be routine in the evaluation of syncope in adults. Arch Intern Med 1990;150;2027–9.
7. Willis J. Syncope. Pediatr Rev 2000;21:201–3.
8. Braden DS, Games CH. The diagnosis and management of syncope in children and adolescents. Pediatr Ann 1997;26:422–6.
9. Lerman-Sagie T, Lerman P, Mukamel M, Blieden L, Mimouni M. A prospective evaluation of pediatric patients with syncope. Clin Pediatr 1994;33:66–70.
10. Scheidt S, Ascheim R, Killip T. Shock after acute myocardial infarction: a clinical and hemodynamic profile. Am J Cardiol 1970;26:556.
11. Califf RM, Bengston JR. Cardiogenic shock. N Engl J Med 1994;330:1724.
12. Wackers FJ, Lie KI, Becker AE, et al. Coronary artery disease in patients dying from cardiogenic shock or congestive heart failure in the setting of acute myocardial infarction. Br Heart J 1976;38:906.
13. Page DL, Caulfield JB, Kastor JA, et al. Myocardial changes associated with cardiogenic shock. N Engl J Med 1971;285:133.

14. Waksman R, Weiss AT, Gotsman MS, Hasin Y. Intraaortic counterpulsation improves survival in cardiogenic shock complicating acute myocardial infarction. Eur Health J 1993;14:1–74.
15. Sanborn TA, Sleeper LA, Bates ER, et al, for the SHOCK Investigators. Impact of thrombolysis, aortic counterpulsation, and their combination in cardiogenic shock: a report from the SHOCK Trial registry. J Am Coll Cardiol 2000;36:1123–9.
16. Hochman JS, Sleeper LA, Godfrey E, et al, for the SHOCK Investigators. Should we emergently revascularize occluded coronaries for cardiogenic shock? An international randomized trial of emergency PTCA/CABG-Trial design. Am Heart J 1999;137:313–21.
17. Myerburg RJ, Kessler KM, Castellanos A. Sudden cardiac death: epidemiology, transient risk, and intervention assessment. Ann Intern Med 1993;119:1187.
18. Bigger JT, Fleiss JL, Kleiger R, et al. The relationships among ventricular arrhythmias, left ventricular dysfunction and mortality in the 2 years after myocardial infarction. Circulation 1984;69:250.
19. Driscoll DJ, Edwards WD. Sudden unexpected death in children and adolescents. J Am Coll Cardiol 1985;5:118B–21B.
20. Anderson KR, Hill RW. Occlusive lesions of the cardiac conduction tissue arteries in sudden infant death syndrome. Pediatrics 1982;69:50.
21. Schwartz PJ, Stramba-Badiale M, Segantini A, et al. Prolongation of the QT interval and the sudden infant death syndrome. N Engl J Med 1998;338:1709–14.
22. Maron BJ, Epstein SE, Roberts WC. Causes of sudden death in competitive athletes. J Am Coll Cardiol 1986;7:240.
23. Maron BJ, Roberts WC, McAllister HA, et al. Sudden death in young athletes. Circulation 1980;62:218–29.
24. Fananapazir L, Cannon RO III, Tripodi D, et al. Impact of dual chamber permanent pacing in patients with obstructive hypertrophic cardiomyopathy with symptoms refractory to verapamil and beta adrenergic blocker therapy. Circulation 1992;85:2149.
25. Robbins RC, Stinson EB. Long term results of left ventricular myotomy and myectomy for obstructive hypertrophic cardiomyopathy. J Thorac Cardiovasc Surg 1996;111:586.
26. Packer M. Sudden unexpected death in patients with congestive heart failure: a second frontier. Circulation 1985;72:681.
27. Konishi Y, Matsuda K, Nishiwaki N, et al. Ventricular arrhythmias late after aortic and/or mitral valve replacement. Jpn Circ J 1985;49:576.
28. The Antiarrhythmics Versus Implantable Defibrillators (AVID) Investigators. A comparison of antiarrhythmic drug therapy with implantable defibrillators in patients resuscitated from near fatal ventricular arrhythmias. N Engl J Med 1997;337:1569–75.
29. Moss AJ, Hall WJ, Cannon DS, et al. Improved survival with an implanted defibrillator in patients with coronary disease at high risk for ventricular arrhythmia. N Engl J Med 1996;335:1933–40.
30. Dajani AS, Taubert KA, Wilson W, et al. Prevention of bacterial endocarditis. Recommendations by the American Heart Association. JAMA 1997;277:1794.

31. O'Nunain S, Perez I, Roelke M, et al. The treatment of patients with infected implantable cardioverter defibrillator systems. J Thorac Cardiovasc Surg 1997;133:121–9.
32. Braun TC, Hagen NA, Hatfield RE et al. Cardiac pacemakers and implantable defibrillators in terminal care. J Pain Symptom Manag 1999;18:126–131.
33. Ballew KA, Philbrick JT. Causes of variation in reported in-hospital CPR survival: a critical review. Resuscitation 1995;30:203–15.
34. Guidelines 2000 for cardiopulmonary resuscitation and emergency cardiovascular care: international consensus on science. Circulation 2000;102(suppl 1):1–138.
35. Eisenberg MS, Mengert TJ. Cardiac resuscitation. N Engl J Med 2001;344:1304–13.

10
Medical Care of the Surgical Patient

Mel P. Daly

Family physicians are frequently called on for consultations and medical management of patients who require surgical procedures. Advances in surgical techniques and anesthesia have significantly reduced the risk of death and serious morbidity from intraoperative and postoperative complications.[1] Factors that increase the risk for adverse outcomes have been more clearly defined, and interventions to address and treat known risk factors before surgery have contributed to declines in morbidity and mortality. Notwithstanding these advances, up to 20% of all surgical patients have at least one perioperative complication. Most surgical morbidity and mortality occurs as a result of cardiac (5%), pulmonary (10%), or infectious complications (15%).[2]

There are 25 million patients who undergo noncardiac surgery in the United States annually. Up to 7 million of them have cardiac disease or are at risk of developing cardiac disease during the operative period. About 50,000 patients sustain perioperative myocardial infarctions (MIs); 50% die as a result of their MI. Whereas cardiac problems are the major cause of mortality, most morbidity results from pulmonary complications, sepsis, or renal failure. Overall risk is related to individual patient factors (coexistent medical illness, age, pathology requiring surgery) and the type and urgency of the surgical procedure.[3]

The goal of the medical consultant is to identify prohibitive or potentially treatable risk factors so that the patient can be taken to the operating room in the best possible condition within the time available. Prior to surgery, patients, families, and surgeons should be aware of the potential medical risks of the procedure and if this risk can be reduced by preoperative interventions. It is imperative that family physicians become involved in the medical care of their patients during this most physiologically stressful time of their life.

Preoperative Assessment

History

The preoperative medical history should be comprehensive and focus on uncovering factors that may affect outcome. Previous surgery or anesthetic mishaps should be documented. It is important to take a menstrual history to prevent elective surgery on a pregnant woman inadvertently. For pediatric patients, particular attention must be paid to recent or current infectious conditions to ensure that they are infection free at the time of surgery. Seriously chronically ill pediatric patients with congenital anatomic anomalies (especially those children with cardiac disease) should be referred to specialists, when appropriate, prior to surgery.

A list of prescription and nonprescription medications should be obtained. Cardiac medications (digoxin, antiarrhythmic agents), antihypertensives (beta-blockers and alpha-blockers), major tranquilizers, and monoamine oxidase inhibitors can result in life-threatening arrhythmias. All currently taken medications should be documented and strategies developed for their use before, during, and after surgery. Patients should be asked about their use of corticosteroids within the previous 6 months to a year, as there are reports of patients failing to mount an adequate intraoperative stress response to surgery as a result of iatrogenic hypothalamic-pituitary-adrenal axis suppression.[4] All patients should be asked about their use of alcohol, cigarettes, and recreational drugs.

A major determinant of outcome for patients undergoing noncardiac operations is baseline functional capability. This is especially true for older patients, and patients with cardiac and pulmonary conditions. All patients should be asked about their daily routines and how well they are able to perform activities of daily living. Patients who can climb a flight of stairs without difficulty or who can mow their lawn, play golf without a cart, or do housework are likely to have good physiologic reserve and will usually tolerate most surgical procedures. For older patients, this assessment is also likely to be useful in predicting how much help will be required after surgery that will result in functional impairment after discharge (e.g., hip or knee replacement surgery, or trauma surgery).

Physical Examination

A comprehensive physical examination is always indicated. Anesthesiologists appreciate knowing about a deviated nasal septum, loose teeth, and the patient's ability to open his or her mouth. The examiner should pay particular attention to the cardiac and pulmonary systems. The heart rhythm, presence of significant murmurs, and added sounds (particularly an S_3) should be noted. It is important to note signs of congestive heart failure (rales, jugular venous pressure, edema) and aortic stenosis (murmur, pulse pressure). A careful respiratory examination, observing for lung expansion and diaphragmatic excursion and listening for wheezing or rhonchi, may identify the presence and severity of emphysema, asthma, or chronic obstructive lung disease. Patients with rheumatoid arthritis have a high incidence of atlantoaxial joint involvement and may be at risk of spinal cord compression with hyperextension during intubation. Range of motion should be tested and cervical spine radiographs considered. A mental status examination should be done for all elderly patients prior to surgery, because of the high incidence of postanesthesia delirium among elderly surgical patients.

Laboratory Testing

Many studies cite the lack of data supporting the routine use of laboratory testing before surgery. Many screening tests are ordered, but few are abnormal and rarely is surgery or anesthesia changed as a result.[5] This is especially true for patients who are to have low-risk surgical procedures (e.g., cataract surgery, breast biopsy, podiatric procedures, outpatient procedures, hernia repair).[6] Thus, routine preoperative laboratory testing is not justified; selective testing should be done instead if there are specific clinical indications. From a primary care perspective, routine testing may be indicated if a broader focus on long-term, otherwise neglected health care needs is appropriate. In many instances surgery is necessary and may be the only reason for someone to see a physician. This may present an opportunity for primary care assessment and maintenance.

It has been estimated that it costs in excess of $2 million for screening tests to identify an abnormal prothrombin time if it is not suspected by the history and physical examination. It is unusual to detect renal abnormalities on preoperative laboratory testing unless there is a suspicion based on risk factors for renal insufficiency (e.g., diabetes mellitus, hypertension, use of nephrotoxic medications). Similar data have revealed low yields for detecting abnormal results by doing a routine complete blood count (CBC), urinalysis, and liver function tests in asymptomatic patients. Thus laboratory testing must relate to the medical history, the proposed surgical procedure, and the potential for morbidity and mortality.[7]

In most centers patients are required to have a CBC prior to surgery, yet a strong argument can be made not to obtain this test, especially for men under age 60, as the incidence of anemia is low. Surgeons are unwilling to operate without knowing their patient's hemoglobin level, prothrombin time (international normalized ratio, INR), and partial thromboplastin time (PTT) because of potential bleeding risks; however, there is little indication for doing these tests unless there is a specific indication.

There is a high incidence of unsuspected abnormal electrocardiograms (ECGs) among presurgical patients, yet whether it changes the anesthesiologist's approach to surgery has not been studied. Because most deaths after surgery result from cardiac complications, it is worthwhile to order an ECG prior to surgery for people over age 40. After age 70, a measure of renal function (blood urea nitrogen, creatinine) is indicated because of age- and disease-related changes in creatinine clearance.

The likelihood of finding abnormal laboratory tests is increased in patients with underlying pathologic conditions and those taking prescription medications. Patients who have a history of bleeding disorders or bruiseability/excessive bleeding or who are currently taking anticoagulant medications should have a prothrombin time, INR, PTT, and platelet count determined. Those with renal disease should have their renal function measured, and patients with diabetes or who are currently taking corticosteroids should have serum electrolyte and glucose levels determined. Patients taking digitalis should have serum digoxin and potassium levels measured. Previously ordered laboratory tests rarely need to be repeated; tests done up to 4 months prior to surgery that were normal are rarely abnormal on repeat testing and usually do not affect anesthesia or surgical outcomes. Thus it is reasonable to accept laboratory testing and ECGs done within 4 months of elective surgery.[8]

Preoperative Report

Surgery should be postponed if a patient's medical condition can be improved and surgery safely delayed (elective and semielective procedures). If, in the opinion of the medical consultant, surgery ought to be postponed, it should first be communicated to the surgeon. The written preoperative report should identify medical conditions that place the patient at increased risk of adverse outcomes and make suggestions about how risk may be reduced in the time available.

It is tempting to make recommendations about the type and route of anesthesia. There is, however, little evidence to suggest that the type or route of anesthesia is important for predicting adverse outcomes.[9] General anesthetic agents are myocardial suppressants and peripheral vasodilators. Spinal anesthesia induces a sympathectomy at the level at which it is administered and causes levels of hypotension similar to those seen with general anesthetic agents. Furthermore, spinal anesthesia induces motor muscle paralysis that may interfere with forced expiration. Patients may have a heightened level of anxiety because they are awake, which increases myocardial oxygen demand. There is a greater likelihood of aspiration pneumonitis among patients given spinal anesthesia because the airway is unprotected. Occasionally, particularly in elderly patients, it is not possible to administer spinal anesthesia because of thoracolumbar spondylosis. Thus if a patient is "cleared" for spinal anesthesia and the anesthesiologist is technically unable to administer spinal anesthesia, general anesthesia may be the only option.

Assessment of Risk

The risk of mortality or morbidity is low and is individualized and related to the presence and severity of comorbid medical illnesses (especially cardiac and pulmonary pathology), the surgical procedure, and whether the procedure is emergent or elective. The risk of an adverse outcome can be estimated in a number of ways. The American Society of Anesthesiologists (ASA) physical status classification, first described during the 1950s, is widely used today.[10] Patients are classified based on their physical health status to somewhat qualitatively determined classes, ranging from class 1 (healthy) to class 5 (moribund). In large studies describing outcomes of thousands of operations, the ASA classification system has proved useful for predicting risk of complications and death. Limitations of the ASA system are that assignment of risk is subject to observer bias, and the inherent risk of the surgical procedure is not considered. Emergency operations are associated with a two- to fourfold risk of adverse outcomes when compared to elective surgery. True surgical emergencies (perforated organ, peritonitis, trauma, aortic aneurysm) rarely allow time for a comprehensive preoperative medical evaluation. In most other instances, the risk of adverse outcomes can be estimated by assessing clinical predictors in the context of the hemodynamic physiologic stress (alterations in heart rate, blood pressure, volume, hemoglobin, oxygenation, thrombogenicity) of the proposed operation. Major surgery can be long (intrathoracic, vascular, or neurosurgical procedures) and associated with a greater likelihood of adverse outcomes. Moderate-risk operations include extremity operations lasting 2 hours or longer (e.g., orthopedic surgery), and surgery that is less likely to result in adverse medical outcomes includes distal extremity operations, hernia repair, thoracoscopy, and transurethral resection of the prostate (Table 10.1).

Another commonly used risk assessment instrument is the Goldman Cardiac Risk Index, which was first published during the late

Table 10.1. **Surgical Procedure Risk**

High risk (reported cardiac risk ≥ 5%)
 Coronary artery bypass graft surgery
 Pneumonectomy
 Trauma surgery
 Neurosurgery
 Major vascular procedure
 Ruptured abdominal viscus
 Emergency surgery
 Anticipated prolonged surgery, with hemodynamic instability

Moderate risk (reported cardiac risk usually ≤ 5%)
 Abdominal surgery (open cholecystectomy, colon resection, etc.)
 Orthopedic surgery
 Urogynecologic surgery (prostatectomy, hysterectomy, cesarean
  section)
 Splenectomy
 Cancer staging procedures
 Peripheral vascular procedures (endarterectomy, femoral-popliteal
  bypass)
 Prostate surgery

Low risk (generally <1%)
 Cataract surgery
 Podiatry procedures
 Endoscopy and biopsy
 Breast biopsy
 Mastectomy
 Herniorrhaphy
 Vasectomy
 Appendectomy
 Dermatologic procedures

Source: Modified from Eagle et al,[16] with permission.

1970s and has been widely used subsequently.[11] More than 1000 patients admitted to Massachusetts General Hospital for surgical procedures underwent comprehensive preoperative physical assessments and were followed postoperatively to identify major cardiac complications and death. A multivariate discriminate risk analysis identified factors significantly associated with these outcomes, and each risk factor was assigned a weighted point score based on its relative association with adverse outcomes. Based on point scores, patients were retrospectively assigned to a level of risk associated with serious cardiac complications (ventricular tachycardia, death, MI, pulmonary edema) (class I, 0.7%, to class IV, 22.0%) and mortality (class I, 0.2%, to class IV, 50.0%). Factors not found to increase the risk of serious cardiovascular morbidity and mortality were controlled hypertension, the presence of an S_4, diabetes mellitus, hyperlipidemia, and stable angina pectoris. The latter was defined as angina that had not changed over the previous year in patients able to ambulate a distance of two blocks. Some of these factors (congestive heart failure and general medical condition) are potentially reversible preoperatively.

Lower reinfarction rates for patients operated on within 6 months of the original MI have been reported more recently and reflect an increased awareness of risk and more experience using invasive hemodynamic monitoring, pressors, and beta-blockers.[12] Perhaps more important for estimating the risk of reinfarction is the extent of prior myocardial damage and whether the patient has myocardium that is at risk because of coronary artery stenosis. Patients who have had non–Q-wave MIs may be at a greater risk of reinfarction than patients who have survived a transmural infarction. These patients frequently have borderline zones of potential ischemia that may be in jeopardy during anesthesia. Symptom-linked exercise testing to assess the extent of previous damage and identify at-risk myocardium is indicated in all patients who have had recent MIs requiring noncardiac surgery.

More recently published cardiac risk indices have taken these and other factors into consideration. Subsequent modifications (Table 10.2) of the Goldman Risk Index and includes point ratings for unstable angina (class III angina after one to two blocks of ambulation; class IV angina at rest) and critical aortic stenosis.[13] Each of the published cardiac risk indices has been studied and shown to accurately predict the risk (class III or IV) of having an adverse cardiac outcome (pooled data: 16% for class III and 56% for class IV). A higher than expected serious complication rate for class I and II patients has been reported among those operated on for abdominal aortic

Table 10.2. **Cardiac Risk Assessment (Modified Multifactorial Risk Index)**

Criteria, points
Coronary artery disease, 10
Myocardial infarction ≤6 months
Myocardial infarction >6 months
Canadian Cardiovascular Society angina
Class 3, 10
Class 4, 20
Unstable angina within 3 months, 10
Alveolar pulmonary edema
Within 1 week, 10
Ever, 5
Valvular disease
Critical aortic stenosis, 20
Arrhythmias
Sinus plus atrial premature beats or rhythm other than sinus on preoperative ECG, 5
More than 5 PVCs/min at any time prior to surgery, 5
Medical status, 5
Poor general medical status
PO_2 <60 or PCO_2 >50
K <3.0 or HCO_3 <20 mEq/L
BUN >50 mg/dL or creatinine >3 mg/dL
Abnormal SGOT
Chronic liver disease
Bedridden due to noncardiac cause
Age >70 years, 5
Operation: emergency, 10

Source: Modified from American College of Physicians,[17] with permission.

ECG = electrocardiogram; PVCs = premature ventricular contractions; BUN = blood urea nitrogen; SGOT = serum glutamate oxolic acid.

aneurysms, probably reflecting a high incidence of asymptomatic cardiac disease among these patients, resulting in their being misclassified as low-risk class I patients.[14]

Cardiac Risk

Coronary Artery Disease

Patients with a history of a documented MI have a greatly increased likelihood of having an intra- or postoperative cardiac complications (see Chapter 2). This is especially true for patients who have sustained their infarction within 3 months of their noncardiac surgery. Patients who have sustained a recent MI and who have evidence of residual ischemic risk (unstable or severe angina, poorly controlled ischemic-mediated congestive heart failure, or severe valvular heart disease) should be considered at prohibitively high risk for adverse perioperative cardiac complications. These patients should be referred to cardiologists for further evaluation and potential cardiac surgical interventions prior to considering noncardiac elective surgery.[15]

Patients with mild angina, prior MI (older than 1 month), history of congestive heart failure, diabetes mellitus, and elderly patients should be classified at intermediate risk for having perioperative cardiac-related complications. Patients with underlying peripheral vascular disease should also be considered at intermediate risk because of the high incidence of coexisting cardiac pathology (often "silent").[16] Patients without cardiac disease have a low incidence of postoperative MI and other cardiac complications (Table 10.3).

An important component of the preoperative cardiac evaluation for all patients is an assessment of how well a patient can perform functional activities. This may be helpful in deciding whether further cardiac testing is necessary, especially for intermediate-risk patients who are scheduled to have major surgery. Patients who can participate in strenuous activities such as running, playing basketball, or long-distance swimming have excellent functional reserve capacity, while sedentary patients who have difficulty carrying groceries up a flight of stairs have poor functional capacity. Patients with excellent functional capacity usually can tolerate major surgery, while patients with poor functional capacity are at much greater risk for adverse outcomes. Patients with moderate functional capacity should be further evaluated if they have intermediate- or high-risk clinical profiles or if they are to have major surgery.

Further testing and recommendations about how best to proceed can be made by carefully evaluating the preoperative clinical risk profile, functional capacity, and the proposed procedure. This is outlined by the American College of Cardiology/American Heart Association (ACC/AHA) Task Force, which suggests a progressive stepwise approach to preoperative cardiac assessment (Fig. 10.1).

The goal of the preoperative assessment is to evaluate not only the risk of the immediate surgery but also the long-term cardiac risk. Thus this may be an ideal time to consider further testing (noninvasive or invasive) if this is likely to improve outcome. Noninvasive testing (see below) should be considered for patients who are at intermediate clinical risk and are to undergo a major procedure. Exer-

Table 10.3. **Clinical Predictors of Increased Perioperative Cardiac Risk**

High risk
　Recent myocardial infarction (within 1 month)
　Congestive heart failure (unstable)
　Valvular heart disease (esp. aortic stenosis)
　Unstable angina
　Significant cardiac arrhythmias (ventricular tachycardia with
　　ischemia, supraventricular arrhythmias with uncontrolled
　　ventricular response)

Intermediate risk
　History of myocardial infarction
　Stable congestive heart failure
　Stable/mild angina pectoris
　Diabetes mellitus
　Age over 70 years
　Rhythm other than normal sinus rhythm on the preoperative ECG
　Uncontrolled hypertension
　Peripheral vascular disease
　Mitral valve prolapse ± regurgitation

Low risk
　Age over 70 years
　Controlled hypertension
　History of cerebrovascular disease
　Cardiac murmur
　"Minor" ECG abnormalities (premature atrial contractions,
　　nonspecific STT changes)
　Controlled atrial fibrillation
　History of stroke
　Low functional capacity

STT = serial thrombin time.
Source: Modified from Eagle et al,[16] with permission.

cise stress testing, echocardiography (resting, stress), or perfusion imaging (dipyridamole, dobutamine) can further assist in stratifying risk; however, there is as yet no evidence that this type of testing improves perioperative care. Invasive testing (arteriography) should be reserved for high-risk patients with suspected left main disease, triple vessel disease, or unstable angina in whom angioplasty or coronary artery bypass grafting would be indicated. Patients at low risk should have no further testing.[17]

The peak time of occurrence of postoperative MI is 3 to 6 days after surgery; it is due to increased activity, pain, and shifts of third-

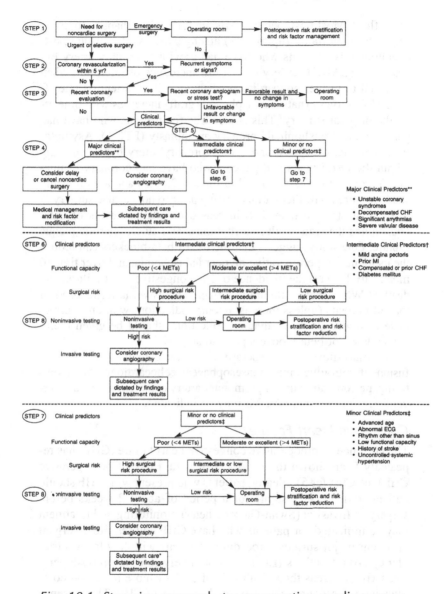

Fig. 10.1. Stepwise approach to preoperative cardiac assessment. Steps are discussed in text. *Subsequent care may include cancellation or delay of surgery, coronary revascularization followed by cardiac surgery, or intensified care. (From Eagle et al,[16] with permission.)

space fluid. Most postoperative MIs are "silent," perhaps accounting for the high mortality (up to 50%) among patients who sustain postoperative MIs. Patients who have had previous coronary artery bypass graft (CABG) surgery have a low incidence of infarction when subjected to further noncardiac procedures.[18] The restenosis rate after CABG surgery (native or saphenous graft) increases with time after the original surgery. This is also true for patients who have had percutaneous transluminal coronary angioplasty (PTCA). Asymptomatic patients who have undergone coronary artery bypass grafting within the last 5 years and patients who have had coronary evaluation (cardiac stress testing) within the last 2 years and are clinically stable require no further cardiac testing prior to noncardiac surgery.[16]

Surgical stress can lead to increased circulating levels of catecholamines that can result in arrhythmias and atherosclerotic plaque rupture. One study suggests that the use of beta-blockers can reduce the incidence of perioperative myocardial ischemia, and over time (6 months to 2 years) the incidence of MI, congestive heart failure, and death.[19] While these data are less than conclusive, it seems prudent that all patients (unless there is a contraindication) with an intermediate or high risk for cardiac complications should be given therapeutic doses of beta-blockers prior to surgery.[20]

In certain situations, preoperative intensive care, intraoperative infusion of nitroglycerine, transesophageal echocardiographic monitoring, perioperative use of pulmonary artery catheterization, and surveillance for perioperative MI may be indicated.

Congestive Heart Failure

The presence of preoperative congestive heart failure (CHF) has repeatedly been shown to be associated with a risk of postoperative CHF (see Chapter 5). Ideally, patients who present with CHF should be hemodynamically stable for a period of about 2 weeks before surgery.[21] Invasive (Swan-Ganz catheter) monitoring and treatment may be indicated for patients who have CHF and require emergent or urgent major surgical procedures. Patients with low left ventricular ejection fractions (EFs) are more likely to develop postoperative CHF, whereas those with EFs of 50% or more have low complication rates, even if they have had a history of CHF. The presence of jugular venous distention, current pulmonary edema, or an S_3 gallop places a patient at risk for perioperative cardiac complications. If possible, surgery is postponed until the CHF has been treated with a goal of euvolemia for a period of 2 weeks or more prior to surgery.

Hypertension

Poorly controlled hypertension is associated with perioperative cardiac complications, blood pressure lability, and renal failure (see Chapter 1). Severe hypertension may occur especially during induction of anesthesia, intubation, and emergence from anesthesia. Diastolic blood pressure readings of more than 120 mm Hg and systolic blood pressures of more than 200 mm Hg are associated with a greater likelihood of adverse cardiac outcomes.[22] Patients with well-controlled hypertension are not at increased risk during surgery. Patients taking antihypertensive medications such as beta-blockers, angiotensin-converting enzyme (ACE) inhibitors, clonidine, and calcium channel blockers show attenuated blood pressure responses to intubation and induction of anesthesia. Of greater importance for patients with mild to moderate hypertension is the effect of anesthesia on mean arterial blood pressure (MAP) levels. Large reductions in MAP (>30% for more than 10 minutes) are associated with a greater likelihood of intraoperative MI, CHF, and renal insufficiency. The goal of treatment prior to surgery is to achieve consistent systolic blood pressure readings below 170 mm Hg and diastolic blood pressures below 110 mm Hg.

Cardiac Arrhythmias

The significance of cardiac arrhythmias identified preoperatively is somewhat controversial (see Chapter 3), as it has become clear that the presence of nonsustained premature ventricular contractions (PVCs) is not a risk factor for ventricular tachycardia or sudden death unless associated with underlying cardiac ischemia (suggesting the presence of severe coronary artery disease).[23] Prophylaxis with antiarrhythmic medications is indicated for patients with sustained ventricular tachycardia, especially if they have had a recent MI. Atrial fibrillation is an important rhythm during the perioperative period, because when the ventricular response rate is rapid, the ability to increase cardiac output is compromised. This situation occurs because of reduced left ventricular filling volume as a result of a shorter diastolic filling time and loss of the presystolic "atrial kick." New-onset atrial fibrillation, particularly in patients with fixed outflow tract obstruction (aortic stenosis, asymmetric septal hypertrophy) may result in severe CHF and an inability to increase cardiac output. Thus control of the ventricular rate becomes important during anesthesia to allow adequate end-diastolic filling volumes and cardiac output. There is a higher incidence of atrial fibrillation during anesthesia in patients who undergo long surgical procedures, those with thoracic or neurosurgical procedures, and the elderly. Digoxin, beta-blockers, or calcium channel blockers should be continued up to and including the day of surgery. Most patients undergoing anesthesia (especially those with a history of arrhythmias) develop some kind of arrhythmia on induction of anesthesia, usually isolated occasional ectopic ventricular or atrial beats. Supraventricular arrhythmias may exacerbate underlying cardiac disease by increasing myocardial oxygen demand. These arrhythmias may also be a manifestation of noncardiac problems such as electrolyte abnormalities, or infection.

It is rare that patients need to have a pacemaker inserted prior to a major surgical procedure.[24] Placement of a pacemaker should be considered in patients who have long sinus pauses, high-grade second-degree heart block, or complete heart block. There is no indication for pacemaker placement in patients with first-degree atrioventricular (AV) block or asymptomatic bifascicular block, as these patients rarely develop complete heart block. The use of the electrocautery machine during surgery may interfere with "demand" pacemaker function; if the earth lead is placed away from the pacemaker magnet and the surgeon administers short bursts of electrocautery, this effect is reduced. However, it may be necessary to convert the pacemaker function to the fixed-rate mode when "demand" pacemaker responses are suboptimal.

Valvular Heart Disease

Valvular heart disease (especially hemodynamically significant aortic stenosis) is associated with an increased risk for perioperative mortality[25] (see Chapter 4). Severe and symptomatic aortic stenosis may require valve replacement or valvuloplasty if high-risk noncardiac surgery is to be done safely. Mitral stenosis is not associated with increased mortality, but these patients are sensitive to preload volume changes especially when tachycardia results in a reduction in diastolic filling time. Patients with aortic regurgitation and mitral regurgitation are less sensitive to volume changes but require adequate left ventricular contractility, as regurgitation takes place during both diastole and systole. Bradycardia is less well tolerated because of increased potential for regurgitation during prolonged diastole. Prosthetic valves increase the risk of bacterial endocarditis and thrombotic complications. Asymmetric septal hypertrophy may be difficult to manage perioperatively because the degree of outflow tract obstruction is variable. Certain medications exacerbate outflow tract obstruction; diuretics and nitrates reduce preload and intravascular volume; inotropes may increase obstruction because of increased contractility; and tachycardia may cause similar effects because of decreased diastolic filling time.

Peripheral Vascular Disease

There is a high incidence of occult coronary artery disease among patients with peripheral vascular disease (PVD) (see Chapter 2). Up to 60% have severe coronary artery disease; many have no clinical symptoms and frequently have normal ECGs. Patients with PVD have a high incidence of postoperative mortality, mostly because of intraoperative and postoperative MIs.[26] Additional cardiac testing should be considered for patients with PVD scheduled for major surgery.[27] Exercise stress testing (EST), if positive, can identify patients at increased risk of having a cardiac event, but the positive predictive value is low. The negative predictive value is high (i.e., a negative test makes it unlikely that a patient will develop a postoperative cardiac complication). Many patients cannot tolerate EST because of intermittent claudication, deconditioning, rest ischemia, or amputations. Furthermore, many patients with PVD have ECG changes of the left bundle branch block or left ventricular hypertrophy, or they are currently taking digoxin, making exercise test ECG readings uninterpretable.

Evidence has suggested that perioperative ECG monitoring may be useful in patients with PVD.[28] Preoperative ischemia and silent ischemia are good predictors of perioperative and postoperative ischemia and cardiac events. Furthermore, patients without signs of ischemia preoperatively are unlikely to have ischemic events. Again, the positive predictive value of silent ischemia is low because few patients with PVD and positive tests develop postoperative cardiac complications.

Perhaps even more useful is chemical stress testing using nuclear medicine imaging or echocardiography.[29] Dipyridamole is a coronary vasodilator; hence, stenotic arteries do not dilate, and infarcted areas remain unperfused. In normal hearts thallium is evenly distributed throughout the myocardium, with no distribution distal to stenosed arteries. These areas show up as "cold spots" on thallium imaging studies. If thallium redistributes on delayed imaging (4 hours later) to a previously imaged "cold spot," it may be an indication of underperfused myocardium. Thus redistribution on late imaging with thallium may be an important factor for determining the risk of intraoperative ischemia in a patient with PVD. The advantages of dipyridamole thallium testing are that patients do not have to exercise and increase their target heart rate, and there are few complications associated with infusing dipyridamole.

When dipyridamole thallium scintigraphy results are considered in conjunction with important clinical parameters (angina, CHF, Q wave on ECG, diabetes mellitus, PVCs), they add significant weight when predicting adverse outcomes for patients with PVD.[30] Risk stratification may be further enhanced by quantifying the number of areas on thallium imaging that show evidence of redistribution on delayed imaging studies.

A strategy for patients with PVD scheduled for a major vascular procedure may be to conduct a noninvasive stress test, which if negative suggests that surgery can proceed without further testing.[31] If the imaging study shows evidence of thallium redistribution, the size of the defect should be measured. If in the opinion of the radiologist or cardiologist the defect is small, the risk is low; but if it is moderate to large, the patient may be a candidate for cardiac catheterization and revascularization before having major noncardiac surgery. If the patient is not a candidate for coronary artery revascularization, the previously planned surgery or an alternative surgical procedure should be considered. If the patient is a candidate for coronary vascularization, coronary angiography may be indicated.

It is important to consider the cumulative and relative risks of having these procedures[32] (Table 10.4). The risk of mortality from coronary angiography is about 1%, and the risk for CABG or PTCA in a patient with PVD is in the range of 6% to 10%. The risk of delaying noncardiac surgery for testing depends on the reason for the delay and the urgency of the proposed procedure (e.g., a limb that is ischemic or in jeopardy). The risk of mortality for noncardiac surgery after a revascularization procedure is still in the range of 2% to

Table 10.4. **Relative Risk for Further Investigation Versus Proceeding with Noncardiac Surgery in Patients with PVD**

No revascularization prior to noncardiac surgery
Risk of noncardiac procedure
Long-term outcome

Revascularization prior to noncardiac surgery
Risk of cardiac catherization (1% risk)
Risk of CABG/PTCA (6–10%)
Risk of delaying surgery
Risk of surgery after revascularization (2–3%)
Long-term outcome
Perioperative risk without revascularization must be ≥15% for CABG or PTCA to be of benefit.

PVD = peripheral vascular disease; CABG = coronary artery bypass grafting; PTCA = percutaneous transluminal coronary angioplasty.

3%, together with unknown long-term risks of morbidity and mortality. Thus the potential risk of death by further investigating and treating patients with PVD is in the range of about 10% to 15%. If the risk of the noncardiac procedure without further testing is less, it may be appropriate to proceed with surgery and inform the patient, anesthesiologist, and surgeon of the increased risk.[33]

Medications

In general, all medications should be continued up to the day of surgery. Monoamine oxidase inhibitors interfere with autonomic function and may cause perioperative hypertension and hypotension. These agents may prolong neuromuscular blockade, inhibit hepatic enzymes, and prolong the action of narcotic drugs. If possible, the medication is discontinued a few weeks before surgery. Beta-blockers and clonidine should be continued until the day of surgery, as there is a possibility of postwithdrawal rebound hypertension. The surgeon should order antibiotic prophylaxis. Most surgeons prefer first-generation cephalosporins (usually cefazolin), starting with the preanesthetic dose and continuing for 24 hours.

Management of anticoagulants may be problematic during the perioperative period. For patients taking Coumadin, the risk of discontinuing anticoagulation must be assessed. For patients with metallic heart valves, Coumadin discontinuation is risky, although continuing Coumadin up to the time of surgery is contraindicated. If it is reasonable to discontinue the Coumadin, it is stopped 3 days before surgery and then reinstituted after surgery. If it is necessary to anticoagulate the patient up to surgery, Coumadin can be stopped 3 days before the operation and the patient treated with intravenous heparin. The heparin infusion is stopped 6 hours before surgery, and Coumadin is reinstituted after surgery. Alternatively, low molecular weight heparin (LMWH) may be used in doses of ~1 mg/hr every 12 hours adjusted to renal function for 3 days prior to surgery with the last dose administered 12 hours prior to the operation. LMWH or Coumadin may then be reinstituted after surgery. Aspirin, which irreversibly inhibits cyclooxygenase and affects platelet adhesiveness, should be discontinued 7 days before surgery. Other nonsteroidal and nonsalicylate products may be continued up to surgery.

Patients who are at risk for bacterial endocarditis (patients with prosthetic heart valves, previous endocarditis, congenital malformations, hypertrophic cardiomyopathy, and mitral valve prolapse with mitral regurgitation) should receive prophylactic antibiotic coverage (Table 10.5). Bacterial endocarditis prophylaxis is recommended for

Table 10.5. **Bacterial Endocarditis Prophylaxis**

Dental, Oral, Respiratory Tract, or Esophageal Procedures (Follow-up dose no longer recommended.) Total children's dose should not exceed adult dose.

I. Standard general prophylaxis for pateints at risk:
Amoxicillin: Adults, 2.0 g (children, 50 mg/kg) given orally one hour before procedure.

II. Unable to take oral medications:
Ampicillin: Adults, 2.0 g (children, 50 mg/kg) given IM or IV within 30 minutes before procedure.

III. Amoxicillin/ampicillin/penicillin allergic patients:
Clindamycin: Adults, 600 mg (children, 20 mg/kg) given orally one hour before procedure. **-OR-**
   Cephalexin* or Cefadroxil*: Adults, 2.0 g (children, 50 mg/kg) orally one hour before procedure. **-OR-**
   Azithromycin or Clarithromycin: Adults, 500 mg (children 15 mg/kg) orally one hour before procedure.

IV. Amoxicillin/ampicillin/penicillin allergic patients unable to take oral medications:
Clindamycin : Adults, 600 mg (children, 20 mg/kg) IV within 30 minutes before procedure. **-OR-**
   Cefazolin*: Adults, 1.0 g (children, 25 mg/kg) IM or IV within 30 minutes before procedure.

*Cephalosporins should not be used in patients with immediate-type hypersensitivity reaction to penicillins.

Genitourinary/Gastrointestinal Procedures
I. High-risk patients:
Ampicillin plus gentamicin: Amplicillin (adults, 2.0 g; children 50 mg/kg) plus gentamicin 1.5 mg/kg (for both adults and children, not to exceed 120 mg) IM or IV within 30 minutes before starting procedure; 6 hours later ampicillin (adults, 1.0 g; children, 25 mg/kg) IM or IV, or amoxicillin (adults, 1.0 g; children, 25 mg/kg) orally.

II. High-risk patients allergic to ampicillin/amoxicillin:
Vancomycin plus gentamicin: Vancomycin (adults, 1.0 g; children, 20 mg/kg) IV over 1–2 hours plus gentamicin 1.5 mg/kg (for both adults and children, not to exceed 120 mg) IM or IV. Complete injection/infusion within 30 minutes before starting procedure.

III. Moderate-risk patients:
Amoxicillin: Adults, 2.0 g (children, 50 mg/kg) orally one hour before procedure **-OR-**
   Ampicillin: Adults, 2.0 g (children, 50 mg/kg) IM or IV within 30 minutes before starting procedure.

Table 10.5. (Continued)

IV. Moderate-risk patients allergic to ampicillin/amoxicillin:
Vancomycin: Adults, 1.0 g (children 20 mg/kg) IV over 1–2 hours.
Complete infusion within 30 minutes of starting the procedure.

NOTE: For patients already taking an antibiotic, or for other special situations, please refer to the full statement referenced below.

Adapted from *Prevention of Bacterial Endocarditis: Recommendations by the American Heart Association* by the Committee on Rheumatic Fever, Endocarditis, and Kawasaki Disease. *JAMA* 1997, 277:1794–1801, *Circulation* 1997, 96:358–366, and *JADA* 1997, 128:1142–1150. Health Care Professionals—Please refer to these recommendations (endorsed by the American Dental Association and American Society for Gastrointestinal Endoscopy) for more complete information as to which patients and which procedures need prophylaxis.

Source: Reproduced with permission.
http://www.americanheart.org/presenter.jhtml?identifier=11086
© 2004, American Heart Association.

cardiac conditions that are high (prosthetic valves) or intermediate risk (mitral valve prolapse with regurgitation), for developing endocarditis; and for procedures that may result in bacteremia. Simplified prophylaxis regimens are recommended for dental, gastrointestinal, and genitourinal procedures. There is no need to institute endocarditis prophylaxis for patients with atrial septal defects, post-CABG patients, or patients with pacemakers.[34]

Pulmonary System

Pulmonary complications are the most common reasons for morbidity among patients undergoing noncardiac surgery (25–50% of major surgical procedures). Pneumonia, lobar collapse, pneumonitis, atelectasis, and respiratory failure can occur. These complications frequently result in prolonged hospital stays and increased mortality.

A number of reproducible physiologic changes occur with general anesthesia that place patients (especially those with underlying pulmonary disease) at risk of developing a respiratory complication. Predictable changes occur in patterns of ventilation, lung volumes, gas exchange, and pulmonary defense mechanisms.[35] These changes occur as a result of the procedure itself, the anesthesia, altered sensorium, analgesia, immobility, restrictive bandages, and relative imn·obility. General anesthesia results in a 20% decrease in tidal volume, but a compensatory increase in respiratory rate occurs, such that the minute ventilation changes minimally. Lung compliance de-

Table 10.6. **Major Risks for Adverse Pulmonary Outcomes**

Forced expiratory volume in 1 second (FEV_1) <1 L
Maximum voluntary ventilation <50% of predicted
P_{CO_2} >90 mm Hg
P_{CO_2} <50 mm Hg
Relative hypoxemia
Upper abdominal and intrathoracic procedures
Prolonged anesthesia (>3 hours)
Cigarette abuse
Obesity (>30% above ideal body weight)
Chronic obstructive pulmonary disease
American Society of Anesthesiologists (ASA) class IV
Age >70 years

creases by 33%, and sighing is abolished by the effects of narcotic medications. Total lung capacity and all subdivisions of lung volumes decrease. Vital capacity decreases by half and lasts for 2 weeks after general anesthesia. Most importantly, functional residual capacity (FRC) decreases by up to 40% after upper abdominal and thoracic procedures. Closing volume (CV, the volume at which airway flow stops during expiration) increases significantly. Under normal circumstances FRC is about 50% and CV is about 30% of total lung capacity, and when these volumes decrease because of general anesthesia the lungs become subject to airway closure, atelactasis, and pneumonia.[36]

General anesthesia results in relative hypoxia because of ventilation-perfusion mismatches. Nondependent areas of lung are relatively overventilated and underperfused (dead space), whereas dependent parts of the lung are relatively perfused and underventilated (shunts). Normal pulmonary defense mechanisms (cough and ciliary action) are also impaired during general anesthesia.

Factors that further increase the likelihood of developing pulmonary complications (Table 10.6) include the site of the incision (thoracic and upper abdominal incisions), supine position, prolonged anesthesia (>3 hours), a history of productive cough, cigarette smoking, and fluid overload. Obesity, defined as weighing more than 30% over ideal body weight, is associated with an increased work of breathing, reduced lung volumes, and hypercapnia; all are associated with an increased risk of complications.

The limits of pulmonary operability have never been clearly defined. There are no studies that demonstrate the level of forced expiratory volume in 1 second (FEV_1) below which a person is at increased risk, nor is there consensus about indications for preoperative pulmonary function testing.[37] An FEV_1 of less than 2 L is associated with an increased risk of pulmonary complications, and patients with an FEV_1 value as low as 1 L may be more likely to require ventilator support and develop pulmonary complications.

There are no clear guidelines for estimating potential risk of developing pulmonary complications prior to surgery. Chest radiographs may be useful in high-risk patients. There are no clear indications for ordering pulmonary function tests. These tests may help in defining the severity of underlying pulmonary disease, and thus may help estimate the potential risk for complications. For patients who are to have cardiac surgery, pneumonectomy, or esophagectomy, more sophisticated testing such as quantitative ventilation-perfusion scanning, diffusing capacity studies, and estimation of maximum oxygen consumption during exercise may be indicated.

For patients with pulmonary disease, it may be possible to reduce complications by instructing them to stop cigarette smoking at least 8 weeks before surgery,[38] which results in enhanced mucociliary transport mechanisms, reduced secretions, less bronchospasm, and reduced levels of circulating carboxyl hemoglobin. Optimal bronchodilation prior to surgery may require home or inpatient nebulizer treatments and use of steroids for patients with asthma. Incentive spirometry has been shown to reduce the incidence of pulmonary complications and the length of hospital stay. Emphasis is placed on general conditioning, nutrition, and psychological preparation if a person is likely to spend some time in the intensive care unit after surgery. Anesthesiologists are aware of the need to minimize anesthesia time, use intermittent hyperinflation, and control secretions. Postoperatively, patients should be encouraged to get out of bed early, take deep breaths, use the incentive spirometer, and cough. Narcotic and analgesic medications should be administered in doses titrated to obtain analgesic effects without clouding the sensorium. Because cardiac and pulmonary complications occur for up to 7 days after surgery, medical consultants should closely monitor patients during this stressful time.

Hematologic System

Hemoglobin and Hematocrit

The optimal levels of hemoglobin and hematocrit for surgery traditionally have been ≥ 10 g/dL and 30%, respectively. Consensus conference reports have now recognized the increasing evidence of the safety of transfused blood products and the excellent outcomes of surgery on anemic patients; it is therefore concluded that no single criterion can be used to support preoperative blood transfusion.[39] There is good evidence that surgical procedures can be done in patients with hemoglobin levels above 8 g/dL and in patients with hemoglobin levels as low as 6 g/dL if blood loss is less than 500 mL. The risks associated with blood transfusion are low; there is a less than 1% risk of transfusion mortality associated with the human immunodeficiency virus (HIV) and a less than 0.3% risk of acquiring hepatitis C (since testing became available during the 1990s); the risk of hemolytic reactions or congestive cardiac failure is also low.

Higher hemoglobin levels are advisable for older patients, those likely to experience significant blood loss, and patients with coronary artery or cerebrovascular disease. Lower levels of hemoglobin are acceptable for patients with chronic anemia with compensated intravascular volumes. When possible, transfusion is done preoperatively, as transfusion reaction signs may be obliterated under general anesthesia. The more widespread use of autologous blood, cell savers, and erythropoietin has greatly reduced the need for transfusion with banked blood.[40] The hematocrit level for optimal oxygen delivery to tissues and rheology is around 45%. Patients with polycythemia and erythrocytosis are more likely to bleed or have blood clots and should be phlebotomized to hematocrits of around 45% to 50% before elective surgery.

Platelets

Patients with thrombocytopenia rarely bleed until platelet counts are below 100,000 cells/μL, and the risk of bleeding is procedure-dependent for patients with platelet counts between 50,000 and 100,000/μL.[41] Platelet counts below 50,000/μL are associated with an increased risk of bleeding. Qualitative platelet functioning can be impaired even when platelet counts are normal. Medications including nonsteroidal antiinflammatory drugs (NSAIDs), aspirin, tricyclic antidepressants, alcohol, and even beta-blockers can impair platelet adhesion. Patients with uremia, liver disease, alcoholism, and leukemia may also develop qualitative platelet disorders. For these patients it may be useful to determine the bleeding time prior to surgery.

Coagulation Disorders

Coagulation disorders are rare, as a loss of 80% of clotting factor levels is required to prolong the prothrombin time (PT) or partial thromboplastin time (PTT). The most common disorder affecting clotting factor production is severe liver disease. Patients with prolonged PTs and PTTs can be managed intraoperatively with transfusions of fresh frozen plasma and whole blood. For patients with known or suspected acquired factor deficiency, a hematologist should be consulted for further investigation, recommendations, and treatment perioperatively.

Deep Venous Thrombosis

All surgical patients are at risk for developing deep venous thrombosis (DVT) (see Chapter 7). This risk is increased for elderly patients, the obese, cigarette smokers, cancer patients, patients who are having long procedures, those with previous venous disease, and those with a history of CHF. The risk of developing a postoperative DVT depends on the type of surgical procedure and the presence of risk factors. The optimal modality for DVT prophylaxis is controversial. LMWH (40 mg/day or 30 mg q12h) significantly reduces the incidence of DVT and pulmonary embolism in patients undergoing general surgical procedures, such as urologic or gynecologic surgery, surgery for elective hip or knee replacement or hip fracture, and other orthopedic procedures including trauma surgery. LMWH in doses of 40 mg per day or 30 mg every 12 hours significantly reduces the incidence of postoperative DVT.[42] It is unclear if LMWH is superior to warfarin (Coumadin) for prophylaxis of DVT for major surgical procedures, including orthopedic surgery. LMWH is expensive and not without side effects (thrombocytopenia, bleeding). Dosing of LMWH must be adjusted according to creatinine clearance. Elderly patients should be carefully monitored for bleeding complications. LMWH prophylaxis is not recommended for patients who are to have neurosurgical procedures or spinal anesthesia, because of an increased risk of bleeding that may compromise neurologic functioning.[43] Neurosurgical patients or patients undergoing spinal cord surgical procedures should have prophylaxis with intermittent compression or elastic stockings, as there is no risk for hemorrhagic complications. A decision to institute pharmacologic prophylaxis should be made by the neurosurgeon.

Multicenter trials comparing warfarin and LMWH are currently under way. Consensus conference opinion supports the use of LMWH (30 mg enoxaparin SC q12h), heparin (5000 IU SC q12h), or warfarin (10 mg po on the night of surgery followed by 5 mg po qhs, titrating the dose to achieve an international normalized ratio of 2–3) for prophylaxis of DVT for general surgery and orthopedic surgical patients. The optimal duration of DVT prophylaxis is controversial. Some would recommend that LMWH or warfarin be continued for 6 weeks to 2 months after surgery. At a minimum DVT prophylaxis should be continued until the patient is ambulatory for functional distances.

Liver Disease

For patients with liver disease, the likelihood of developing complications is related to the degree of hepatic compromise.[44] Patients with acute viral hepatitis and elevated liver enzyme levels, determined by liver function tests (LFTs), should not have surgery until about 4 weeks after the LFTs are normalized. Most surgical procedures cause elevated LFTs because of hypoxia, hypercarbia, traction, reduced blood flow, and portal hypotension induced by anesthetic agents. The major perioperative complications in patients with liver disease are bleeding, infection, and renal insufficiency (especially in patients with obstructive jaundice secondary to malignant disease). Patients with liver disease are likely to have a poor prognosis if they have hypoalbuminemia, a prolonged prothrombin time, ascites, esophageal varices, or encephalopathy. These patients should be managed aggressively with the help of a gastroenterologist using mannitol, lactulose, hyperalimentation, fresh frozen plasma, vitamin K, spironolactone, and other diuretics.

Endocrine Disorders

The most common endocrine disorder encountered during the perioperative period is diabetes mellitus. Surgical mortality for patients with diabetes is greater among those who have concomitant cardiac disease, those who are having peripheral vascular surgery, and those with end-organ damage (autonomic neuropathy or nephropathy) as a result of their diabetes. Autonomic cardiac neuropathy may result in reduced ability to perceive postoperative chest pain, and these patients may be unable to mount an adequate cardiac response to the myocardial suppression due to anesthesia. Patients with diabetes are more likely to develop urinary retention, gastric retention, and pulmonary aspiration. Surgery places an additional strain on the diabetic patient, resulting in wide swings in blood glucose levels, volume shifts, electrolyte abnormalities (most frequently hypo- and hyperkalemia), and changes in acid–base status.[45]

The goal of management is to control blood glucose levels throughout the period of surgical stress. A number of opposing factors are involved. Usually patients are not eating well, which reduces the requirement for insulin, and they are inactive, increasing insulin requirements. During surgery there is an outpouring of catecholamines, glucagon, and cortisol, which dramatically increase insulin requirements. The net effect is the frequently encountered hyperglycemia during surgery. In general, the goal is to keep the blood glucose level below 250 mg/dL. For patients who are insulin-dependent, one half to two thirds of their intermediate-acting insulin should be administered on the morning of surgery and fingerstick glucose levels monitored every 2 hours during surgery, with sliding-scale regular insulin coverage. For patients with "brittle" diabetes, better control may be achieved by starting an insulin infusion a few hours before surgery. The usual rate of infusion is 2 units of insulin per hour, but this dosage can be adjusted depending on the serum glucose levels. To avoid hypoglycemia, a dextrose infusion is administered simultaneously in the other arm. The infusion rates are adjusted based on fingerstick glucose levels. For patients with diabetes taking oral hypoglycemic agents, the oral agent is stopped on the day before surgery and the patient managed with sliding-scale insulin similarly to the patient with insulin-dependent diabetes.

Steroid Use

Patients who are currently taking corticosteroids may be at risk of hypothalamic-pituitary-adrenal axis insufficiency when faced with the stress of surgery. Published case reports describe cardiovascular collapse among patients with steroid-related adrenal insufficiency. Patients who are currently taking steroids, who have used long-acting steroids, or who have taken steroids for more than a week during the previous year may be at increased risk of iatrogenic axis suppression. Consideration should be given to treating these patients with "stress-dose" intravenous steroids during surgery. One critical review of the literature on stress-dose steroids reported that few studies fulfilled the diagnostic criteria for iatrogenic adrenal insufficiency.[46] Furthermore, studies of renal allograft patients who had adrenal functioning testing reported that patients who had been taking prednisone for long periods had normal adrenal responses to adrenocorticotropic hormone (ACTH) stimulation, suggesting that adrenal function was preserved. For patients who are at risk for adrenal axis suppression, it may be useful to assess adrenal gland function. If the patient's cortisol level doubles over a fasting level 1 hour after administering 250 μg of ACTH intravenously or intramuscularly, or if any cortisol level is in the range of 17 to 20 μg/dL, adrenal function is likely to be intact. If it is decided to treat the patient empirically with stress-dose steroids, hydrocortisone sodium succinate (Solu-Cortef) or equivalent 100 mg IV q6h should be given for 24 hours, tapering the dose by 50% until the patient can take the usual dose of steroids.

Renal System

New-onset renal insufficiency during the perioperative period is associated with significant morbidity and mortality. A meta-analysis study reported that the only consistent predictors of postoperative acute tubular necrosis were preoperative elevations of creatinine and blood urea nitrogen (BUN) and patients having a major vascular procedure.[47] Patients who are volume-depleted, elderly, septic, or having a major procedure are at increased risk for developing perioperative acute tubular necrosis. Morbidity and mortality result from sepsis, coagulopathy, and volume and electrolyte disturbances. Anesthesiologists have a heightened level of concern about avoiding this complication, especially in patients with a suspected creatinine clearance of less than 50%. Patients on chronic hemodialysis or peritoneal dialysis can be operated on safely, but dialysis should be completed 6 hours or more before surgery because of the anticoagulant effects of heparin added to the dialysate.

Nutrition

Protein-calorie undernutrition results in increased surgical morbidity and mortality. Surgery may transform mild undernutrition into severe malnutrition, which if it occurs is associated with impaired wound healing, immunodeficiencies, and a reduced ability to resist infection. Older patients are especially at risk for undernutrition after surgery because of coexistent chronic medical illnesses (e.g., congestive heart failure, chronic lung disease), functional impairments, coexistent dementia/postoperative delirium, and surgery-related factors (e.g., nil per mouth, liquid diet).

Patients who have multiple trauma or pancreatitis or who are unable to eat for 7 to 10 days are most likely to develop perioperative malnutrition. The Veterans Administration Parenteral Nutrition Cooperative Study found that mortality and complication rates among patients who received total parenteral nutrition (TPN) were similar to those who did not.[48] The authors concluded that TPN should be considered for severely malnourished patients or those whose gastrointestinal tract was to be rested for 7 to 10 days if previously normally nourished or for 5 days in previously malnourished patients. The exact optimal duration of nutritional support is not well established; however, low-risk nutritional supplementation (oral supplements) make intuitive sense for all perioperative patients until adequate nutritional intake is established.

Conclusion

Family physicians are increasingly being requested to participate in the care of patients during the perioperative period. In general, surgical and anesthesia outcomes have greatly improved, even among elderly patients in good medical condition. There remain, however, categories of patients who are at high risk for adverse outcomes, especially those with comorbid cardiovascular disease, those having peripheral vascular surgery, and those at risk for developing pulmonary complications, sepsis, or renal failure. The medical care of the surgical patient is highly individualized, with a goal of bringing the person to the operating room in the best condition possible and then not abandoning the patient after surgery.

References

1. Milamed DR, Hedley-Whyte J. Contributions of the surgical sciences to a reduction of the mortality rate in the United States for the period 1968 to 1988. Ann Surg 1994;219:94–102.
2. Khuri SF, Daley J, Henderson W, et al. The National Veterans Administration Surgical Risk Study: risk adjustment for the comparative assessment of the quality of surgical care. J Am Coll Surg 1995;180:519–31.
3. King MS. Preoperative evaluation. Am Fam Physician 2000;62:387–93.
4. Adrenal dysfunction and steroid use. In: Adler AG, Merli GJ, McElwain GE, Martin JH, eds. Medical evaluation of the surgical patient. Philadelphia: WB Saunders, 1985;101–17.
5. MacPherson, DS. Preoperative laboratory testing: should any tests be "routine" before surgery? Med Clin North Am 1993;77:289–306.
6. More preoperative assessment by physicians and less by laboratory tests [editorial]. N Engl J Med 2000;342:204–5.
7. Fischer S. Cost-effective preoperative evaluation and testing. Chest 1999;115(suppl 5):96S–100S.
8. MacPherson DS, Snow R, Lofgren RP. Preoperative screening: value of previous tests. Ann Intern Med 1990;113:969–73.
9. Farrow SC, Fowkes FGR, Lunn JN, et al. Epidemiology in anesthesia. II. Factors affecting mortality in hospital. Br J Anaesth 1982;54:811–7.
10. Dripps RD. A new classification of physical status. Anesthesiology 1963;24:111.
11. Goldman L. Cardiac risks and complications of non-cardiac surgery. Ann Intern Med 1983;98:504–13.
12. Belzberg H, Rivkind AI. Preoperative cardiac preparation. Chest 1999; 115(suppl 5):82S–95S.
13. Detsky AS, Abrams HB, McLaughlin JR. Predicting cardiac complications in patients undergoing noncardiac surgery. J Gen Intern Med 1986;1:211–9.
14. Jeffrey CC, Kunsman J, Cullen DJ, Brewster DC. A prospective evaluation of cardiac risk index. Anesthesiology 1983;58:462–4.
15. Hollenberg SM. Preoperative cardiac risk assessment. Chest 1999; 115(Suppl 5):51S–7S.
16. Eagle KA, Brundage BH, Chaitman BR, et al. Guidelines for perioperative cardiovascular evaluation for noncardiac surgery; report of the

American College of Cardiology/American Heart Association Task Force on Practice Guidelines (Committee on Perioperative Cardiovascular Evaluation for Noncardiac Surgery). J Am Coll Cardiol 1996;27: 910–48.

17. American College of Physicians. Clinical guideline, Part I. Guidelines for assessing and managing the perioperative risk from coronary artery disease associated with major noncardiac surgery. Ann Intern Med 1997;127:309–12.

18. Crawford ES, Morris GC, Howell JF, Flynn WF, Moorhead DT. Operative risk in patients with previous coronary artery bypass. Ann Thorac Surg 1978;26:215–21.

19. Mangano DT, Layug EL, Wallace A, Tateo I. Effect of atenolol on mortality and cardiovascular morbidity after noncardiac surgery. N Engl J Med 1996;335:1713–20.

20. Higham H, Handa A, Hands LJ, et al. Slowing the heart saves lives: advantage of perioperative beta-blockade. Br J Surg 2000;87(12):1736–7.

21. Weitz HH. Non-cardiac surgery in the elderly patient with cardiovascular disease. Clin Geriatr Med 1990;6:511–29.

22. Wolfsthal SD. Is blood pressure control necessary before surgery? Med Clin North Am 1993;77:349–63.

23. O'Kelly B, Browner WS, Massie B, Tubau J, Ngo L, Mangano DT. Ventricular arrhythmias in patients undergoing noncardiac surgery. JAMA 1992;268:217–21.

24. Weitz HH, Goldman L. Non-cardiac surgery in the patient with heart disease. Med Clin North Am 1987;71:413–32.

25. O'Keefe JH, Shub C, Rettke SR. Risk of non-cardiac surgical procedures in patients with aortic stenosis. Mayo Clin Proc 1989;64:400–5.

26. Wong T, Detsky AS. Having peripheral vascular surgery. Ann Intern Med 1992;116:743–53.

27. Fleisher LA, Barash PG. Preoperative evaluation of the cardiac patient for noncardiac surgery. Yale J Biol Med 1993;66:385–95.

28. Mangano DT, Hollenberg M, Fegert G, et al. Perioperative myocardial ischemia in patients undergoing noncardiac surgery. I. Incidence and severity during the 4 day perioperative period. J Am Coll Cardiol 1991;17:843–50.

29. Botvinick EH, Dae MW. Dipyridamole perfusion scintigraphy. Semin Nucl Med 1991;21:242–65.

30. Lette J, Waters D, Cerino M, Picard M, Champagne P, Lapointe J. Preoperative coronary artery disease risk stratification based on dipyridamole imaging and a simple three-step, three-segment model for patients undergoing noncardiac vascular surgery or major general surgery. Am J Cardiol 1992;69:1553–8.

31. Fleisher LA, Barash PG. Preoperative cardiac evaluation for noncardiac surgery: a functional approach. Anesth Analg 1992;74:586–98.

32. Potyk DK. Cardiac evaluation and risk reduction in patients undergoing major vascular operations. West J Med 1994;161:50–6.

33. Goldman L. Cardiac risk for vascular surgery (editorial comment). J Am Coll Cardiol 1996;27(4):799–802.

34. Dajani AS, Taubert KA, Wilson W, et al. Prevention of bacterial endo-carditis. Recommendations of the American Heart Association. JAMA 1997;277:1794–801.
35. Tisi GM. Preoperative identification and evaluation of a patient with lung disease. Med Clin North Am 1987;71:399–412.
36. Ferguson MK. Preoperative assessment of pulmonary risk. Chest 1999;115(suppl 5):58S–63S.
37. Zibrak JD, O'Donnell CR. Indications for preoperative pulmonary function testing. Clin Chest Med 1993;14:227–36.
38. Warner MA, Offord KP, Warner ME, Lennon RI, Conover MA, Jansson-Schumacher U. Role of preoperative cessation of smoking and other factors in postoperative pulmonary complications: a blinded prospective study of coronary artery bypass patients. Mayo Clin Proc 1989;64:609–16.
39. Carson JL, Willett LR. Is a hemoglobin of 10 g/dl required for surgery? Med Clin North Am 1993;77:335–47.
40. Konishi T, Ohbayashi T, Kaneko T, Ohki T, Saitou Y, Yamato Y. Pre-operative use of erythropoietin for cardiovascular operations in anemia. Ann Thorac Surg 1993;56:101–3.
41. Hematology. In: Adler AA, Merli GJ, McElwain GE, Martin JH, eds. Medical evaluation of the surgical patient. Philadelphia: WB Saunders, 1985;44–50.
42. Ament PW, Bertolino JG. Enoxaparin in the prevention of deep venous thrombosis. Am Fam Physician 1994;50:1763–8.
43. Clagett GP, Anderson FA, Geerts W, et al. Prevention of venous throm-boembolism. Chest 1998;114(suppl 5):531S–60S.
44. Brown FH, Shiau YF, Richter GC. Anesthesia and surgery in the patient with liver disease. In: Goldmann DR, Brown FH, Levy WK, et al, eds. Medical care of the surgical patient: a problem-oriented approach to management. Philadelphia: Lippincott, 1982;326–42.
45. Ockert DBM, Hugo JM. Diabetic complications with special anaesthetic risk. S Afr J Surg 1992;30:90–4.
46. Salem M, Tainsh RE, Bromberg J, Loriaux DL, Chernow B. Perioper-ative glucocorticoid coverage: a reassessment 42 years after emergence of a problem. Ann Surg 1994;219:416–25.
47. Novis BK, Roizen MF, Aronson S, Thisted RA. Association of preop-erative risk factors with postoperative acute renal failure. Anesth Analg 1994;78:143–9.
48. Buzby GP. Overview of randomized clinical trials of total parenteral nu-trition for malnourished surgical patients. World J Surg 1993;17:173–7.

11

Selected Disorders of the Cardiovascular System

David E. Anisman

Pericarditis

Pericarditis may be divided into two types—acute and constrictive. Acute pericarditis (AP), which is an inflammatory condition of the membranes lining the heart, affects men more frequently than women, and is seen with increasing frequency with advancing age. While AP is diagnosed in less than 1% of hospital admissions, it has an estimated prevalence of 2% to 6% in the general population, underscoring the frequency with which it is either clinically not apparent or not considered in the differential diagnosis.[1] The most common etiologies are idiopathic, viral (which may actually account for most idiopathic cases), and in association with cardiac ischemia (Table 11.1). Indeed, the chest pain associated with AP may make it difficult to distinguish from acute myocardial ischemia. Constrictive pericarditis (CP), formerly known as Pick's disease, is characterized by a thickened, adherent, and fibrous pericardium that impairs diastolic filling, leading to the gradual onset of symptoms consistent with systemic venous congestion, such as congestive heart failure (CHF). It is a postinflammatory sequela of many of the same etiologies as AP, but the clinician should always maintain a high suspicion for tuberculosis, which is still the leading cause of CP in developing countries.[2]

Table 11.1. **Etiologies of Pericarditis**

Infectious
  Bacterial: pneumococcus, staphylococcus, *Neisseria meningitidis*,
    streptococcus, mycoplasma, tuberculosis, *Haemophilus*
    influenzae, rickettsia
  Viral: coxsackie, echovirus, adenovirus, influenza, varicella-zoster,
    HIV
  Fungal: histoplasmosis, aspergillosis, blastomycosis,
    coccidioidomycosis
Trauma: blunt chest trauma, post-thoracic surgery
Medications: procainamide, phenytoin, isoniazid, penicillin, heparin,
  warfarin, cromolyn sodium, methysergide
Cardiac: AMI, Dressler's syndrome, endocarditis, aortic dissection
Radiation therapy
Neoplastic: breast, bronchogenic lung, lymphoma, leukemia
Uremia: poorly controlled or while on hemodialysis
Autoimmune: systemic lupus erythematosus, rheumatoid arthritis,
  inflammatory bowel, acute rheumatic fever, scleroderma,
  polyarteritis nodosa, dermatomyositis
Other: sarcoidosis, amyloidosis

AMI = acute myocardial infarction.

Presentation and Diagnosis

Acute pericarditis may be heralded by a viral prodrome, and classically presents with a triad of chest pain, pericardial friction rub, and
characteristic electrocardiographic (ECG) changes. The chest pain is
usually rather abrupt in onset, retrosternal in location, and made worse
with recumbency, deep inspiration, and swallowing. It is often eased
by sitting up and leaning forward. The pain may radiate to the trapez-
ius ridge, or may mimic the pain of acute myocardial ischemia with
radiation into the left arm. Respiratory symptoms are generally the
result of secondary pleural irritation rather than a primary effect of
AP on cardiac function. The pathognomonic pericardial friction rub
is classically described as triphasic (atrial systole, ventricular systole,
and diastole), with the ventricular systolic component most readily
and most often heard. The rub is scratchy or "Velcro-like" and best
heard with the patient sitting upright and leaning forward, with res-
pirations interrupted, and by placing the diaphragm over the left lower
sternal border and cardiac apex. Confusion with murmurs can be
avoided by recognizing that the rub does not radiate or vary in either
loudness or timing with maneuvers that typically are used for murmur identification.

The four classic stages of ECG changes in AP are summarized in
Table 11.2; not all phases need be present to confirm the diagnosis.

Table 11.2. **Electrocardiographic Findings for the Four Stages of Acute Myopericarditis**

Stage	Duration	Electrocardiographic finding
I	Days–2 weeks	Diffuse PR segment depression (I, II, III, aVL, V2–6) (with reciprocal PR segment elevation in aVR, V1) Diffuse ST segment elevation (I, II, III, aVL, V2–6) (with reciprocal ST segment depression in aVR, V1)
II	1–3 weeks	ST segment normalization T wave flattening with decreased amplitude
III	3–several weeks	T wave inversion
IV	Several weeks	Normalization and return to baseline ECG

Source: Chan et al,[3] with permission.

Because PR segment depression may coexist with ST segment elevation, it is crucial to use the TP segment as a baseline.[3] Acute pericarditis may be differentiated from acute myocardial infarction (AMI) by the diffuseness of ST changes, the absence of Q waves, and the characteristically concave up-sloping morphology of the ST segment. Benign early repolarization (BER) also may present with diffusely elevated ST segments, but use of the ST/T ratio (Fig. 11.1) is helpful in making the distinction.

Because of the wide variety of presenting signs and symptoms, CP is difficult to diagnose solely on history and physical examination.[2] Symptoms of right-sided CHF, such as abdominal distention, peripheral edema, and anorexia reflect impaired diastolic filling and chronically depressed cardiac output. Left-sided CHF symptoms such as dyspnea and orthopnea also occur, but are less frequent.[4] Common ex-amination findings include Kussmaul's sign (jugular venous pressure *increasing* with inspiration), ascites, cachexia, hepatomegaly, and a pericardial knock (an early diastolic sound heard best with the diaphragm and increased with squatting). Though rarely normal, the ECG findings are nonspecific, revealing generalized low voltage, T-wave inversions, conduction delays, and atrial dysrhythmias (especially atrial fibrillation).[4,5] When the presentation suggests constrictive or restrictive pathophysiology, a chest x-ray showing pericardial calcification argues for CP over other etiologies. Better still, magnetic resonance imaging (MRI) and computed tomography

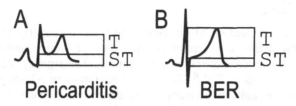

Fig. 11.1. This PR segment–ST segment discordant ratio may also help in discriminating between the ST segment elevation resulting from benign early repolarization (BER) and acute myopericarditis. It is objectively assessed by comparing the heights of the ST segment and T wave in lead V6: the ST segment/T wave magnitude ratio. Using the PR segment as the baseline for the ST segment and the J point as the beginning of the T wave, the heights are measured with calculation of the ratio. If the ratio is 0.25 or greater, pericarditis is the likely diagnosis; with results less than 0.25, one should consider BER. (From Chan et al,[3] with permission.)

(CT) are the preferred methods for identifying the pericardial thickening of CP. Echocardiography is often helpful in evaluating ventricular function and documenting the impaired diastolic filling characteristic of CP. Cardiac catheterization is the gold standard for resolving the diagnostic dilemmas via demonstration of equalized diastolic pressures between atria and ventricles.

Differential Diagnosis

Differential considerations for AP include AMI, pulmonary embolus, aortic dissection, cardiac contusion, mediastinitis, esophageal spasm, esophagitis, and pneumonia. A thorough history, examination, ECG analysis, and selected diagnostic testing and imaging will usually address these concerns, but the distinction between AP and AMI may remain difficult, complicating subsequent therapy. Constrictive pericarditis must be differentiated from tamponade, restrictive cardiomyopathy, intraabdominal malignancy, and hepatic cirrhosis. Liver function tests in CP patients are typical for passive congestion (elevated alkaline phosphatase and γ-glutamyl transpeptidase), while cirrhotic patients show diminished albumen and increased prothrombin times. Echocardiogram, CT, and MRI are also helpful in making these distinctions. Where confusion between constrictive and restrictive etiologies persists, catheterization with endomyocardial biopsy is indicated.[1,5]

Intervention

Initial management of AP focuses on treating the underlying cause, if possible. Purulent pericarditis requiring IV antibiotics must be documented by pericardiocentesis and is a medical emergency, with mortality rates of up to 77%.[6] Clinicians should monitor AP for pericardial effusion and the development of cardiac tamponade, requiring emergent pericardiocentesis. Analgesia for AP is critical, and is best achieved with nonsteroidal antiinflammatory drugs (NSAIDs) such as aspirin (650 mg po q4h) or indomethacin (25 to 50 mg po q6h). Intravenous ketorolac (30 mg IM or IV q6h) is also effective. Since the high doses of corticosteroids needed for pain control have both immune and adrenal suppressive effects, it is prudent to withhold them for at least 48 hours to determine if NSAIDs will be effective for symptom management. When the patient is pain free for 5 to 7 days, all antiinflammatory agents should be tapered. Recurrent pericarditis is treated by reinstituting high-dose NSAIDs, followed by tapering these agents over several months. Colchicine has also been used with some success. Even though the presence of AP is a relative contraindication to administration of thrombolytics, the incidence of post-AMI AP can be decreased by the appropriate use of thrombolytic therapy for the AMI, since decreasing the size of the AMI will decrease the likelihood for development of AP.

The progressive nature of CP demands referral to a cardiovascular surgeon for all symptomatic patients, since the earlier stage at which pericardiectomy is performed, the better the outcome. Improvement is usually dramatic and sustained. Temporizing measures include the use of diuretics. Rate-slowing drugs should be used with caution, if at all, since maintaining an adequate cardiac output in CP is often rate-dependent.

Prevention

The most common etiologies of AP do not lend themselves to effective preventive efforts, and prevention of CP is usually dependent on prevention of AP. Focusing efforts on preventable etiologies, such as coronary artery disease (CAD), malignancy, management of uremic conditions, and judicious use of certain medications are most likely to be productive measures.

Myocarditis

Occurring most commonly in 20- to 50-year-old men, myo-carditis is the inflammation of cardiac myocytes and associated structures

Table 11.3. **Etiologies of Myocarditis**

Infectious
  Bacterial: clostridia, diphtheria, gonococcus, haemophilus,
    legionella, meningococcus, mycobacteria, mycoplasma,
    salmonella, staphylococcus, streptococcus (especially
    pneumococcus)
  Spirochetes: borrelia, leptospira, syphilis
  Fungal: actinomyces, aspergillus, candida, coccidioides,
    histoplasma
  Protozoal: toxoplasma, trypanosoma
  Rickettsia: Q fever, Rocky Mountain spotted fever, scrub typhus,
    typhus
  Viral: adenovirus, Coxsackie, cytomegalovirus, Epstein-Barr,
    hepatitis, herpes simplex, HIV, influenza A and B, rabies,
    respiratory syncytial virus, varicella zoster
Medications: hydrochlorothiazide, lithium, penicillins,
  sulfamethoxazole/trimethoprim, tetracycline
Physical agents: radiation therapy
Autoimmune: rheumatoid arthritis, systemic lupus erythematosus
Other: giant cell myocarditis, hypersensitivity reactions, Kawasaki
  disease, peripartum myocarditis, rheumatic fever, sarcoidosis

(vascular, interstitium, and pericardium). Viral infection in general, and Coxsackie B virus in particular, is the most common cause in North America (Table 11.3). Myocyte damage during the first 3 days appears to be due to a direct viral effect, which is terminated by antibody-mediated viral clearance. A persistent T-cell–mediated response in a subset of patients seems to underlie the evolution of abnormal ventricular architecture and the eventual development of dilated cardiomyopathy (DCM).[7,8] While most cases of myocarditis are asymptomatic and resolve spontaneously, one third of patients have residual cardiac abnormalities ranging from subtle ECG changes to CHF, which may be acute and life-threatening. The more mild cases generally respond well to conventional CHF management, whereas the more severe cases may require mechanical ventricular assist devices or even transplant. Cases of sudden death have been reported, presumably secondary to ventricular dysrhythmia.

Presentation and Diagnosis

Symptomatic patients often note a nonspecific flu-like prodrome, occasionally accompanied by palpitations. One third note chest pain that may mimic ischemia, and a small number present with symptoms of CHF. Examination may reveal tachycardia, a muffled first heart sound, or a murmur of tricuspid or mitral regurgitation. Severe cases will have findings consistent with CHF. Electrocardiogram commonly reveals a sinus tachycardia with nonspecific ST and T wave changes (often superimposed on those of pericarditis). Conduction delays are not uncommon, and intraventricular delays often denote more serious myocardial damage and a worse prognosis. White blood count is elevated in a quarter of patients, and the erythrocyte sedimentation rate (ESR) is increased in up to 60%. Serology is rarely clinically useful. Echocardiography may show increased left ventricular (LV) wall thickness similar to that seen in other forms of cardiomyopathy, and is very important in identifying ventricular wall motion abnormalities, detecting ventricular thrombus, and measuring LV ejection fraction (LVEF). A near-normal baseline LVEF is currently the best predictor of a good outcome; findings on light microscopy from biopsy specimens have not correlated well with prognosis.[9,10]

Myocardial biopsy is most useful if performed within the first 3 to 4 days when the diagnostic yield is highest. Even then, however, it is uncommon that biopsy findings will significantly change management decisions. Some authorities consider biopsy to be the gold standard in the diagnosis of myocarditis and recommend it in all cases of ventricular dysfunction where the cause is unclear.[11] Others question this recommendation, noting the low yield of biopsy due to the patchy nature of inflammatory infiltrates, and the difficulty with which current pathologic criteria are employed.[9]

Differential Diagnosis

Several serious cardiac conditions must be differentiated from myocarditis. These include AMI, CHF due to other causes (e.g., ischemia, hypertension), dysrhythmias, and pericarditis. Complicating the evaluation is the fact that all of these conditions may coexist with myocarditis.

Intervention

If an infectious agent is identified, appropriate therapy should be instituted immediately. Most patients with mild to moderate symptoms require supportive measures specific to their presentation. Bed rest is critical to limit continued damage to the myocardium. Treatment of the systemic symptoms typical of viral infection with analgesics and antipyretics is indicated, but NSAIDs should be avoided in the first 2 weeks due to the potential for myocardial cell damage. Conventional treatment with digoxin, diuretics, nitrates, and angiotensin-converting enzyme inhibitors (ACEIs; especially when ejection fraction is less than 40%) is appropriate when CHF is present.[7,11] Temporary cardiac pacing is indicated in cases of third-degree or symptomatic second-degree type II atrioventricular block. Anticoagulation may be warranted for ventricular thrombus or to prevent development of thrombus in the presence of atrial fibrillation. Cardiac transplantation is used only as a last ditch effort, often after intraaortic balloon pump or LV assist device have failed. Antiviral therapies such as interferon-α and polyclonal immunoglobulin (Ig) are rarely useful, since they are only of benefit when started before or during viral infection.[12] Alpha-, beta-, and calcium channel blocking drugs may be of benefit due to their vasodilating properties, but as yet remain investigational.[12] Steroids and other immunosuppressive agents have not been found to produce a significant benefit in clinical outcomes. In fact, they may be harmful in the acute phase of viral myocarditis, possibly due to decreased antibody-mediated clearance of virus. Their use is suggested only in biopsy-proven cases after other treatments have failed, and prior to transplant.[7,9,12] One exception is in the treatment of autoimmune causes such as giant cell myocarditis or systemic lupus, where it is the treatment of choice. Future therapies may include immunomodulating agents if such can be found to target T cells only.[8]

Prevention

The majority of viruses that constitute the most common causes of myocarditis are not amenable to effective prevention measures. Less common causes such as sexually transmitted diseases are preventable through counseling on risk-limiting behavioral mechanisms. Others causes such as pneumococcus, influenza, hepatitis, and diphtheria may be prevented through immunization, though the risk of myocarditis in the general population does not warrant a change in current immunization strategy.

Endocarditis

Infectious endocarditis (IE) is an infection of the endocardial surface mainly due to bacteria, but rarely may be caused by fungi and protozoa. The interaction between the infecting organisms and the host's immune response gives rise to the classic though not universally found lesion of IE: the valvular vegetation. These vegetations may interfere with valvular function leading to CHF, and may embolize to produce a wide variety of focal and systemic signs and symptoms. Acute bacterial endocarditis (ABE) is a subset of IE in which the clinical course may become fulminant in as little as 3 to 5 days, tends to be caused by more virulent organisms such as *Staphylococcus aureus*, and generally affects patients with previously normal valves, intravenous drug users (IVDUs), and those with prosthetic valves. Because of its aggressive course, the complications of ABE tend to be severe. In contrast, subacute bacterial endocarditis (SBE) is more gradually progressive, often taking weeks to months before being diagnosed. The subacute form of IE is caused by less virulent organisms (e.g., *Streptococcus viridans*), has severe complications less often than ABE, and primarily affects patients with abnormal valvular architecture, either congenital or prosthetic. The overall incidence of IE in the United States is estimated at between 1.6 and 6.0 cases per 100,000 population, with a slight male predominance and a median age of 50 years.[13] This demographic is changing due to the decreased prevalence of rheumatic heart disease, advances in the surgical management of children with congenital cardiac disease, and a steady rise in intravenous drug abuse. As a result, children and IVDUs make up an increasing proportion of those with IE. Untreated, IE is almost uniformly fatal. Therefore, if IE is suspected, aggressive evaluation and treatment, to include early surgery in some cases, is essential. Such a strategy has decreased mortality rates to as low as 40% in nonaddicts with *S. aureus* ABE and 0% to 10% in IVDUs.[14]

Effective management of IE relies on targeting treatment to specific organisms. Gram-positive bacteria are the most common cause of IE, with over 80% of cases due to staphylococcal and streptococcal species.[13,14] Gram-negative bacteria account for 10% to 20% of cases, with *Pseudomonas* occurring primarily in IVDUs and those with prosthetic valve endocarditis (PVE), and the HACEK group (*Haemophilus* species, *Actinobacillus actinomycetemcomitans, Cardiobacterium hominis, Eikenella corrodens,* and *Kingella kingae*) occurring most commonly in native valve, non-IVDUs. While IE is rare in children overall, those with congenital cardiac disease most often have *S. viridans* or *S. aureus* as causative agents.[15] More than half of IE in IVDUs is due to *S. aureus,* but gram-negative bacteria, especially *Pseudomonas,* and fungi are common as well. In addition, IVDUs have a very high incidence of right-sided valvular involvement, especially the tricuspid valve. Prosthetic valve endocarditis is most often due to *S. viridans, S. aureus,* and *Staphylococcus epidermidis,* as well as *Pseudomonas* and other gram-negative bacilli. As a general rule, a normal vaginal delivery poses little increased risk of IE. However, bacteremia during delivery carries an increased risk of enterococcal, group B streptococcal, and *S. aureus* IE.[13] Nosocomial IE is most commonly due to staphylococcal species, enterococci, fungi, and *Pseudomonas*, and is seen in patients with burns, extended intensive care unit stays, and placement of intravascular and intracardiac devices or urinary catheters.

Presentation and Diagnosis

Though the primary lesion in IE is in the heart itself, many of its presenting signs and symptoms reflect the systemic nature of the disease. Fever, myalgias, fatigue, headache, and abdominal pain are common in all types of IE, but are more severe and persistent in ABE. Findings consistent with CHF develop in up to 60% of all cases of IE, and are often a poor prognostic sign as CHF carries a mortality of up to 80% and is the most common cause of death in all types of IE.[16] Vegetations can embolize to almost any location, causing distant infection or infarction; such embolization occurs in about 12% to 40% of patients with SBE and 40% to 60% of patients with ABE.[13] Right-sided embolic events may lead to specific complaints of chest pain, cough, and hemoptysis. Left-sided embolic events can present as mental status changes, stroke, myocardial infarction, splenic infarction, and renal abscess. Up to 90% of patients with *Streptococcus pneumoniae* ABE have an associated meningitis. Other complications of IE include osteomyelitis, septic arthritis, and mycotic aneurysms.

With the exception of Janeway lesions, which are found most commonly with ABE, few physical findings are highly specific for IE. Nonetheless, Roth spots, Osler's nodes, petechiae, splinter hemorrhages, and splenomegaly occur in up to 25% of cases of IE, and when more than one occur together it is strongly suggestive of the diagnosis. Cardiac murmurs in IE are most often regurgitant, but frequently are not present on initial evaluation. While a change in a preexisting murmur is of uncertain significance, a new aortic regurgitant murmur in association with fever is strongly associated with IE.[13] Laboratory evaluation is frequently of less value in making the early diagnosis of IE than are the history and examination, but usually shows granulocytosis, especially in ABE. In SBE, anemia, a positive rheumatoid factor, elevated Veneral Disease Research Laboratory (VDRL) titers, and circulating immune complexes are common. Other laboratory findings and imaging may reflect other complications as mentioned above. Electrocardiogram may reveal conduction abnormalities, indicating the extension of an aortic valve infection to a valve-ring abscess, which carries a worse prognosis.[13]

Table 11.4. **Criteria for Diagnosis of Infective Endocarditis**

Definite infective endocarditis
  Pathologic criteria
    Microorganisms: demonstrated by culture or histology in a
      vegetation, *or* in a vegetation that has embolized, *or* in an
      intracardiac abscess, *or*
    Pathologic lesions: vegetation or intracardiac abscess present,
      confirmed by histology showing active endocarditis
  Clinical criteria, using specific definitions listed in Table 11.5
    2 major criteria, *or*
    1 major and 3 minor criteria, *or*
    5 minor criteria
Possible infective endocarditis
  Findings consistent with infective endocarditis that fall short of
    "definite," but not "rejected"
Rejected
  Firm alternate diagnosis for manifestations of endocarditis,
    or
  Resolution of manifestations of endocarditis, with antibiotic therapy
    for 4 days or less, *or*
  No pathologic evidence of infective endocarditis at surgery or
    autopsy, after antibiotic therapy for 4 days or less

Source: Durack et al,[17] with permission.

In 1994, with the goal of increasing the proportion of definite diagnoses of IE correctly identified, Durack and colleagues[17] proposed a revised set of diagnostic criteria patterned after the Jones criteria for rheumatoid arthritis. Under these so-called Duke criteria, the diagnosis of definite IE is arrived at either through one of two pathologic criteria or through one of several combinations of major and minor clinical criteria (Table 11.4). The clinical criteria emphasize two main areas: positive blood cultures and evidence of endocardial involvement (Table 11.5). The latter clinical criterion takes advantage of both transthoracic (TTE) and transesophageal (TEE) echocardiography as safe yet highly sensitive means for identifying endocardial lesions.[16] It is recommended that TTE be the initial study of choice for most patients. However, where TTE is negative and clinical suspicion remains high, or in cases involving a prosthetic valve, possible abscess, or valve perforation, TEE is preferable, as it has higher sensitivity in such cases. In spite of a negative predictive value of 80%, a negative TEE should be repeated frequently in high-risk patients.[16] The Duke criteria have been extensively studied and found to have sensitivity ranging from 75% to 100% while maintaining ex-

Table 11.5. **Definitions of Terminology Used in the Diagnostic Criteria of Infective Endocarditis**

Major criteria
  Positive blood culture for infective endocarditis
    Typical microorganism for infective endocarditis from two
      separate blood cultures
        Viridans streptococci,[a] *Streptococcus bovis,* HACEK group, *or*
        Community-acquired *Staphylococcus aureus* or enterococci, in
          the absence of a primary focus, *or*
    Persistently positive blood culture, defined as recovery of a
      microorganism consistent with infective endocarditis from
      Blood cultures drawn more than 12 hours apart, *or*
    All of three or a majority of four or more separate blood
      cultures, with first and last drawn at least 1 hour apart
  Evidence of endocardial involvement
    Positive echocardiogram for infective endocarditis
      Oscillating intracardiac mass, on valve or supporting
        structures, *or* in the path of regurgitant jets, *or* on implanted
        material, in the absence of an alternative anatomic
        explanation, *or*
      Abscess, *or*
      New partial dehiscence of prosthetic valve, *or*
    New valvular regurgitation (increase or change in preexisting
      murmur not sufficient)
Minor criteria
  Predisposition: predisposing heart condition or intravenous drug
    use
  Fever: ≥38.0°C (100.4°F)
  Vascular phenomena: major arterial emboli, septic pulmonary
    infarcts, mycotic aneurysm, intracranial hemorrhage,
    conjunctival hemorrhages, Janeway lesions
  Immunologic phenomena: glomerulonephritis, Osler's nodes, Roth
    spots, rheumatoid factor
  Microbiologic evidence: positive blood culture but not meeting
    major criterion as noted previously[b] *or* serologic evidence of
    active infection with organism consistent with infective
    endocarditis
  Echocardiogram: consistent with infective endocarditis but not
    meeting major criterion as noted previously

HACEK = *Haemophilus* spp., *Actinobacillus actinomycetemcomitans, Cardiobacterium hominis, Eikenella* spp., and *Kingella kingae.*

[a]Including nutritional variant strains.

[b]Excluding single positive cultures for coagulase-negative staphylococci and organisms that do not cause endocarditis.

Source: Durack et al,[17] with permission.

cellent specificity (92–99%) and a negative predictive value of at least 92%.[17–20] These criteria have also been validated for both the adult and pediatric populations, as well as special groups such as those with PVE.[21–23] However, since an adequate amount of clinical data must be collected before the Duke criteria can be applied, early empiric therapy should not be delayed if IE is suspected. In this regard, the criteria are best used to assist in sculpting medical therapy and determining a need for surgical intervention.

Differential Diagnosis

Virtually any systemic infection should be considered in the differential diagnosis of IE. These include, but are not limited to, pneumonia, meningitis, pericarditis, abscess, osteomyelitis, tuberculosis, and pyelonephritis. Noninfectious etiologies to be considered include stroke, myocardial infarction, rheumatic fever, vasculitis, malignancy, and fever of unknown origin.

Intervention

Because bacteria in valvular vegetations are relatively protected from host immune defenses, antibiotics chosen to treat IE must be bactericidal, and regimens for their administration must be aggressive and of adequate duration to completely eradicate the organism and prevent relapse (Tables 11.6 to 11.9).[24,25] Repeat blood cultures should be negative within 48 hours of beginning antibiotic therapy, especially for staphylococcal infection. Cultures should also be repeated at 4 and 8 weeks after completion of antibiotic therapy. If positive, those with native valve IE should receive a repeat course of antibiotics; those with PVE or resistant enterococcus should receive both repeat antibiotics and possible surgical intervention.[25] Careful attention should be given to identifying and treating complications. CHF in particular must be treated aggressively, since there is a dramatic worsening of prognosis as CHF becomes more severe.[26] Therapy of CHF should be initiated with conventional medications (ACEIs and diuretics), but the timing of surgical intervention should be given particular emphasis. To that end, early surgical, infectious disease, and cardiology consultations are warranted for all patients with suspected IE.

In general, surgery should not be delayed because of active IE. Indications for surgical intervention include CHF that is progressive despite appropriate antibiotic and medical management, periannular or myocardial abscess, valvular obstruction, persistent bacteremia despite appropriate antibiotics, dehiscence of a prosthetic valve, fungal

Table 11.6. **Treatment Regimens for Viridans Streptococci[a] Bacterial Endocarditis**

Penicillin susceptibility	Antibiotics	Duration
High (MIC $\leq$0.1 μg per mL)	Aqueous penicillin, 12 to 18 million U day	4 weeks
	or	
	Ceftriaxone, 2 g daily	4 weeks
	or	
	Penicillin, 12 to 18 million U per day, plus gentamicin, 1 mg per kg every 8 hours[b]	2 weeks
Moderate (MIC >0.1, <0.5 μg per mL)	Penicillin, 18 million U per day	4 weeks
	plus	
	Gentamicin, 1 mg per kg every 8 hours[b]	2 weeks
Low (MIC $\geq$0.5 μg per mL)	Penicillin, 18 million U per day, plus gentamicin, 1 mg per kg every 8 hours[b]	4 to 6 weeks
In patients with penicillin allergy		
MIC <0.5 μg per mL	Vancomycin, 15 mg per kg every 12 hours[b]	4 weeks
MIC $\geq$0.5 μg per mL	Vancomycin, 15 mg per kg every 12 hours,[b] plus gentamicin, 1 mg per kg every 8 hours[b]	4 to 6 weeks

MIC = minimal inhibitory concentration.

[a]These regimens also apply to treatment of endocarditis caused by *Streptococcus bovis*.

[b]Dosages need to be adjusted based on renal function.

Source: Giessel et al,[24] as adapted from Wilson et al.[25] with permission.

Table 11.7. **Treatment Regimens for Enterococcal Bacterial Endocarditis**

Penicillin-allergic patient	Penicillin-susceptible organism	Antibiotics	Duration
No	Yes	Penicillin, 18 to 30 million U per day, plus gentamicin, 1 mg per kg every 8 hours[b] *or*	4 to 6 weeks[a]
No	No	Ampicillin, 12 g per day, plus gentamicin, 1 mg per kg every 8 hours[b]	4 to 6 weeks
		Vancomycin, 15 mg per kg every 12 hours,[b] plus gentamicin, 1 mg per kg every 8 hours[b]	4 to 6 weeks
Yes	No or yes	Vancomycin, 15 mg per kg every 12 hours,[b] plus gentamicin, 1 mg per kg every 8 hours[b]	4 to 6 weeks

[a]Six-week course of therapy for endocarditis involving a prosthetic valve or when symptoms have been present for longer than 3 months.

[b]Dosages need to be adjusted based on renal function.

Source: From Giessel et al,[24] as adapted from Wilson et al,[25] with permission.

Table 11.8. **Treatment Regimens for Staphylococcal Bacterial Endocarditis**

Penicillin-allergic patient	Methicillin-susceptible organism	Involved valve	Antibiotics	Duration
No	Yes	Native	Nafcillin, 2 g every 4 hours,[a] or oxacillin, 2 g every 4 hours	4–6 weeks
			plus	
			(Optional) Gentamicin, 1 mg per kg every 8 hours[a]	3–5 days
Yes[b]	Yes	Native	Cefazolin, 2 g every 8 hours[a]	4–6 weeks
			plus	
			(Optional) Gentamicin, 1 mg per kg every 8 hours[a]	3–5 days
Yes[c]	No or yes	Native	Vancomycin, 15 mg per kg every 12 hours[a]	4–6 weeks
No or yes	No	Native		
No	Yes	Prosthetic	Nafcillin, 2 g every 4 hours,[a] or oxacillin, 2 g every 4 hours	≥6 weeks
			plus	
			Rifampin, 300 mg every 8 hours	≥6 weeks
			plus	
			Gentamicin, 1 mg per kg every 8 hours[a]	2 weeks
No	No	Prosthetic	Vancomycin, 15 mg per kg every 12 hours[a]	≥6 weeks
				(continued)

Table 11.8 (Continued).

Penicillin-allergic patient	Methicillin-susceptible organism	Involved valve	Antibiotics	Duration
Yes[c]	No or yes	Prosthetic	*plus* Rifampin, 300 mg every 8 hours	≥6 weeks
			plus Gentamicin, 1 mg per kg every 8 hours[a]	2 weeks
Yes	No	Prosthetic	Cefazolin, 2 g every 8 hours[a]	≥6 weeks
			plus Rifampin, 300 mg every 8 hours	≥6 weeks
			plus Gentamicin, 1 mg per kg every 8 hours[a]	2 weeks

[a]Dosages need to be adjusted based on renal function.

[b]History of allergy that does not involve immediate-type hypersensitivity.

[c]History of immediate-type hypersensitivity.

Source: Giessel et al,[24] as adapted from Wilson et al,[25] with permission.

Table 11.9. **Treatment Regimens for Bacterial Endocarditis caused by HACEK Organisms**

Antibiotic	Dosage and route	Duration
Ceftriaxone[a]	2 g once daily IV or IM	4 weeks
Ampicillin[a] plus	12 g per day IV, either continuously or in 6 equally divided doses	4 weeks
Gentamicin[b]	1 mg per kg IM or IV every 8 hours	4 weeks

HACEK = *Haemophilus* spp., *Actinobacillus actinomycetemcomitans, Cardiobacterium hominis, Eikenella* spp., and *Kingella kingae.*

[a]Experience in treating HACEK organisms with other than β-lactam antibiotics is limited; for patients unable to tolerate β-lactam antibiotics, consult an infectious disease specialist.

[b]Dosages need to be adjusted based on renal function.

Source: Wilson et al,[25] with permission.

infection, conduction delay or heart block, enlarging vegetations, and recurrent emboli.[13,14,26]

Once the diagnosis of IE is suspected, antibiotic therapy should be instituted without delay. Until culture results and sensitivities are available to guide antibiotic selection, choice of empiric therapy should primarily rely on whether the clinical scenario is acute or subacute.[13] Other factors to be considered include nosocomial vs. community-acquired infection, presence of prosthetic material, and intravenous drug use. In the acute setting, nafcillin (2.0 g IV q4h) plus ampicillin (2.0 g IV q4h) plus gentamicin (1.5 mg/kg IV q8h) should be used; vancomycin (1.0 g IV q12h) should replace nafcillin when methacillin-resistant *S. aureus* is a concern. For SBE, ampicillin (2.0 g IV q4h) plus gentamicin (1.5 mg/kg IV q8h) is indicated.

Prevention

Prevention of IE in those with abnormal valvular architecture is covered in detail in Chapter 1. In those with normal valves, prevention is mainly an issue of education on the avoidance of IV drug use.

Cardiomyopathies

In 1995, the World Health Organization's classification of cardiomyopathies (CMs) recognized two main groupings.[27] The *functional* CMs describe anatomic and hemodynamic changes, and include dilated, hypertrophic, and restrictive forms, as well as the less common arrhythmogenic right ventricular CM. The *specific* CMs describe particular etiologies, and include ischemic, hypertensive, valvular, inflammatory, metabolic, general system disease, muscular dystrophies, neuromuscular disorders, toxic reactions, and peripartal. The specific CMs generally have the clinical features of one or more functional types. Indeed, many CMs previously labeled idiopathic are now known to be primary disorders of the myocardium caused by well-defined genetic mutations. In general, the clinician first recognizes a particular functional type of CM, and then proceeds to search for a specific etiology, since treatment of an underlying cause may arrest the cardiomyopathic process. Management of all the CMs should include early consultation with a cardiologist well versed in the pertinent and complex issues surrounding diagnosis and treatment.

Most CMs present with some manifestations of CHF, and so have two primary underlying pathogenic mechanisms: activation of the renin-angiotensin system and of the adrenergic nervous system. As a result, treatment with ACEIs and beta-blocking agents are often a mainstay of treatment. Diuretics are used for volume overload states, with digoxin as a second- or third-line agent for symptom control. Anticoagulation is indicated for a history of embolic phenomena and the dysrhythmias that might predispose to them, or significantly depressed LVEF.

Dilated Cardiomyopathy

Dilated cardiomyopathy (DCM) is characterized by an increase in LV diastolic and systolic volumes with an associated reduction in LVEF, and is the leading cause of CHF. The idiopathic form is the most common subtype, demonstrating myocyte hypertrophy and interstitial fibrosis on histology, and may be due to chronic myocarditis, either viral or autoimmune. Etiologies of DCM include primary genetic abnormalities (which are often autosomal dominant, making family history very important), toxic (including alcohol induced), and drug related (e.g., anthracyclines, cocaine). It may also be secondary to systemic conditions such as myocardial ischemia, hypertension, and valvular abnormalities.[28]

Patients with DCM often present with generalized symptoms of fatigue and dyspnea worsening over months to years; sudden death and embolic phenomena are less common. Physical examination reveals pulmonary and, less often, systemic venous congestion. When atrial fibrillation occurs, the presentation is often one of acute decompensation. Screening laboratory tests include ESR; creatinine kinase (to screen for inherited muscular dystrophies); renal, liver, and thyroid function studies; iron studies (to identify hemochromatosis); and, if the presentation is acute, viral serologies. The ECG may be normal, but often shows T wave changes, septal Q waves, atrioventricular conduction abnormalities, and bundle branch blocks. Sinus tachycardia and supraventricular dysrhythmias are common, and nonsustained ventricular tachycardia occurs in 20% to 30%.[28] Echocardiogram is essential to demonstrate the diagnostic criteria of ejection fraction <0.45, fractional shortening <25%, and LV end diastolic volume >112%. If diastolic dysfunction is demonstrated, endomyocardial biopsy should be performed to rule out infiltrative disease.

Treatment follows the basic precepts for CHF, with several notable caveats. In DCM secondary to hypertension or valvular disease, afterload reduction is best achieved by adding hydralazine or nitrates to the standard CHF regimen. Recent studies have suggested that the combination of angiotensin II receptor antagonists with ACEIs may be more effective than either agent alone.[29] In patients with New York Heart Association class IV failure and an LVEF <35%, adding 25 mg of spironolactone to the standard CHF regimen has been shown to decrease overall mortality by 30%.[30] Transplantation may be the only option for select, severely symptomatic patients, especially those with idiopathic DCM.

Hypertrophic Cardiomyopathy

Hypertrophic cardiomyopathy (HCM) is defined as increased LV wall thickness, either symmetric or asymmetric, and either global or regional, with overall normal (or slightly reduced) LV chamber size. Twenty-five percent of patients with HCM have dynamic outflow tract obstruction due to ventricular septal hypertrophy and anterior displacement of the papillary muscles, with associated abnormal mitral valve formation.[31,32] This obstruction may be a cause of sudden death, and is increased by activities that increase myocardial contractility (e.g., strenuous exercise), or by maneuvers or agents that decrease venous return (e.g., Valsalva, diuretics). Conversely, obstruction is decreased by agents that decrease myocardial contractility (e.g., beta-blockers) or by maneuvers that increase venous return (e.g., squatting). The risk for sudden death is highest in children and young adults, and may be the initial presentation. Possible risk factors for sudden death include recurrent syncope, prior cardiac arrest, sustained ventricular tachycardia, massive LV hypertrophy, and a family history of sudden death from HCM.[32] Hypertrophic CM is a primary, heterogeneous disease of the sarcomere, with autosomal dominant inheritance demonstrated most commonly.[32,33]

In addition to the common CHF symptoms such as fatigue, dyspnea, and orthopnea, patients with HCM often complain of palpitations (due to atrial fibrillation caused by left atrial enlargement), presyncope, and syncope. Since most HCM is nonobstructive, auscultation generally reveals no murmur. Patients with outflow tract obstruction often demonstrate a 3–4/6 systolic murmur heard over both the left sternal border (due to outflow obstruction) and the axilla (due to mitral regurgitation). An S_4 is often heard due to increased filling from the enlarged atria. Pulmonary congestion is rare except with severe outflow obstruction or end-stage HCM (when systolic and diastolic dysfunction become manifest), or with atrial fibrillation. The ECG usually reveals a wide array of nonspecific changes including LV hypertrophy, ST changes, T wave inversion, left atrial enlargement, and Q waves. The chest radiograph is often normal or suggestive of atrial enlargement. As with DCM, echocardiogram with Doppler studies is essential, with the transesophageal approach useful to define subtle mitral valve abnormalities. Nuclear angiography and MRI may yield additional information on myocardial dysfunction.

There is no consensus on the utility of prophylactic treatment of asymptomatic patients with HCM, but avoiding strenuous exercise is critical for all patients, as is antibiotic prophylaxis for SBE.[31] For symptomatic patients with obstruction, beta-blocking agents are essential to decrease outflow obstruction by increasing diastolic filling time and decreasing filling pressures. Other negative inotropic agents may be used to similar effect, but the vasodilating properties of many calcium antagonists (especially verapamil) may counter this effect, leading to decreased filling, increased obstruction, and sudden death. Oral disopyramide at 600 to 800 mg per day is the drug of choice according to some authors.[32] In symptomatic patients with obstruction who have failed medical management, dual-chamber pacing has been shown to be effective.[33] Restoration and maintenance of sinus rhythm in patients with atrial fibrillation is usually achieved with either sotalol or amiodarone. In end-stage HCM, systolic and diastolic dysfunction may necessitate the use of standard CHF drug regimens, with particularly cautious use of digitalis and diuretics. Myectomy and valve replacement are often effective at resolving obstruction, but the relief may be temporary, due to surgically induced dysrhythmias and progression of the underlying primary myopathic process.

Restrictive Cardiomyopathy

Diastolic dysfunction is the hallmark of restrictive cardiomyopathy (RCM); LV size and shape, and systolic function are either normal or nearly so. The least common of all functional cardiomyopathies, restrictive pathophysiology may be seen in both HCM and hypertensive CM. Other etiologies include infiltrative diseases such as hemochromatosis and amyloid (the most common systemic cause of RCM), scleroderma, carcinoid, sarcoidosis, radiation therapy, and anthracycline use. Idiopathic RCM also occurs and may be an autosomal-dominant condition associated with skeletal myopathies.[34]

The pathophysiology is characterized by decreased cardiac output, increased jugular venous pressure, and pulmonary congestion. Biatrial enlargement accounts for frequent thromboembolic events, a presenting symptom in up to one third of patients with RCM.[34] Both right- and left-sided CHF symptoms are common presenting scenarios. Examination reveals increased jugular venous pulse and decreased pulse pressure. An S_3 due to abrupt cessation of early rapid filling is common. The ECG is invariably abnormal, showing left bundle branch blocks more commonly than right, decreased voltage (especially in amyloidosis), and a wide variety of dysrhythmias (particularly in the infiltrative diseases). Chest radiograph reveals evidence of pulmonary and venous hypertension and congestion. Echocardiogram is essential to rule out other causes of the patient's symptoms, and to assess filling rates and pressures. CT and MRI are often very helpful in distinguishing RCM from its most important differential consideration—constrictive pericarditis. Cardiac catheterization is critical to define hemodynamic parameters and to perform endomyocardial biopsy. If the distinction between RCM and constrictive pericarditis remains unclear, exploratory surgery and empiric pericardectomy are often attempted.

Treatment with diuretics is indicated for congestive symptoms, but caution must be exercised to avoid decreasing preload to the extent that cardiac output is compromised further. Because of its proarrhythmic effects, digitalis should be avoided if systolic function is normal; amiodarone is preferred for maintenance of sinus rhythm. For clinically significant conduction abnormalities that are refractory to medical therapy, pacemaker implantation is indicated. As a last resort, transplantation may be considered in idiopathic RCM, but has a poor prognosis in amyloidosis and sarcoidosis, as these diseases tend to recur in the transplanted heart.[34]

Prevention

Because so many instances of CM are secondary to treatable causes, early and appropriately aggressive prevention and treatment of hypertension, CAD, and alcohol and illicit drug abuse, as well as optimizing control of the host of metabolic conditions that may predispose to CM, form the mainstay of preventive strategy. While little can be done to prevent the types of CM having a primarily genetic etiology, it is imperative to perform careful screening of all first-degree relatives with a thorough history, physical examination, and echocardiogram.

Pulmonary Hypertension

Pulmonary hypertension (PH) is a rare disease with a universally fatal outcome if untreated. It is defined by a mean pulmonary artery (PA) pressure >25 mm Hg at rest and >30 mm Hg during exercise.[35] The incidence of primary pulmonary hypertension (PPH) is one to two cases per million population, with a female predominance (1.7:1), a mean age at diagnosis in the mid-30s, and a median survival of 2 years after diagnosis; the 5-year survival is less than 40%. It has been shown that 6% to 10% of PPH is familial, with autosomal-dominant inheritance and incomplete penetrance.[36] Many common congenital cardiac defects as well as a long list of acquired conditions may also lead to the development of PH. The final common pathway for all causes of PH is right ventricular failure (RVF). With recent advances in the characterization and management of PH, early diagnosis is imperative since starting therapy before pulmonary vasculature has lost its responsiveness increases the likelihood of therapeutic success.

All etiologies of PH are felt to have one or more underlying pathophysiologic mechanisms: vascular injury (PA plexogenic arteriopathy of PPH), an alteration in the balance of vasodilatation and vasoconstriction normally controlled by local vascular factors, and thrombotic changes in the pulmonary vasculature. Numerous secondary etiologies of PH have been identified. Atrial and ventriculoseptal defects (ASD and VSD) and patent ductus arteriosus lead to a hyperkinetic state with increased flow to the right heart. Pulmonary venous hypertension may be caused by mitral stenosis, pulmonary obstruction (tumor, pulmonary embolism, sickle cell disease), or LV failure. If detected early, hyperkinetic states and pulmonary venous hypertension are often reversible, as is the pulmonary arterial hypertension that results. Pulmonary hypertension secondary to other causes is often less reversible, and these causes include parenchymal lung disease, obstructive sleep apnea, chest wall deformities and neuromuscular disorders that impair the mechanics of ventilation, CREST syndrome (calcinosis, Raynaud's phenomenon, esophageal dysmotility, sclerodactyly, and telangiectasias), pulmonary vasculidities (Raynaud's, dermatomyositis, rheumatoid arthritis, systemic lupus erythematosus), hepatic cirrhosis with portal hypertension, and human immunodeficiency virus (HIV) disease. Conditions less strongly associated with PH include hypothyroidism and the use of appetite suppressants.

Presentation and Diagnosis

Because the presentation can be so nonspecific, the physician's challenge is to be aware of the risk factors for PH and to have an appropriate index of suspicion. The goal of the evaluation and early consultation is to identify an underlying cause and to define the extent of pulmonary vascular pathology and RV dysfunction. The most common presenting symptoms include dyspnea (initially only with exertion), angina due to RV ischemia, and syncope or near-syncope due to reduced cardiac output. Examination may reveal increased jugular venous distention, RV heave, and a prominent P_2. Significant RVF may be evidenced by an S_4, peripheral edema, hepatomegaly, and ascites. With more severe PH one may appreciate an S_3, the holosystolic murmur of tricuspid regurgitation, or the early diastolic murmur of pulmonic regurgitation (the Graham Steell murmur). Chest radiograph may show increased hilar structures and enlarged RV and right atrium. Electrocardiogram usually reveals a normal sinus rhythm, right chamber enlargement, and a strain pattern. Transthoracic echocardiogram with Doppler is the screening method of choice,[37] allowing measurement of RV systolic pressures and morphologic abnormalities, LV function, valvular assessment, and identification of intracardiac shunts.

Definitive diagnosis requires right heart catheterization and measurement of PA pressures. Specific studies that are useful for the evaluation of specific causes of PH include TEE for selected intracardiac abnormalities; polysomnography for obstructive sleep apnea; pulmonary function testing for parenchymal lung disease; serologic tests for connective tissue disorders (e.g., lupus anticoagulant, anticardiolipin and antinuclear antibodies); platelet count and liver functions for cirrhosis and portal hypertension; HIV screening; hemoglobin electrophoresis for sickle cell disease; serum coagulation tests; and ventilation-perfusion scan and possibly CT for chronic pulmonary emboli (PE). If chronic PE is suspected, pulmonary angiography is indicated.

Differential Diagnosis

Coronary artery disease and cardiomyopathies leading to RV dysfunction may account for the presenting symptoms and signs of PH.

This broad diagnostic overlap often results in nearly a 2-year delay in diagnosing PH.[36]

Intervention

Due to the invasive means necessary to diagnose and treat PH, early consultation is a must to determine the feasibility and timing of surgical therapies for potentially reversible causes (e.g., ASD, VSD, mitral stenosis). General measures to be recommended include supplemental oxygen on airplanes, and avoiding high altitudes, pregnancy (a hemodynamically high flow state), and oral contraceptive drugs (due to clotting risk).[35] Supplemental oxygen is otherwise only useful for documented hypoxemia, which is usually found only with exertion, though patients with parenchymal lung disease may need it at rest. Digoxin may be used for overt RV failure, but other agents commonly used for LV failure (e.g., beta-blockers and ACEIs) are contraindicated due to their tendency to depress RV function. Diuretics should be used only for signs of systemic congestion, and then with extreme caution as RV function is preload dependent. Anticoagulation is associated with increased survival times, and warfarin is indicated to achieve an international normalized ratio of 2.0. Approximately one third of patients respond to vasodilating agents with a decrease in PA pressures and resistance, and can be placed on oral dihydropyridine calcium antagonists. However, empiric trials of these agents should never be undertaken, since nonresponders may decompensate precipitously. Responder status is best determined during right heart catheterization with the administration of potent, short-acting IV vasodilators while monitoring PA pressure and resistance. Those who do not respond may benefit from epoprostenol, a prostacyclin administered continuously via a Hickman catheter. Originally used as a temporizing measure while awaiting organ donation, epoprostenol allowed many such patients to avoid the need for transplant altogether. In addition to its vasodilating action, it is believed that epoprostenol's antiplatelet and vascular remodeling effects may underlie its success.

Except for repairing the underlying defects mentioned earlier, surgical interventions are generally options of last resort. Pulmonary thromboendarterectomy is indicated in severe PH caused by a clot that is proximal enough in the pulmonary vascular tree to be amenable to removal. Atrial septostomy, which creates a right to left shunt, thereby unloading the RV and increasing cardiac output, may be used in patients with recurrent syncope or RV failure when medical therapy has failed, and generally only as a bridge to transplant. Single or bilateral lung, and heart–bilateral lung transplant yields up to a 44% 5-year survival without recurrence of PH, though bronchiolitis obliterans is common.[37]

Prevention

Early repair of anatomic defects causing either a hyperkinetic state or pulmonary venous hypertension is paramount. Efforts to prevent or effectively manage parenchymal lung disease are also important. All first-degree relatives of patients with either PPH or a congenital cardiac anomaly should be screened with TTE at the time of diagnosis of the index case.

Peripheral Vascular Disease

While the prevalence of peripheral vascular disease (PVD) in the general population is 30%, only 5% have symptoms of claudication.[38] Coronary artery disease and stroke occur 2 to 4 times more often in symptomatic patients with PVD than in those without symptoms, and 2 to 3 times more often in patients with asymptomatic PVD compared to those without PVD. In addition, 70% to 80% of patients with symptomatic PVD are stable over 5 to 10 years. Amputation rates range from 0.8% to 1.0% per year, and are higher in smokers and diabetics. Therefore, the primary importance in diagnosing PVD lies in its role in identifying patients at risk for CAD morbidity and mortality.

Atherosclerosis is the most common cause of PVD, just as it is for CAD and stroke. Risk factors for PVD parallel those for CAD and include smoking, diabetes, hypertension, hyperlipidemia, age over 50 years, male gender, obesity, and postmenopausal status. Putative risk factors whose link to PVD is less well established include homocystinemia, elevated fibrinogen and uric acid levels, and chlamydia infection.[39]

Presentation and Diagnosis

The cardinal symptom of PVD is claudication, although patients may also present with complaints of poorly healing ulcerations. Numbness, paresthesias, and rest pain are often associated with severely compromised circulation. Aortoiliac disease is heralded by low back and buttock pain, and when accompanied by impotence is termed Leriche's syndrome. Thigh pain indicates iliac or common femoral artery disease, whereas foot pain is usually due to infrapopliteal dis-

ease. Calf pain is most commonly caused by superficial femoral arterial disease, but may be the result of occlusion at any level above
this. However, since 83% of PVD patients are asymptomatic, findings on physical examination may be the only clinical clue to the
presence of disease. Significant signs include diminished pulses and
increased capillary refill time; atrophic changes such as muscle wasting, changes in skin color, and hair loss; and decreased warmth and
dependent rubor. A bruit found with a decreased pulse indicates a
hemodynamically significant obstruction, but does not quantify its
severity. Evaluation of collateral circulation carries important treatment implications and is performed by placing the patient in the
supine position and elevating the limb to 45 degrees; pallor in the
distal extremity indicates inadequate collateral circulation.

The key diagnostic study is the ankle-brachial index (ABI), normally 1.0 to 1.1. An ABI <0.8 indicates significant PVD, and <0.5
indicates multilevel disease. In either case, further imaging is indicated with either duplex ultrasound and Doppler color flow (which
localizes diseased segments and grades lesion severity) or MR angiography (especially good for evaluation of arterial dissection and
wall morphology). Where noninvasive techniques are inadequate and
surgery is indicated, fluoroscopic angiography is the test of choice.

Differential Diagnosis

The most common differential considerations include neurogenic
claudication due to either disk disease, spinal stenosis, or osteophytic
changes, and shin splints (in younger persons). Less common causes
are Buerger's disease (thromboangiitis obliterans) and congenital anatomic abnormalities such as popliteal artery entrapment.

Intervention

As smokers with PVD have a tenfold risk of amputation, tobacco
cessation is essential. Other nonspecific interventions include diets
low in cholesterol and fat and high in fruits and vegetables, keeping
the feet warm and dry and nails trimmed, and inspecting the feet daily
and reporting any trauma to the physician immediately. Graded exercise programs improve exercise tolerance in up to 30% of patients.
Pharmacologic measures to decrease blood pressure and serum lipid
levels are also indicated, with similar end points to those for treating
CAD. Aspirin (75–325 mg po qd) with or without dipyridamole
(150–400 mg po qd) has been shown to decrease CAD and stroke
risk, and is indicated for PVD as well. Ticlopidine (250 mg po bid

with meals) and clopidogrel (75 mg po qd) have both been shown to be effective in decreasing the incidence of vascular morbidity in general, and ticlopidine has also been shown to improve symptoms and objective measures of PVD. However, ticlopidine is associated with significant adverse hematologic effects which may limit its utility.[40] Pentoxifylline (400 mg po tid) offers no consistently significant clinical benefit, but may be considered in severely impaired patients for whom even small symptomatic improvements would be meaningful. Vasodilator and anticoagulant therapy have not been shown to be useful in chronic PVD. Surgical consultation is indicated for occupation or lifestyle limiting symptoms where nonsurgical therapy has failed or for signs or symptoms of ischemia at rest.

References

1. Lorell BH. Pericardial diseases. In: Braunwald E, ed. Heart disease: a textbook of cardiovascular medicine, 5th ed. Philadelphia: WB Saunders, 1997;1478–505.
2. Myers RBH, Spodick DH. Constrictive pericarditis: clinical and pathophysiologic characteristics. Am Heart J 1999;138(2):219–32.
3. Chan TC, Brady WJ, Pollack M. Electrocardiographic manifestations: acute myopericarditis. J Emerg Med 1999;17(5):865–72.
4. Vaitkus PT, LeWinter MM. Pericardial disease. In: Bone RC, Alpert JS, eds. Current practice of medicine. Philadelphia: Churchill Livingstone, 1996;II:21.1–8.
5. Osterberg L, Vagelos R, Atwood JE. Case presentation and review: constrictive pericarditis. West J Med 1998;169(4):232–9.
6. Sagrista-Sauleda J, Barrabes JA, Permanyer-Miralda G, Soler-Soler J. Purulent pericarditis: review of a 20-year experience in a general hospital. J Am Coll Cardiol 1993;22:1661–5.
7. Caforio ALP, McKenna WJ. Recognition and optimum management of myocarditis. Drugs 1996;52(4):515–25.
8. Kawai C. From myocarditis to cardiomyopathy: mechanisms of inflammation and cell death. Circulation 1999;99(8):1091–100.
9. Pisani B, Taylor DO, Mason JW. Inflammatory myocardial diseases and cardiomyopathies. Am J Med 1997;102(5):459–69.
10. Mendes LA, Picard MH, Dec GW, Hartz VL, Palacios IF, Davidoff R. Ventricular remodeling in active myocarditis. Am Heart J 1999;138(2):303–8.
11. Parrillo JE. Myocarditis: How should we treat in 1998? J Heart Lung Transplant 1998;17(10):941–4.
12. Rezkalla SH, Raikar S, Kloner RA. Treatment of viral myo-carditis with focus on captopril. Am J Cardiol 1996;77(8):634–7.
13. Durack DT. Infective endocarditis. In: Alexander RW, Schlant RC, Fuster V, eds. Hurst's the heart, arteries and veins, 9th edition. New York: McGraw-Hill, 1997;2205–39.

14. Cunha BA, Gill MV, Lazar JM. Acute infective endocarditis: diagnostic and therapeutic approach. Infect Dis Clin North Am 1996;10(4): 811–34.
15. Brook MM. Pediatric bacterial endocarditis: treatment and prophylaxis. Pediatr Clin North Am 1999;46(2):275–87.
16. Kemp WE, Citrin B, Byrd BF. Echocardiography in infective endocarditis. South Med J 1999;92(8):744–54.
17. Durack DT, Lukes AS, Bright DK. New criteria for diagnosis of infective endocarditis: utilization of specific echocardiographic findings. Am J Med 1994;96(3):200–9.
18. Cecchi E, Parrini I, Chinaglia A, et al. New diagnostic criteria for infective endocarditis: a study of sensitivity and specificity. Eur Heart J 1997;18(7):1149–56.
19. Hoen B, Beguinot I, Rabaud C, et al. The Duke criteria for diagnosing infective endocarditis are specific: analysis of 100 patients with acute fever or fever of unknown origin. Clin Infect Dis 1996;23(2):298–302.
20. Dodds GA, Sexton DJ, Durack DT, Bashore TM, Corey GR, Kisslo J. Negative predictive value of the Duke criteria for infective endocarditis. Am J Cardiol 1996;77(5):403–7.
21. Stockheim JA, Chadwick EG, Kessler S, et al. Are the Duke criteria superior to the Beth Israel criteria for the diagnosis of infective endocarditis in children? Clin Infect Dis 1998;27(6):1451–6.
22. Del Pont JM, De Cicco LT, Vartalitis C, et al. Infective endocarditis in children: clinical analyses and evaluation of two diagnostic criteria. Pediatr Infect Dis J 1995;14(12):1079–86.
23. Nettles RE, McCarty DE, Corey GR, Li J, Sexton DJ. An evaluation of the Duke criteria in 25 pathologically confirmed cases of prosthetic valve endocarditis. Clin Infect Dis 1997;25(6):1401–3.
24. Giessel BE, Koenig CJ, Blake RL. Management of bacterial endocarditis. Am Fam Physician 2000;61(6):1725–32.
25. Wilson WR, Karchmer AW, Dajani AS, et al. Antibiotic treatment of adults with infective endocarditis due to streptococci, enterococci, staphylococci, and HACEK microorganisms. JAMA 1995;274(21): 1706–13.
26. Moon MR, Stinson EB, Miller DC. Surgical treatment of endocarditis. Prog Cardiovasc Dis 1997;40(3):239–64.
27. Richardson P, McKenna W, Bristow M, et al. Report of the 1995 World Health Organization/International Society and Federation of Cardiology Task Force on the definition and classification of cardiomyopathies. Circulation 1996;93(5):841–2.
28. Elliott P. Diagnosis and management of dilated cardiomyopathy. Heart 2000;84(1):106–12.
29. McKelvie RS, Yusuf S, Pericak D, et al. Comparison of candesartan, enalapril and their combination in congestive cardiac failure. Randomized evaluation of strategies for left ventricular dysfunction (RESOLVD) pilot study. Circulation 1999;100(10):1056–64.
30. Pitt B, Zannad F, Remme WJ, et al. The effect of spironolactone on morbidity and mortality in patients with severe heart failure. N Engl J Med 1999;341(10):709–17.

31. Louie EK, Edwards LC III. Hypertrophic cardiomyopathy. Prog Cardiovasc Dis 1994;36(4):275–308.
32. Wigle ED, Rakowski H, Kimball BP, Williams WG. Hypertrophic cardiomyopathy: clinical spectrum and treatment. Circulation 1995;92(7): 1680–92.
33. Maron BJ. Hypertrophic cardiomyopathy. In: Alexander RW, Schlant RC, Fuster V, eds. Hurst's the heart, arteries and veins, 9th edition. New York: McGraw-Hill, 1997;2057–74.
34. Kushwaha SS, Fallon JT, Fuster V. Restrictive cardiomyopathy. N Engl J Med 1997;336(4):267–76.
35. Barst RJ. Recent advances in the treatment of pediatric pulmonary artery hypertension. Pediatr Clin North Am 1999;46(2):331–45.
36. Peacock AJ. Primary pulmonary hypertension. Thorax 1999;54: 1107–18.
37. Krowka MJ. Pulmonary hypertension: diagnostics and therapeutics. Mayo Clinic Proc 2000;75:625–30.
38. Fowkes FGR. Epidemiology of peripheral vascular disease. Atherosclerosis 1997;131(suppl):29–31.
39. Powers KB, Vacek JL, Lee S. Noninvasive approaches to peripheral vascular disease: what's new in evaluation and treatment? Postgrad Med 1999;106(3):52–64.
40. Jackson MR, Clagett GP. Antithrombotic therapy in peripheral arterial occlusive disease. Chest 1998;114(5 suppl):666S–82S.

Index